# Immigrant Women's Health

# Immigrant Women's Health

## Problems and Solutions

Elizabeth J. Kramer,

Susan L. Ivey, and

Yu-Wen Ying,

Editors

Jossey-Bass Publishers • San Francisco

Jossey-Bass books and products are available through most bookstores. To contact Jossey-Bass directly, call (888) 378-2537, fax to (800) 605-2665, or visit our website at www.josseybass.com.

Substantial discounts on bulk quantities of Jossey-Bass books are available to corporations, professional associations, and other organizations. For details and discount information, contact the special sales department at Jossey-Bass.

 Manufactured in the United States of America on Lyons Falls Turin Book. This paper is acid-free and 100 percent totally chlorine-free.

**Library of Congress Cataloging-in-Publication Data**
Immigrant women's health : problems and solutions / Elizabeth J. Kramer, Susan L. Ivey, and Yu-Wen Ying, editors. — 1st ed.
    p.    cm.
Includes bibliographical references and indexes.
ISBN 0-7879-4294-4 (cloth : acid-free paper)
1. Women immigrants—Health and hygiene—United States.  I. Kramer, Elizabeth Jane.  II. Ivey, Susan L.  III. Ying, Yu-Wen.
RA448.5.I44 I44 1999
613'.04244'08691—dc21

                                                                98-40198
                                                                CIP

FIRST EDITION
*HB Printing* 10 9 8 7 6 5 4 3 2 1

# Contents

Exhibits and Tables     xi

Foreword     xiii

Preface     xv

The Editors     xvii

The Contributors     xix

**Part One: Background**     **1**

1    **Demographics, Definitions, and Data Limitations**     3
Elizabeth J. Kramer, Lisa C. Tracy, Susan L. Ivey

2    **Culture and Multicultural Competence**     19
Ernesto Ferran, Lisa C. Tracy, Francesca M. Gany,
Elizabeth J. Kramer

3    **Linguistic Issues**     35
Sherry Riddick

4    **Health Services Utilization and Access to Care**     44
Susan L. Ivey

5    **Utilization of Mental Health Services**     54
Kevin M. Chun, Phillip D. Akutsu

6    **The Impact of Recent Legislation on the Delivery
of Health Care to Immigrants**     65
*Welfare and Immigration Reforms in 1996 and 1997*
Susan L. Ivey
*Proposition 187: California's Anti-Immigrant Statute*
Nobuko Mizoguchi

**Part Two: Health Problems and Concerns** 79

7 **Screening, Infectious Diseases,
and Nutritional Concerns** 81

*Initial Assessment, Screening, and Immunizations*
Susan L. Ivey, Shotsy Faust

*Infectious Diseases*
Robin K. Avery

*Nutritional Assessment and Dietary Intervention*
Marion M. Lee, Shirley Huang

8 **Prenatal and Reproductive Health Care** 121
Francesca M. A. Taylor with Ruby Ko and Marilyn Pan

9 **Chronic Diseases** 136

*Cardiovascular Disease*
Susan L. Ivey, Gerrie Gardner

*Hypertension*
Dina Lieberman, Mary L. Del Monte, Eugenia L. Siegler

*Diabetes Mellitus*
Elizabeth J. Kramer, William B. Bateman

*Breast and Cervical Cancer*
Barbara A. Wismer

*Osteoporosis*
Eugenia L. Siegler, Elizabeth J. Kramer

**Part Three: Emotional, Psychosomatic, Behavioral,
and Mental Health Problems** 175

10 **Domestic and Sexual Violence** 177

*Domestic Violence*
Shobha Srinivasan, Susan L. Ivey

*Sexual Violence, Rape, and War*
Kaila Morris Compton, Deanna Chechile

*Female Genital Mutilation*
Kaila Morris Compton, Deanna Chechile

11    **Depression and Anxiety Disorders**                              205
      Lisa C. Tracy, Sandra Mattar

12    **Posttraumatic Stress Disorder**                                 220
      Lisa C. Tracy

13    **Somatization, Neurasthenia, and Culture-Bound
      Syndromes**                                                       232
      *Somatization Disorders*
      Cora R. Hoover
      *Neurasthenia*
      Pamela Yew Schwartz
      *Culture-Bound Syndromes*
      Anthony T. Ng

**Part Four: Meeting the Health Care Needs of Immigrant
Women: Model Programs and Tools**                                        257

14    **Applications of Linguistic Strategies in Health Care
      Settings**                                                        259
      Sherry Riddick

15    **A Model Posttraumatic Stress Disorder Support
      Group for Cambodian Women**                                       271
      Judith Shepherd

16    **An Educational Program for Families on
      Intergenerational Conflict**                                      282
      Yu-Wen Ying

17    **The Korean Breast and Cervical Cancer Screening
      Demonstration**                                                   295
      Barbara A. Wismer, Arthur M. Chen, Stella Jun,
      Soo H. Kang, Rod Lew, Katya Min, Joel M. Moskowitz,
      Thomas E. Novotny, Ira B. Tager

18    **A Case Study of Asian Health Services**                         305
      Sherry M. Hirota

19    **A Cultural Competence Curriculum**                              322
      Elizabeth J. Kramer, William B. Bateman

**20 Cultural Competence Assessment of Practices, Clinics, and Health Care Facilities** 330

Dennis P. Andrulis

**Epilogue** 336

Elizabeth J. Kramer, Susan L. Ivey, Yu-Wen Ying

References 343

Name Index 397

Subject Index 408

# Exhibits and Tables

## Exhibits

7.1   Screening Protocol for Refugee Women at
      San Francisco General Hospital's Refugee Clinic   87
7.2   Screening Protocol for All Refugees from Countries
      with High Prevalence of Hepatitis B Carriers   88
7.3   Questions for a Dietary History   117
10.1  Screening Protocol for Domestic Violence   187
10.2  Medical Clues Raising the Suspicion of Domestic
      Violence   188

## Tables

1.1   Where New Immigrants Settle   7
7.1   Recommended Primary Immunization Schedule
      in the United States, 1998   94
7.2   Recommended Adult Immunization Schedule in
      the United States, 1998   95
7.3   Geographic Distribution of Major Infectious Diseases   99
7.4   Medical History and Review of Systems for Infectious
      Diseases in Immigrants   101
7.5   Some Causes of Acute Febrile Illness in Immigrants   101
7.6   Physical Examination of the Immigrant   102
9.1   Age-Adjusted Mortality Rates for Ischemic Heart
      Disease and Stroke in Women, by Race   139
9.2   Age-Adjusted Mortality Rates for Ischemic Heart
      Disease and Stroke in Women, by Hispanic/Non-
      Hispanic Origin   139

9.3     Age-Adjusted Mortality Rates for Cardiovascular
        Disease in Women, by Race, 1995                             140

9.4     Age-Adjusted Mortality Rates of Women, by API
        Subgroups Compared to Other Races, 1992                     141

9.5     Average Annual Age-Adjusted Breast and Cervical
        Cancer Rates per 100,000 Women, California,
        1989–1993                                                   163

9.6     Women Age Fifty and Older Reporting
        Mammogram, California, 1993–1994                            164

9.7     Women Reporting Mammogram or Pap Test,
        Behavioral Risk Factor Survey, Hawaii, 1993                 165

9.8     Women Reporting Mammogram or Pap Test,
        Behavioral Risk Factor Survey, Florida, 1996                166

9.9     Bone Loss Categories                                        171

18.1    Ethnic Distribution of the Population
        in Alameda County                                           307

# Foreword

As Lance Morrow (1985) wrote, "Everyone is an immigrant in time, voyaging into the future.... The immigrant who travels both in time and geographical space achieves a neat existential alertness, the dimension of time and space collaborate. America, a place, becomes a time, the future" (p. 25).

Beyond the hard statistics of immigration are personal stories of those who have made America their home, whether as transients, permanent residents, or naturalized citizens. As immigration to the United States from all parts of the globe has increased, we have become a country of many diverse cultures. Although many immigrants are assimilated, not all acculturate. Furthermore, as evidenced by a recent three-part series in the *New York Times,* there is a strong movement toward biculturalism to the point that immigrants and their children move freely between their culture of origin and the United States, keeping the country of origin's cultural mores, beliefs, and traditions alive for succeeding generations.

Margaret Sanger, a staunch feminist and social reformer, went to jail in 1917 for distributing contraceptives to immigrant women from a makeshift clinic in Brooklyn, New York. Her work in the birth control movement benefited women from all over the world. Shortly before her death in 1966, Sanger said she hoped to be remembered for helping women as "they take care of culture and tradition and preserve what is good."

Women traditionally are and have been the health caregivers, as well as the brokers and protectors of their families' health. They also use health care services more frequently than men, particularly during their childbearing years. The burden of these functions is an even greater challenge for immigrant women, many of whom face multiple barriers to obtaining access to health care, among them linguistic, financial, legal, cultural, and in many instances, geographic and temporal.

As health care providers, we are frequently thwarted in our efforts to provide adequate, effective, and culturally competent services to the immigrant women in our communities. We encounter legal, financial, and regulatory constraints, and we lack understanding of others' cultures and the knowledge, attitudes, beliefs, and practices they bring with them from their countries of origin.

*Immigrant Women's Health* builds the bridge that connects the health problems of immigrant women to actual or potential solutions. Part of the solution is understanding *cultural competency,* a term that recently evolved as the lingua franca to describe the process of integrating cultural knowledge and expertise into systems, be they educational, scientific, or institutional. The California Cultural Competency Task Force defined *cultural competency* as "a process that requires individuals and systems to develop and expand their ability to know about, be sensitive to, and have respect for cultural diversity."

The time has come for health care providers, health care organizations, institutions, the government, and the communities in which they are located to address the inequities in the delivery of health care to all who reside in the United States, regardless of race, creed, national origin, or source of payment for services. To do this, we must be willing to listen to and learn from individuals from diverse cultures and to provide services and information in appropriate languages at comprehension and literacy levels that meet their cultural, psychosocial, and educational needs.

This book goes a long way toward achieving that goal by providing a solid background on the major clinical, behavioral, and policy issues, problems, and prospects, as well as potential solutions and examples of programs that can be replicated. It comes to the marketplace not a moment too soon!

*Kansas City, Kansas*     LILLIAN PARDO-GONZALEZ
*September 1998*

# Preface

The women whose faces appear on the dust jacket—Helena Cheung from Hong Kong, Noris Douglas from Panama, Levia Ivis Gomez from Puerto Rico, Noemi Mascarenes from the Philippines, and Coreen Parks from Guyana are not models. They are Liz's co-workers and friends. They represent the many immigrant women whose struggles and courage, hopes and dreams have inspired this book. The picture was taken on the Lower East Side of Manhattan, about a mile from Battery Park where the ferries to the Statue of Liberty and Ellis Island depart. Liz's parents were born there in the early 1900s. The faces have changed, the languages are different, but New York City remains a significant entry point for new immigrants.

*Immigrant Women's Health* is about cultural diversity and delivering culturally competent health care to women who come to the United States from all over the world in search of a better life. The three of us have different perspectives on this vast field. Liz works in a clinic that has served new immigrants for over 100 years; today approximately 90 percent of the patients are recently arrived, primarily from China and the Dominican Republic. Yu-Wen immigrated to New York from Taiwan via Germany with her parents in the 1960s. She became a psychologist to better understand her own cross-cultural experiences, to heal the pain associated with them, and to help others, especially immigrants from Asia, to do the same. Although Susan's family has been in this country for many generations, her clinical experience as an emergency physician has included countless encounters with recent immigrants, often—in a given shift—from several different countries. Together we have attempted to address a wide range of health and mental health challenges facing immigrant women today. We hope this book will contribute to the development and implementation of effective, culturally competent solutions in an era of diminishing resources.

Research was supported in part by grants from Pfizer Women's Health to Liz, and the Committee on Research, University of California, Berkeley, to Yu-Wen, and by Cooperative Agreement #U48/CCU909706 between the Centers for Disease Control and Prevention and the Center for Family and Community Health, University of California, Berkeley.

Many individuals have helped with the preparation of this manuscript. Francesca Gany suggested the idea for the book. In addition to our contributors, to whom we owe a great debt of gratitude, we thank Barry Bateman, Angelina Borbon, Loren Brewster, Andrew Delp, Lucy Fisher, Anthony Grieco, Andrea Jones, Eva Lu, Francis Lu, Eric Mannheimer, Ann Morse, Joel Moskowitz, Annette Ramirez, Susan Resnik, Michael Tanner, Heike ThieldeBocanegra, Lisa Tracy, Frances Wong, James Zazzali, Fontaine Zhang, and the anonymous peer reviewer for their support and feedback, which greatly strengthened the final manuscript. Special thanks to Mary Jane Ruppert, who transformed the many diskettes and more than a thousand references into the final product, and to our colleagues, patients, students, families, and friends from whom we continue to learn.

*September 1998*

Elizabeth J. Kramer
*York, Pennsylvania*

Susan L. Ivey
*Berkeley, California*

Yu-Wen Ying
*Berkeley, California*

# The Editors

*Elizabeth J. Kramer,* a clinical epidemiologist and medical writer, is a research scientist in the Division of Primary Care Internal Medicine at New York University School of Medicine. Her interests include women's health, immigrant health and the delivery of culturally competent care to immigrant patients, patient education, and the interface of medical education and medical care. She is an alumna of New York University College of Arts and Sciences and the Johns Hopkins University School of Hygiene and Public Health.

*Susan L. Ivey* is a board-certified family and emergency physician and a health policy research specialist in the Center for Family and Community Health at the University of California at Berkeley School of Public Health. Her research interest is access to medical care by the underserved. She graduated from the University of Southern California, St. George's University School of Medicine, and George Washington University.

*Yu-Wen Ying* is a clinical psychologist and professor at the School of Social Welfare, University of California at Berkeley. She also has a small private practice serving Asian Americans in the San Francisco Bay Area. Her research interests include Asian American mental health, immigrant and refugee adaptation, acculturation and ethnic identity formation, family relationships in migrant families, and culturally competent mental health prevention and treatment interventions. She is an alumna of Barnard College and the University of California at Berkeley.

# The Contributors

Phillip D. Akutsu, Ph.D.
Assistant Professor
Pacific Graduate School of Psychology
San Francisco, California

Dennis P. Andrulis, Ph.D.
Head, Office of Urban Populations
New York Academy of Medicine
Adjunct Associate Professor
Health Services Management and Policy
George Washington University
Washington, D.C.

Robin K. Avery, M.D.
Staff Physician
Cleveland Clinic Foundation
Cleveland, Ohio

William B. Bateman, M.D.
Medical Director
Gouverneur Diagnostic and Treatment Center
Associate Clinical Professor of Medicine
New York University School of Medicine
New York, New York

Deanna Chechile, J.D.
Attorney
Sherman & Sterling
Berkeley, California

Arthur M. Chen, M.D.
Health Officer
Alameda County (California) Health Care Services Agency
Oakland, California

Kevin M. Chun, Ph.D.
Assistant Professor
Department of Psychology
University of San Francisco
San Francisco, California

Kaila Morris Compton, Ph.D.
Joint Medical Program
University of California at Berkeley and San Francisco
Berkeley and San Francisco, California

Mary L. Del Monte, M.D.
Clinical Assistant Professor, Medicine
New York University School of Medicine
Chief, Nephrology
Brooklyn Hospital
Brooklyn, New York

Shotsy Faust, M.S.N., F.N.P.
Nurse Practitioner
San Francisco General Hospital Refugee Clinic
Associate Clinical Professor
Department of Family Health Nursing
University of California, San Francisco
San Francisco, California

Ernesto Ferran, M.D.
Assistant Professor of Psychiatry
New York University School of Medicine
New York, New York

Francesca M. Gany, M.D.
Executive Director
New York Task Force on Immigrant Health

Assistant Professor of Medicine
New York University School of Medicine
New York, New York

Gerrie Gardner, D.O.
Private Practice, Cardiology
Carson City, Nevada

Sherry M. Hirota
Executive Director
Asian Health Services
Oakland, California

Cora R. Hoover, M.S.
Joint Medical Program
University of California at Berkeley and San Francisco
Berkeley and San Francisco, California

Shirley Huang, B.A.
University of California at San Francisco School of Medicine
San Francisco, California

Stella Jun, B.A.
Community Health Specialist
Asian Health Services
Oakland, California

Soo H. Kang, Dr. P.H.
Consultant
Asian Health Services
Oakland, California

Ruby Ko, C.N.M., M.S.N.
Nurse Midwife
New York University Medical Center
Gouverneur Diagnostic and Treatment Center
New York, New York

Marion M. Lee, Ph.D.
Associate Professor, Epidemiology
University of California at San Francisco
San Francisco, California

Rod Lew, M.P.H.
Associate Director, External Programs
Association for Asian Pacific Community Health Organizations
Oakland, California

Dina Lieberman, M.D.
Brooklyn Hospital
Brooklyn, New York

Sandra Mattar, Psy.D.
Consultant, Cultural Competence
Walnut Creek, California

Katya Min, B.A.
Program Coordinator
Asian Health Services
Oakland, California

Nobuko Mizoguchi, M.P.H., M.P.P.
University of California School of Public Health
and Richard and Rhonda Goldman School of Public Policy
Berkeley, California

Joel M. Moskowitz, Ph.D.
Associate Director
Center for Family and Community Health
University of California School of Public Health
Berkeley, California

Anthony T. Ng, M.D.
Clinical Instructor, Psychiatry
New York University School of Medicine
Associate Medical Director
Project Renewal
New York, New York

Thomas E. Novotny, M.D., M.P.H.
Centers for Disease Control and Prevention Liaison
World Bank
Washington, D.C.

Marilyn Pan, C.N.M., M.S.N.
Nurse Midwife
New York University Medical Center
Gouverneur Diagnostic and Treatment Center
New York, New York

Sherry Riddick, R.N., M.P.H.
Cross Cultural Health Care Consultant
Seattle, Washington

Pamela Yew Schwartz, Ph.D.
Psychologist
Manhattan Psychiatric Center
New York, New York

Judith Shepherd, D.S.W.
Executive Director
Nobiru-Kai Japanese Newcomers Services
San Francisco, California

Eugenia L. Siegler, M.D.
Associate Professor of Clinical Medicine
New York University School of Medicine
Chief, Geriatrics
The Brooklyn Hospital
Brooklyn, New York

Shobha Srinivasan, Ph.D.
Researcher
Center for Asian Studies
University of California
Davis, California

Ira B. Tager, M.D., M.P.H.
Director, Center for Family and Community Health
Professor of Epidemiology
University of California School of Public Health
Berkeley, California

Francesca M. A. Taylor, M.D.
Assistant Professor of Family Medicine
University of Southern California School of Medicine
Codirector, University of Southern California—California
   Hospital Medical Center Family Medicine Residency Program
Los Angeles, California

Lisa C. Tracy, M.S.W.
Researcher
Center for Asian Studies
University of California
Davis, California

Barbara A. Wismer, M.D., M.P.H.
Assistant Clinical Professor, Medicine
University of California San Francisco
Research Specialist
Center for Family and Community Health
University of California School of Public Health
Berkeley and San Francisco, California

# Immigrant Women's Health

# Part One

# Background

# Chapter One

# Demographics, Definitions, and Data Limitations

*Elizabeth J. Kramer,*
*Lisa C. Tracy, and*
*Susan L. Ivey*

Carmen is a fifty-three-year-old, overweight, Mexican American woman who moved to the United States from rural Mexico to live with her daughter. She presents to a primary care provider complaining of recent nausea and fatigue. Her symptoms are particularly pronounced when she walks up and down a flight of stairs in her apartment building to get her mail. She does not smoke and eats a traditional Mexican diet with high daily intake of beans cooked with lard, rice, raw vegetables, and fresh fruit. She has given up walking outdoors since she moved to the United States because of fear of the urban setting. *"Me duele en pecho"* ("It hurts in my chest"), she tells the physician. *"En su corazon?"* ("In your heart?"), is the response. After puzzling for a moment, she replies, *"No me duele el corazon, yo estoy contenta"* ("My heart doesn't hurt, I am happy").

This book focuses on the health and mental health of immigrant women and the provision of culturally competent services to them. The 1990s have been a decade of significant advances in women's health. With the creation of the Office of Women's Health within the U.S. Public Health Service (USPHS) and the implementation of the Women's Health Initiative, the largest randomized,

Many thanks to Francesca Gany for her input in this chapter.

3

controlled clinical trial in history, the uniqueness of women as biological and psychological human beings finally has received due recognition. Immigrant women are a substantial subgroup of women who reside in this country. They experience the same problems as their American-born sisters and, like them, often are the health care decision makers for their entire families. However, they also encounter unique problems in obtaining access to and receiving health care services.

The book is not intended to be a definitive treatise on the physical and mental health of immigrant women. Rather, its purpose is to introduce readers to the health status and health care problems of immigrant women, the mores and belief systems they bring with them from their countries of origin, and some of the many barriers they face in their efforts to obtain health care services in the United States. Our goal is to build cultural competence among providers, suggest possible solutions, and, in the process, pave the way for a more competent delivery system.

We begin with a series of operational definitions and delineation of the issues and problems from the perspective of both the patient and the health care delivery system. From there we move on to some common health problems immigrant women may bring to this country, a discussion of prenatal care and childbirth issues, and some of the chronic diseases acculturated immigrant women are likely to acquire. Part Three discusses mental health and psychosocial problems. Finally, Part Four looks at some exemplary programs and food for thought on topics such as teaching cultural competence to health care providers and improving cultural competence from an institutional perspective.

## Who Are the Immigrants, and Where Do They Come From?

From the late nineteenth century to the early twentieth century, a growing influx of immigrants arrived in the United States, with the wave of immigration peaking between 1900 and 1910. Enactment of a sharply restrictive immigration law, combined with two world wars and the Great Depression, slowed the flood of immigrants from the early 1920s until well into the 1940s.

The interaction of socioeconomic conditions here and abroad and changes in U.S. immigration laws have influenced how many immigrants have entered the United States, as well as the countries from which they came. Nineteenth-century immigrants came primarily from Europe; the first groups originated in northern and western Europe, and later groups came from the southern and eastern parts. By the 1960s migration had shifted from southern Europe to Asia, Central and South America, and the Caribbean islands, a trend that continues today (Bogen, 1987; U.S. Bureau of the Census, 1994).

How does one define an immigrant, or decide that individuals are or are not immigrants? Except for Native Americans, most bona fide residents of the United States theoretically are immigrants or descendants of immigrants. Therefore, we have chosen a broad definition that includes recent arrivals and those who are foreign born. In addition, those who identify strongly with a culture that differs from that of the mainstream in this country, for example, Puerto Ricans and sometimes native Hawaiians and Native Americans (whom we have not for the most part addressed), are operationally defined as immigrants even though they are American citizens. In fact, many existing databases classify them among other ethnic or racial groups.

A March 1997 survey among all segments of the immigrant population in the United States conducted by the Census Bureau found that 25.8 million people (9.7 percent), the largest segment in more than five decades, were foreign born (*Washington Post,* 1998). In fiscal year 1996, of a total of 915,900 immigrants who were admitted to the United States, 493,142 (53.8 percent) were women. Of all the countries from which immigrants came, only Bangladesh, Cuba, Pakistan, and the United Kingdom had larger proportions of men than women. The median age of the women was 28.7 years, with a range of 25.3 (from Bangladesh) to 40.4 (from Iran).

Fifty-seven percent (280,602) of the legal immigrant women came from twelve countries:

| | | |
|---|---|---|
| Mexico | 93,623 | (33.4 percent) |
| Philippines | 33,208 | (11.8 percent) |
| People's Republic of China | 24,406 | (8.7 percent) |
| India | 23,080 | (8.2 percent) |
| Vietnam | 21,918 | (7.8 percent) |
| Dominican Republic | 20,800 | (7.4 percent) |

(*continued*)

| Cuba | 11,350 | (4.0 percent) |
| Ukraine | 11,168 | (4.0 percent) |
| Russia | 10,721 | (3.8 percent) |
| Jamaica | 10,280 | (3.7 percent) |
| Korea | 10,026 | (3.6 percent) |
| El Salvador | 10,022 | (3.6 percent) |

The remaining 212,540 immigrant women came from all over the rest of the world, with sizable numbers from Haiti, Poland, Colombia, Canada, Taiwan, Peru, Iran, the United Kingdom, Pakistan, Yugoslavia, and Nigeria.

The top states that newcomers declared as their intended residence in 1994 were California, New York, Florida, Texas, New Jersey, and Illinois. Other states with significant immigrant influx were Massachusetts, Washington, Maryland, Virginia, Georgia, Connecticut, and Ohio.

Immigrants from most countries tend to cluster in one or two areas of the country. Existing ethnic communities and the presence of family or friends help to influence the decision of where to settle. Table 1.1 shows the distribution of the immigrant women by state and country of origin for the top states based on the 1996 data.

The March 1997 survey found that although distribution has spread, California (nearly 25 percent of residents are foreign born), New York (nearly 20 percent are foreign born), Florida, New Jersey, and Texas continue to be the locations for concentration of new immigrants (*Washington Post,* 1998). New York City remains the major point of entry for new immigrants to the United States. Between 1990 and 1994, 563,000 documented immigrants, or nearly 15 percent of all those entering the United States, settled there. The top three countries of origin for those settling in New York were the Dominican Republic, the former Soviet Union, and China (New York City Department of City Planning, 1990–1994).

Immigrants have a rich cultural, linguistic, and epidemiologic diversity. In fact, substantial differences exist even within groups from one region. For example, East Indian immigrants to the United States represent the diversity in religion, language, and culture that exists in India (Ramakrishna and Weiss, 1992). A study that compared Egyptian, Yemenite, Iranian, Armenian, and Arab

**Table 1.1. Where New Immigrants Settle.**

| Country of Origin | New York | California | Florida | New Jersey | Texas | Illinois | Massachusetts |
|---|---|---|---|---|---|---|---|
| | | | *Resettlement Location* | | | | |
| Mainland China | X | X | | | | | |
| Colombia | X | | X | X | | | |
| Cuba | | | X | | | | |
| Dominican Republic | X | | | | | | |
| El Salvador | | X | | | | | |
| Former Soviet Union | X | X | | | | X | |
| Guatemala | | X | | | | | |
| Guyana | X | | | | | | |
| Haiti | X | | X | | | | |
| India | X | X | | X | | X | |
| Jamaica | X | | X | | | | |
| Korea | | X | | | | | |
| Mexico | | X | | | X | X | |
| Philippines | | X | | | | | |
| Poland | X | | | | | X | |
| Taiwan | | X | | | | | |
| Trinidad and Tobago | X | | | | | | |
| Vietnam | | X | | | X | | X |

U.S. Immigration and Naturalization Service, 1997, Table 17.

immigrants to the United States found significant differences among the five groups on cultural attitudes, social attitudes, family psychological symptoms, perceived health status, and positive morale (Meleis, Lipson, and Paul, 1992).

## Categories of Immigrants

There are a number of categories of immigrants to the United States. Following are the definitions that will be used throughout this book.

*Documented* (or *admitted*) *immigrants* are those who have been granted permanent residence in the United States by the Immigration and Naturalization Service (INS).

*Undocumented immigrants* are those individuals who arrive in the United States as nonimmigrants, for example, as tourists or students, and stay beyond their specified periods of admission (nonimmigrant overstays), and those who enter the United States surreptitiously across land borders that usually are between official ports of entry (such as from Mexico). Nonimmigrant overstays are the most common form of illegal immigration. The INS refers to this part of the population as EWIs (entry without inspection). Immigrants come to the United States by choice and are thus classified as *voluntary migrants.*

*Refugees* are people who have been forced to leave their home of origin due to a well-founded fear of "persecution on account of race, religion, nationality, membership in a particular social group or political opinion" (Refugee Act of 1980, Section 201). Often they are referred to as *involuntary migrants.*

*Asylum seekers* are immigrants who cannot return to their home countries because of likely persecution based on race, religion, nationality, or social or political ties. Asylum seekers differ from refugees in that they already are on U.S. soil when they apply for immigration status.

*PRUCOL* is a commonly used acronym for "permanently residing in the United States, under color of law," and therefore eligible for certain public benefits. In the past, social service laws frequently failed to define which types of immigrants were to be viewed as PRUCOL, thereby creating confusion and conflict over their entitlements. This category was eliminated in the Illegal Immigration Reform Act of 1996.

There are places in this book where the terms *immigrant, migrant,* and *refugee* have been used interchangeably. For the most part, however, we have elected to use the term *immigrant* since refugees are a subset of immigrants.


## Migration

The prior life experiences of, reasons for, and the circumstances under which people migrate vary greatly and hold significant implications for emotional and economic adaptation to life in the United States (Ben-Porath, 1991). Level of education and English-language skill, type of prior occupation, and prior contact with or knowledge of the West, technological societies, and urban lifestyle will have an important impact on the newcomers' adaptation in the United States (Ben-Porath, 1991; Berry, Kim, Minde, and Mok, 1987; Sluzki, 1979). In addition, refugees may have experienced numerous extreme stressors, such as war, rape, torture, reeducation or concentration camps, famine, and loss of family members and communities, with serious implications for their mental health (Ben-Porath, 1991; Sluzki, 1979; Westermeyer, 1987).

Traditional theories of migration present the simple differentiation that refugees migrate because of *push* factors in their home country and immigrants migrate because of *pull* factors in the resettlement country (Boyd, 1989). Refugees may have left home under threat of war, a push factor, and due to the political situation may not be able to return home, although many hold onto the hope of going back (Sluzki, 1979). The search for better employment opportunities, a pull factor, is of major importance in the immigration of both professional workers and seasonal migrant workers (Portes and Rumbaut, 1990), who may come to the United States temporarily and have the choice to return home. Voluntary immigrants tend to have had more time to prepare both psychologically and practically, may come with resources and some level of English-language skill, and have generally experienced less extreme stressors.

More recent migration theories argue that the reasons for migration, and thus the distinction between immigrants and refugees, is more complex than the push versus pull theory (Boyd, 1989). For example, family networks are often significant factors for both refugees and immigrants in the decision to migrate (Boyd, 1989).

Some individuals migrate alone, but many come as families or parts of families, and may join relatives and extended family networks already residing in the United States (Boyd, 1989), a process referred to in immigration policy as *family reunification*. Family, extended family, and ethnic communities provide significant social supports to newcomers, both emotionally and economically (Haines, 1988; Van Arsdale, 1990). Evidence of the importance of such supports includes the development of ethnic communities and the occurrence of secondary migration to locations where relatives reside, when refugees initially have been placed in dispersed or isolated communities (Van Arsdale, 1990).

## Undocumented Immigrants

Despite the clear violation of U.S. law, undocumented immigrants continue to be strongly attracted to the opportunity of higher-paying jobs here. The low wages in their countries of origin make them easy targets of exploitation by American employers, whose offers of relatively low wages and few benefits still are substantially better than those the workers would have received at home. The Immigration Reform and Control Act (IRCA) of 1986 prohibits employers from hiring or recruiting undocumented immigrants. Violators are subject to fines and, in severe cases, even imprisonment.

Undocumented immigrants, who tend to be male, comprise a sizable portion of the immigrant population, and they face the greatest barriers to receiving medical care.

Data from the INS (1997) indicate that Mexico was the country of origin for 1.3 million (39 percent) undocumented immigrants, followed by El Salvador (327,000), Guatemala (129,000), Canada (97,000), Poland (91,000), the Philippines (90,000), and Haiti (88,000). Seven states received 86 percent of the undocumented immigrant population in 1992: California, with 1.4 million (43 percent); New York, with 449,000; Texas, with 357,000; Florida, with 322,000; Illinois, with 176,000; New Jersey, with 116,000; and Arizona, with 57,000.

## Health Status Before and After Migration

Current immigration policy requires documented immigrants and refugees who come into the United States to undergo physical and mental examinations prior to departure from their country of origin. Some individuals are disqualified from entry to the United States on the basis of these examinations. Screening to enter the United States and screening of newly arrived immigrants are described in Chapter Seven.

The health of immigrants is determined by factors in the sending countries, such as underlying health status, exposure to infectious organisms or toxins, nutritional status, their health experiences during migration, and the conditions to which they are subjected on arrival. At the time of arrival, the health status of many new voluntary immigrants is better than that of their U.S.-born "sisters." This is a result of the *healthy migrant effect*, a self-selection process in which only the strongest and healthiest choose to migrate and actually complete the process (Guendelman, Gould, Hudes, and Eskenazi, 1990; Scribner and Dwyer, 1989; Marin, Perez-Stable, and Marin, 1989). However, health status often begins to deteriorate after arrival here. Reasons include poor access to appropriate health care, which may result in delays in seeking care, especially for infectious diseases that are acquired between the initial screening and arrival here.

Adoption of bad health habits, such as a high fat diet, and exposure to environmental risks may accompany acculturation. For example, breast cancer incidence rates in the United States have been four to seven times higher than in China or Japan. Some of the difference is thought to be due to diet and other lifestyle factors, although the reasons remain elusive. When Chinese, Japanese, or Filipino women migrate to the United States, breast cancer risk rises over several generations and approaches that of U.S. whites (Ziegler and others, 1993).

Immigrant women tend to work in the lowest-paying jobs, often in sweatshops and other unhealthy environments, including massage parlors and as prostitutes. Many take positions as home health aides and child care workers that expose them to hazards such as infections (Weitzman and Berry, 1992), while others pursue agricultural work and food packing, which may expose them to toxins and high-injury work environments.

Many women stay in their own ethnic enclaves, disempowered by a lack of language skills and inability to negotiate the complex organizations, including the health care delivery system, of American society. This can result in depression and other psychological problems. Refugee women often have undergone traumatic experiences, including prolonged family separation, torture, rape, genital mutilation, or life in refugee camps under precarious hygienic conditions, which have a negative impact on their health status. Therefore, if we improve the health of immigrants we will improve the health of Americans as well, since they are our family members, our employees, our neighbors, and our friends.

## Existing Data and Their Limitations

Evaluating health and disease in immigrants is complex. Most health statistics include immigrants because nearly 10 percent of Americans are foreign born (*Washington Post*, 1998). However, there are too few published epidemiologic studies of immigrant health due to the lack of an accurate immigrant census, immigrants' fears of participating in studies, the additional resources needed to conduct multilingual studies, lack of inclusion of acculturation variables in surveys, and lack of an accepted classification system for immigrants.

Data usually are not collected by country of origin, length of residence in the United States, self-defined ethnicity, or language. Most studies do not include non-English-speaking participants, in part because of the complexity and expense of translating and administering research instruments. Historically, many medical studies have not included women, although that is now changing. Immigrant women therefore have had a double risk for not being included in research: their gender and their recent immigrant status. This lack of data hampers providers from delivering culturally competent care to immigrant women.

Existing data sets have a range of characteristics that often are missing or incorrectly entered. Hospitals and physicians are relied on to furnish data on reportable conditions, with resultant variation in validity and reliability. Inconsistency of racial and ethnic coding on death certificates is greatest for races other than white or black (Hahn, 1992).

In-person surveys at health care facilities miss immigrants if they are conducted at hospitals or clinics to which immigrants often have limited access. Telephone surveys miss immigrants because a disproportionate number lack telephones, and many have difficulty with English. Mailed surveys miss immigrants because of language and because immigrants are less likely to be literate than the U.S. born. The 1997 immigrant survey by the Census Bureau found that while 16 percent of American-born adults over age twenty-five had not completed high school, this figure was nearly 35 percent among the foreign born (*Washington Post*, 1998).

Often the operational definitions of basic concepts and data collection categories are unclear. For example, *ethnicity* is a group's mutual identification that results from common patterns of behavior, customs, race, and heritage; it refers to cultural features of a given society. *Race* refers to a subdivision of human beings who share a common origin. A race comprises individuals who have a relatively constant combination of physical traits that are transmitted from parents to children. Race therefore has biological as well as cultural components.

Medical records and national data sets classify individuals according to racial and ethnic groups (white, black, Hispanic, Asian), often confusing race and ethnicity, but not according to country of birth or length of residence in the United States. Further, the Census Bureau's definition of race is based on self-identification, and definitions do not denote any clear-cut scientific definition of biological stock. The "white" category in the 1990 census includes all those who indicated their race as white or reported entries such as Canadian, German, Italian, Lebanese, Middle Eastern, Arab, or Polish. Those who reported their race as black or Negro, African American, Afro-American, Black Puerto Rican, Jamaican, Nigerian, West Indian, or Haitian were classified as "black," while Hispanic refers to anyone who self-identifies as Mexican, Puerto Rican, or Cuban, as well as those who came from Spain, the Spanish-speaking countries of Central and South America, or the Dominican Republic, or to those who self-identify in the general categories of Spanish, Spanish American, Hispanic, or Latino.

To complicate the situation, Hispanics are persons who share a common language (Spanish) and a common cultural and ethnic heritage whose roots are in Spain. The term *Hispanic* is distinct from *Iberian,* which encompasses the countries of Spain and Portugal, and *Latin,* which refers to the populations of the countries whose languages have their origin in the Latin language: France, Italy, Spain, and Portugal. Individuals of Hispanic origin may be of any race (Garza-Trevino, Ruiz, and Venegas-Samuels, 1997).

Traditional racial divisions are subject to miscounting and misclassification (Hahn, 1992; Hahn, Mulinare, and Teutsch, 1992). They are especially misleading when dealing with both dark- and light-complexioned people from Africa, Asia, Europe, and the Americas. For example, Fruchter and others (1990) found significant differences in breast and cervical cancer incidence rates among U.S.-born African American, Haitian, and English-speaking Caribbean women living in New York, which remain undetected when all women are classified as black. Data would be more meaningful if they were collected by country of origin, length of stay or generation of residence in the United States, self-defined ethnicity, parents' countries of origin, and primary language spoken.

The 1990 census was underenumerated, particularly among low-income, black, and Hispanic populations and areas where there are many immigrants. Therefore, any immigrant health statistic that has census data in the denominator, such as incidence or prevalence, is likely to be too high because the denominator is too small.

## Barriers to Access

Early entry into primary health care is one of the most effective ways to ensure positive health practices and early diagnosis of diseases, when they can be treated most effectively, at the least expense, and often cured. Approximately 50 percent of newly arrived immigrant women are between the ages of fifteen and forty-four. Obstetrical and pediatric services present a window of opportunity for introducing women into the health care delivery system, especially since until 1997 some states provided access to prenatal services regardless of immigration status. However, this relatively open door for prenatal care faces serious challenges under the 1996–1997 changes in federal law. Immigrant women often face multiple barriers to access, among them linguistic, financial, legal, and cultural ones.

## Linguistic Barriers

In 1980, 23 million U.S. residents did not speak English as their first language. By 1990, the number had increased by 38 percent, to 31.8 million (U.S. Bureau of the Census, 1993). Adult immigrant women may be less likely than men to learn English. On average, they have a lower educational level than immigrant men, they are more likely to be confined to ethnic neighborhoods, and the responsibility to care for their families may impede their attending English as a Second Language classes. Even in places where the provider speaks the same language, there may be major differences in dialect. For example, Puerto Rican and Mexican Spanish are practically two separate languages when it comes to the spoken word. Language and linguistic barriers are discussed in Chapter Three.

A combination of language and cultural barriers presented problems for Carmen, whose case opens the book. Carmen's chest pain was the result of an evolving myocardial infarction. The physician who saw her did not realize that *corazon* ("heart") had a culturally embedded meaning in Mexico, where a happy person has a good heart. The mistake could have been fatal. Cases like these occur every day.

## Cultural Barriers

Cultural barriers to accessing health care include expectations of the health care system, concepts of health and illness, and health care–seeking behaviors. Different gender roles in the United States can be confusing to immigrant women. Concepts of health and illness and health care–seeking behaviors are rooted in cultural systems. The U.S. health care system is itself a cultural system with an explicit structural organization that separates mind and body and implicit expectations about roles for both provider and patient (Friedson, 1961; Szasz and Hollender, 1956; Zola, 1963).

Patients' and providers' health beliefs or explanatory systems are the basis for expectation and behavior within the health care encounter. Cultural barriers to accessing health care by immigrants include differences between patients and providers in health care decision making, role expectations during the health care encounter, and beliefs about the effectiveness of different interventions (Gil, 1982; Harwood, 1981; Kleinman, Eisenberg, and Good, 1978; Maduro, 1983; Snow, 1972; Zola, 1966; Michael and others, 1993; Nguyen, 1985; Schultz, 1982).

Immigrants often come from very different health care systems and have different expectations of medical care. Experiences with the health care system in their home countries can affect the way they seek and experience care in the United States. Gender roles also have an impact on the receipt of care. In some cases, the woman may not be the sole decision maker in her care. Treatment options may be discussed and decided on after conferring with influential members of the extended family or community. For example, Latino husbands may be the ultimate decision makers about whether condoms are used during coitus. For some immigrant groups, the interests of the family as a whole may be more important than those of the individual.

Illnesses associated with stigma, such as human immunodeficiency virus infection or tuberculosis, may not be discussed for fear that they may be a source of family shame or that patients may be rejected by their families (Castro de Alvarez, 1990). Immigrants may not be ready to discuss acquired immunodeficiency syndrome or tuberculosis due to the anxiety that their particular ethnic group is being singled out as causing or spreading the disease (Freudenberg, Jacalyn, and Silver, 1989). Culture and cultural competence are discussed in Chapter Two.

## System Barriers

Although some sterling examples of model services exist, often there is a lack of adequate and appropriate health care services and appropriately trained practitioners to care for immigrants, and community outreach and education may be nonexistent or poor. There is a dearth of training in medical and other health professions schools, and residency programs frequently fail to address these issues as well. For example, a survey of Canadian family practice residencies found that poverty and the health care concerns of Native and immigrant women were included in fewer than 40 percent of the programs (McCall and Sorbie, 1994).

## Financial Barriers

Recently arrived immigrants tend to work in low-paying jobs that often do not provide health insurance coverage and may not pay the employee for time lost due to medical appointments. A trip to the doctor can result in loss of a day's wages, and a woman who needs to make multiple visits to a health care provider for prenatal care or treatment of a complex illness may risk losing her job. These women may not be eligible for entitlement programs; even in localities where they are, they may not be aware that the services exist. Further, foreign-born women may not be assertive in negotiating benefits and demanding their rights.

Immigrant women often have difficulty understanding how to access the fragmented U.S. health care system and where to obtain services at low cost. Copayments, for those who have insurance, and sliding fee scales may be new to them. In many Latin American countries, for example, public health services are provided free without income verification. Women may be surprised and fearful about having to report their incomes.

## Legal Barriers

Perceived legal barriers and an individual's fear of the INS are real barriers. For example, although they do not face deportation for using free medical services or Medicaid, some documented immigrants believe that such utilization might render them "public charges," thereby jeopardizing their chances of becoming citizens and of sponsoring relatives for future immigration. In New York City, municipal employees are prohibited by the city charter from reporting any information on legal status to the INS. However, immigrants often are unaware of this. Patients frequently are asked questions about their income and employment status, as well as other personal information. Such questions strongly deter undocumented immigrants from seeking medical care, even free care in municipal facilities.

Even prior to California's Proposition 187 (1994), which sought to prohibit access to public education and health services by illegal immigrants, a San Francisco study revealed that 75 percent of undocumented Salvadoran and 54 percent of undocumented Mexican women cited fear of deportation as the primary barrier for failure to seek health care (Hogeland and Rosen, 1990). Proposition 187, which has been enjoined, required not only that immigration status be reported, but also that patients be denied services if they were not legal residents of the United States.

Immigrant patients often are surprised by the importance clinicians and institutions give to obtaining informed consent for diagnostic procedures or treatment, and the possible delays that can result in completing a workup or implementing treatment until it is obtained. Health care proxies, durable medical powers of attorney, and living wills can be equally baffling to immigrants, who are accustomed to going to clinics or hospitals and receiving treatment without such procedures.

The anti-immigrant sentiments that are so prevalent in the United States now will only make matters worse. It is not wise economically or socially to deny benefits to immigrants, who want to pay their own way if they can. Because many undocumented immigrants eventually legalize their status, their freshly covered care may cost more if their access to primary care and preventive services was denied.

## Conclusion

The issues that bear on the health care status and treatment of immigrant populations in the United States are complex and vital for all health care providers and others who work with immigrants. Advances in medical technology and improvements in access have been counterweighted by sheer numbers, heterogeneity of new immigrants, and financial barriers that threaten the public health care system.

The numbers of new Americans will only increase, and heightened provider awareness of the issues set forth in this book will enable the second, third, and future generations of immigrant offspring to live healthy and productive lives.

# Chapter Two

# Culture and Multicultural Competence

*Ernesto Ferran,*
*Lisa C. Tracy,*
*Francesca M. Gany,*
*and Elizabeth J. Kramer*

*Webster's College Dictionary* (1997) defines *culture* as "the sum total of ways of living built up by a group of human beings and transmitted from one generation to another." A slightly more sophisticated definition, which we will use in this chapter, is "the integrated pattern of human behavior that includes thoughts, communications, actions, customs, beliefs, values, and institutions of a racial, ethnic, religious or social group" (Cross, Bazron, Dennis, and Isaacs, 1989, p. 3).

Culture defines our relationships to our environment and to one another. Cultural beliefs affect how changes in health status are perceived, recognized, interpreted, and acted on. It is a conservative force that begs us to rely on a traditional response before considering what is perceived to be an alien one. In definitions of culture—and there are more than 175 of them referenced in the anthropologic literature—a common thread is the opinion that for a feature to be part of a cultural belief system, it must be long-standing. That means it has lasted at least three generations and contributes to the survival of a generation.

Cultural competence is "a set of congruent behaviors, attitudes, and policies that come together in a system, agency or among professionals and enables this system, agency or those professionals to work effectively in cross-cultural situations" (Cross, Bazron, Dennis, and Isaacs, 1989, p. iv). "Competence" refers to the acquisition of knowledge, skills, and experience that are needed for the development and implementation of interventions that are adapted to the different groups served. Lavizzo-Mourey and MacKenzie (1995) define cultural competence as "the demonstrated integration of population-specific related cultural values, disease incidence, prevalence, or mortality rates, and population-specific treatment outcomes." They argue that the integration of the three components is as necessary to meet the health care needs of defined populations and subpopulations as are the patients' values and needs.

Provision of culturally competent services requires that clinicians and institutions know the cultural norms for appropriate delivery of services to the various ethnic groups they serve. This includes being responsive to sociopolitical issues, such as the impact of racism, discrimination, immigration, and poverty on patients' health and adapting services to differences in family structure, expectations, preferences, help-seeking behavior, and worldviews. These points help to elucidate why the patient chooses to seek help at a particular time, what coping skills and stresses of daily living the patient brings to the encounter, and what the family strengths and stressors are and how they contribute to the patient's help-seeking behaviors.

Becoming culturally competent is a developmental process in which one learns to recognize, value, and adapt to diversity; assess one's own knowledge, attitudes, and beliefs about others' cultures; and incorporate the patient's beliefs and practices into the health care encounter. Patients perceive services as being culturally competent when they are appropriate for their problems and helpful in achieving desired outcomes according to their explanatory belief models (Dana, 1993).

Culturally competent health care practitioners must be able to differentiate between behavioral and ideological ethnicity. *Behavioral ethnicity* is characterized by traits such as recent immigration to the United States at an older age; frequent trips back to the country of origin; emigration from a rural area; lack of or limited formal education; lower socioeconomic status; segregation in an ethnic subculture in this country; inexperience with Western health care systems; and major differences in language, dress, and diet. *Ideological ethnicity* is characterized by nominal identification with the group of origin (Johnson, Hardt, and Kleinman, 1995, p. 156).

This chapter looks at the cultural issues that affect health care, beliefs about health and illness, health care–seeking behaviors, and effective cross-cultural communication between clinicians and patients.

## Cultural Issues That Affect Health Care

Health care is affected by a number of factors, including gender and gender issues, family structure and intergenerational issues, issues relating to religion and spirituality, occupational issues, and time orientation. These are discussed below.

### Gender Issues, Gender Roles, and Culture

Change in gender roles and expectations is an important factor in immigrants' adaptation to a new country, and it often is a source of family conflict. In most traditional cultures, men and women, and boys and girls have clearly differentiated roles and responsibilities in the family and community (Boyd-Franklin and Garcia-Preto, 1994). Living in a new society in which these roles and responsibilities are questioned, or by necessity changed, can lead to conflict between husbands and wives and between generations (Boyd-Franklin and Garcia-Preto, 1994).

For economic reasons, immigrant and refugee women often must work outside the home (Matsuoka, 1990). In some families, women have an easier time finding work than men do because their skills in housekeeping and sewing are more readily translated into useful services in the United States (Comas-Diaz, 1989). Women may thus gain power and respect in the family while men lose it. In addition, as women and girls are exposed to Western views about male-female equality, they may experience confusion that can lead to personal and familial emotional distress (Boyd-Franklin and Garcia-Preto, 1994). Viewed from a Western perspective, the roles and rights of women and girls in the family can present a complex issue for families from more traditional cultures.

## Family Structure and Intergenerational Issues

In addition to being challenged by changes in gender roles and expectations, many immigrant and refugee families experience intergenerational conflict (Sluzki, 1979). Age, developmental stage, and gender affect the acculturation of individuals and their roles and interactions in the family (Matsuoka, 1990).

Different family members may acculturate in varying ways. Family elders may become vulnerable to loss of status in a new environment when younger members of their family no longer pay heed to their guidance. Because immigrant youth are exposed to mainstream culture in school and are eager to be accepted by their peers, they are more likely to achieve assimilation or integration styles of adaptation than their immigrant parents (Pawliuk and others, 1996), a situation that can lead to disagreements with parents about appropriate behavior and activities (Matsuoka, 1990; Sluzki, 1979). As they learn English more quickly and often serve as interpreter for their parents, the children may take on a dominant role in recent immigrant families, thus reversing the parent-child hierarchy that is so important in many traditional cultures (Ho, 1987).

There are vast differences between middle-class European American parenting practices and those of many traditional cultures (Gray and Cosgrove, 1985; Tseng and Hsu, 1991), where physical discipline and the absolute right of parent over child are the norm (Minuchin, 1974). Concepts such as child abuse and formalized systems to monitor such problems do not exist in some traditional cultures (Tracy, 1998). In some cases, new American children learn about child abuse laws and inform their parents that they will "call the police" if the parents discipline them.

Because of overwhelming stress and isolation from former networks of family and community, the potential for abuse and violence to occur within the family is a genuine concern. Unfortunately, immigrant and refugee families who encounter the child welfare system often are dealt with inappropriately by overworked caseworkers who do not have the time or the inclination to learn about methods of working with and understanding diverse cultures (Gray and Cosgrove, 1985). Some immigrant and refugee families who are uninformed about child welfare law and parenting practices have ended up in tragic encounters with the child welfare system, sometimes inappropriately accused of child abuse (Berger, 1994; Pimental, 1994).

When family members come to the United States at different times, individual members may be at dissimilar stages of acculturation (Ho, 1987). Those who arrive later may speak mostly the language of origin and make little contact with mainstream culture, while those who have been in the United States for many years may have assimilated, and dress, speak, and behave in a manner more typical of mainstream American society (Ho, 1987). Children who were left behind during initial migration may resent the parent and other siblings who went ahead. They may have bonded strongly with other caretakers during the separation and feel divided loyalties. Spouses who have been separated may have developed other intimate relationships and have difficulty returning to the marital relationship.

Relatives who did not migrate may maintain a presence in the lives of immigrants and refugees. Many newcomers send substantial portions of their wages back to family members in the homeland. Receiving news of illness or death about the family members in the country of origin may cause extreme distress. Even pleasant letters may cause sadness, reminding families and individuals of who and what they have left behind.

Any combination of these influences on the family may occur and may result in high levels of anxiety and family conflict. Depression, anxiety, substance abuse, somatic complaints, and marital problems may be seen in adults, while school and behavior problems often are seen in youth. Both the individual and the family are affected, and the interactive effects of both are important to keep in mind. Traumatic stress may be devastating to the individual; it can have an impact on other family members as well.

## Religion and Spirituality

Several studies have indicated that traditional religious beliefs and affiliations among immigrants and refugees are effective coping supports (Canda and Phaobtong, 1992; Kamya, 1997). Clinicians must be aware of and respect these beliefs and practices, provide education about additional alternatives as appropriate, and support and encourage the traditional spiritual practices of their patients.

## Occupational Issues

Immigrants, especially those who are undocumented, face a number of occupational issues. Often professionals and highly skilled technicians find that they cannot access pathways to their normal careers because of language or license and degree verification issues. Some find themselves in positions such as piece-goods workers in garment industry sweatshops, and dishwashers or line cooks in restaurants where they earn less than minimum wage. Many young women find themselves unwittingly working in the sex trade, with all the attendant physical and emotional risks and sequelae. Other women come here with their partners as temporary seasonal workers and then eventually immigrate.

Personality styles that worked in one culture do not necessarily work in another. Tradition or authority may dictate job function in some societies, whereas American workplace culture praises creativity, initiative, and, until recently, individualism.

## Time Orientation

In general, there are three different types of time orientation among cultures: past, present, and future. Asian Americans believe that history is important and we learn from the past; Hispanic Americans and Native Americans tend to live in the present and not worry about tomorrow. Anglo-Americans and African Americans, on the other hand, believe in sacrificing today for a better tomorrow. For example, American health care providers tend to live by the clock and be rigidly inflexible about appointments; Puerto Ricans and Mexican Americans often have a tendency to show up when it suits them. They also are more willing to wait their turn than Anglo-American and often black American patients, who, like their providers, are clock watchers (Lecca, Quervalu, Nunes, and Gonzales, 1998, pp. 23–35).

## Beliefs About Health and Illness and Health Care–Seeking Behaviors

Culture influences explanatory models, what is seen as problematic and why, and how individuals relate to others (Berry, Poortinga, Segall, and Dasen, 1992; Kleinman, 1988; Ying, 1990). Many cultures see health problems as being caused by physical, moral, or spiritual imbalances or relationship problems, whereas European American society heavily emphasizes psychological explanations (Ho, 1987; Kleinman, 1988). Many traditional cultures do not see physical and mental health as distinct. Members may express distress somatically and have no concept of mental health treatment (Lee, 1982; Lee and Lu, 1990; Snowden, 1996; Ying, 1990). In some traditional cultures, shame and stigma strongly inhibit immigrants and refugees from seeking outside help for problems and from openly discussing them with health care providers once they are in a helping setting (Ho, 1987; Lee, 1982; Lee and Lu, 1990). If they cannot resolve a problem on their own, they may seek help from family, physicians, or religious healers. In some cultures, healing is not a solitary process between healer and identified patient; it involves the entire family and other community members.

Culture influences illness and health-seeking behavior by defining symptoms and functioning that are considered normal and abnormal in a given culture; providing people with ideas about causality; determining the health care decision-making hierarchy, as well as who the patient is; and defining the steps that are taken in seeking health care.

## Health Belief Systems

Consider a thirty-year-old woman from rural Senegal who had been in New York, working as a cook, for five months when she presented to the clinic with complaints of fatigue, constipation, and waist and abdominal pain. A complete workup was negative. The patient returned to the clinic increasingly often as her cooking jobs became more scarce. Her frustration mounted as her diagnostic workup was repeatedly negative and no successful treatment could be prescribed.

Eventually it was determined that this patient was suffering from *toy*, a somatization syndrome that does not fit into a Western classification of illness or disease. The symptoms, do, however, correspond to a well-known Senegalese syndrome, which, when viewed in the context of this particular culture, becomes both comprehensible and coherent. *Toy* begins to make sense as one learns about the lives of Senegalese immigrants and the large amounts of daily psychological and physical stress they endure, the urgent economic demands made on them by their families, and the downside of their seemingly reassuring communal lifestyle, which pressures them not to let their brothers and sisters down by failing to pay their share of the bills. Beyond these demands, work has a social and religious importance that is difficult to ignore. Interviews with Senegalese patients have revealed that the ability to work is a central concept in their self-image. In this context, *toy* has a precise and significant place in Senegalese society. The symptoms develop as a consequence of overwork, often in low-skilled jobs, with long hours and poor or no fringe benefits or other protections. The diagnosis of *toy* is one of the few socially acceptable reasons to take life easier.

In Senegal, *toy* is not seen as a "hospital illness." However, there are few, if any, Senegalese healers in the United States. Consequently, health care practitioners and institutions have become the "healers" for the Senegalese, and for many other immigrant groups, and they must learn how to heal this population effectively. For the Senegalese with *toy*, this entails learning about *toy* and treating it with culturally appropriate remedies: permission to rest, talk therapy, and gelatin, because in Senegal *toy* is treated with a gelatinous-like substance called *kell*.

By using an explanatory belief model, providers can assume that all patients who are symptomatic have ideas about the etiology, pathophysiology, severity, prognosis, treatment, and prevention of their symptoms prior to consulting with a practitioner, although the specifics of these explanatory models may be very different from the provider's. Nonetheless, the explanatory belief model can become the basis for negotiation of a diagnostic workup and treatment plan. The extent to which practitioners can meet patients' beliefs about causality and treatment predicts patient adherence to treatment recommendations, patient satisfaction, and effectiveness of care.

Clearly no provider will be able to recognize every culture-bound syndrome or somatization disorder. However, there is a paradigm for eliciting a history that incorporates health explanatory beliefs and cultural orientation. At a minimum, use of it leads to recognition by patients that the consulting clinician is interested in their perception of illness and the significance it has for them.

Kleinman (1986) differentiates between disease, which involves biological deviation from normal, and illness, which refers to the subjective distress patients feel that frequently leads them to seek health care. His explanatory belief model is predicated on the following seven questions:

1. What do you call your problem?
2. What causes your problem?
3. Why do you think it started when it did?
4. How does it work—what is going on in your body?
5. What kind of treatment do you think would be best for this problem?
6. How has this problem affected your life?
7. What frightens or concerns you most about this problem and treatment? [Johnson, Hardt, and Kleinman, 1995, p. 157].

Some African Americans and many Puerto Ricans, Mexicans, and Native Americans may be quick to attribute the etiology of their symptoms to some type of social transgression or emotional state. Members of many cultures, among them Mexican, Puerto Rican, Chinese, and Haitian, believe that illness may be caused by imbalances of "hot" and "cold" forces in the body, which often are attributed to imbalances in the flow of energy or dietary indiscretions and have nothing to do with temperature. Medications, too, may have hot and cold properties. Some cultures also believe that winds or drafts (which are related to the hot and cold theory) are etiologic agents in illness.

The overall goal of culturally competent care should be empathic understanding of the relationships among symptoms, distress, and the interpersonal life of the patient. Understanding the personal meanings of patients' symptoms in the context of their lives also protects practitioners from the frustration and hostility that so often accompany the care of ethnically different patients and that can lead to burnout and iatrogenesis (Kleinman, 1988). For example, Mexican Americans believe that health is a state of feeling well and being able to maintain function. They believe in the here and now and that the future is in God's hands. Mexican Americans see no clear separation of physical and mental illness. Disease is caused by imbalance between the individual and the environment. Emotional, spiritual, physical, and social factors may all play a role. God, spirituality, and interpersonal relationships can contribute to illness.

Russians believe that health is the absence of symptoms. Poor nutrition, not dressing warmly enough, family history, stress, and taking too many medications or not taking care of oneself during pregnancy are thought to be the causes of physical illness, and stress and moving to new environments are believed to be the major causes of mental illness. To Filipinos, good health is related to maintaining balance; illness results from imbalance, although some think it may be punishment for a wrongdoing. They associate health with strength, good food, and freedom from pain. Being overweight is seen as a sign of prosperity. Mental illness is believed to result from a disruption of harmonious function of the whole individual and the spiritual world.

Many immigrants and refugees are likely to choose non-Western medicine prior to or concurrently with seeking Western medical care. The concept of heat and cold, which has its origins in the ancient Chinese tradition of yin and yang, is the basis for both Eastern and Western folk medicine treatment. The Chinese use hot and cold foods to restore balance to the body. Hot foods are thought to give strength and blood, while cold foods reduce temperature, help to cure hot diseases such as fevers and infections, and bring rest and relief. Many Chinese Americans use home remedies for minor ailments but seek the services of Western doctors for more serious illnesses. In making the decision to seek care, patients often ask the advice of relatives and friends.

Chinese Americans are likely to use a combination of folk medicine and modern Western medicine; they believe each is effective, but for different types of disorders. Kleinman (1986) found widespread use of medicinal herbs, often concomitantly with Western medicine, in most Chinese communities.

In an effort to restore the yin-yang balance, the Vietnamese commonly use Chinese herbal medicine and a set of indigenous folk practices referred to as "Southern medicine." Some illnesses are thought to be caused by a bad wind and may be treated by coin rubbing or "scraping out the wind"; others are thought to be caused by spirits or ghosts. Vietnamese patients may delay seeking medical care because of denial, tolerance of physical pain, a tendency to accept illness as part of one's destiny, and a fatalistic attitude toward the illness (Jenkins and others, 1996).

Most Filipinos believe in the concomitant use of folk practitioners and Western medicine. Some believe in the role of healers who can placate or exorcise spirits and ghosts. Russian immigrants usually try home and folk remedies prior to Western medicine. Some may seek medical care as a last resort. Many Mexican Americans will not seek medical care until home remedies have failed and illness interferes with their ability to meet role expectations.

In most Hispanic societies, medical information is passed down from mother to daughter. Home remedies usually are tried first, and approximately 70 to 90 percent of all illnesses are managed outside the formal health care delivery system (Gordon, 1994). This may be because the family feels that it can handle the problem on its own, but it also may result from geographic or financial inaccessibility to physician services. The mother or primary female caretaker is responsible for deciding when an illness is beyond her capacity to treat and requires outside intervention (Reinert, 1986). At that point, the entire family becomes more involved in the decision-making process.

There are at least five major Mexican American folk illnesses that are thought to be incurable with Western medicine and that require folk healers to bring relief (Applewhite, 1995; Mull and Mull, 1983). The first four are considered *males naturales* (natural illnesses): *caida de la mollera* (fallen fontanel in infants), *empacho* (a digestive disorder), *mal ojo* (the evil eye), and *susto* (shock or fright). The fifth is *mal puesto* (sorcery or witchcraft).

Becerra and Iglehart (1995) compared the use of folk remedies or folk medicines among non-Hispanic whites, African Americans, Mexican Americans, and Chinese in Los Angeles and found that 44 percent used them, with prevalence most widespread among the Mexican Americans. Major differences among the groups were that non-Hispanic whites tended to use food rather than herbs, African Americans used herbs more than non-Hispanic whites did, and Chinese Americans used prepared remedies purchased primarily in Chinese stores.

In Cambodia, traditional health practices are the usual form of medical care. In fact, biomedicine is available only in urban centers. In rural Cambodia, medical attention is initially sought from family members, who may suggest herbal supplements or dietary changes. They also may perform dermabrasive techniques such as coining, pinching, cupping, or massage. The advice of a traditional healer, a Kru Khmer, often is sought if symptoms are not relieved at home. Allopathic medical care usually is employed only after traditional methods have failed (Shimada, Jackson, Goldstein, and Buchwald, 1995).

In some areas of the Caribbean, organized health care is sought only after self-treatment has failed and the person remains very ill (Gany and Thiel-deBocanegra, 1996). Hispanics traditionally turn to family and community for help and advice, including advice on health issues. The element of *personalismo,* or the personal relationships that are established and developed over time, is very important to Hispanic patients, who may avoid seeking care from providers and institutions that they perceive as valuing impersonality and efficiency.

Puerto Ricans and Mexican Americans expect their health care providers to show *respecto,* or concern for them as people, rather than just as cases. They expect the social distance between the providers and themselves to be reduced and that the providers will display *personalismo* and *respecto,* and spend substantial time with them discussing their health.

Mexican Americans and Hmong might include their entire extended kinship system in reaching a consensus about appropriate treatment. The antithesis of this approach occurs among the Indochinese, where the eldest member of the family often decides if another family member should seek medical care and, if so, whether to seek traditional or biomedical care (Coll and Magnuson, 1996).

Vietnamese may prefer to seek care from Chinese herbalists, acupuncturists, sorcerers, fortune tellers, mediums, and Buddhist priests rather than from Western physicians. They also may wear amulets to ward off disease (Jenkins and others, 1996).

## Use of Traditional Practitioners

Mexican Americans are perceived as being quite likely to seek the services of folk healers, who may be *curanderos, yerberos* (herbalists), *hueseros* and *sobadores* (respectively, bone and muscle therapists), and *parteras* (midwives). Curanderos usually are highly respected people who project great personal concern for patients and their families, as well as a firm belief in the efficacy of their treatments. They use a variety of modalities, including native herbs, ritualistic prayers, "white magic," massage, and raw eggs (Mull and Mull, 1983).

The extent of folk healing within any community varies with the strength of the traditional belief system and the availability of folk practitioners (Applewhite, 1995). Folk healers are quite prevalent in border towns. Higginbotham, Trevino, and Ray (1990) found that satisfaction with conventional medical care, language, self-perceived health status, and income were more likely to affect the use of these practitioners than the size of the community. Some elderly Mexican Americans use folk healers because they cannot afford modern health care; others use them because they find the U.S. health care delivery system too efficient and impersonal (Applewhite, 1995).

Chinese immigrants are likely to employ several traditional therapies, including acupuncture, herbs, nutrition, meditation, and qi gong, a form of moving meditation that is used to improve the flow of energy (Williams, 1995). Traditional oriental medical doctors, who can be found in most Chinese communities, may prescribe decoctions (beverages) and dispense the herbs themselves, or they may send patients to the local herb shop to obtain the items. Traditional Chinese pharmacies that dispense herbs are readily available in most large and even medium-sized cities with sizable Chinese or Vietnamese populations. Many Chinese also obtain herbs from China.

## Cross-Cultural Communication Between Clinicians and Patients

Physician and patient miscommunication often occurs, not only because of lack of a spoken common language but because the patient and physician do not have the same cultural framework and therefore do not share the same illness concepts or language of distress.

Three elements of language are important in the establishment of patient-provider rapport: linguistic (spoken), ethnocentric (perception-based on foreign accent), and idiosyncratic (the perception that a person has expressed interest through inflections, tones, rate of speech, and so forth). Immigrants often come from health care systems that are different from those of clinicians. Hence, they have very different expectations of medical

care. Women may be unfamiliar with procedures such as gynecological exams and may be embarrassed if they are asked to un-
dress, especially if the request comes from a male practitioner. Any
hesitancy the patient exhibits may be a sign that there is a cultural
practice the practitioner needs to explore to effect a compromise
satisfactory to both parties.

The practitioner needs to be mindful of gender, age, and class
issues that can affect the establishment of a therapeutic alliance.
The health care provider should assess the patient's cultural identity. A series of items may prove valuable to the clinician when
making assessments or treatment recommendations.

*Assessment of ethnicity.* It is vital that the provider not simply label a patient as Asian or Hispanic or African. People take great
pride in their countries of origin and may immediately become
offended if it is assumed that they are natives of another country.
Koreans do not want to be called Chinese, Dominicans do not
want to be called Puerto Ricans, and Ukrainians do not want to be
called Russians.

*Language.* An assessment of a person's abilities in his or her native language and in English is vital for ongoing communication.
If a provider is able to speak the patient's native language, that is
always preferable if it is what the patient desires. To assume that it
is better for the patient to communicate in English, however non-
dominant it may be, is simply another variant of an English-only
movement that serves to hurt rather than to help.

*Migration history.* Knowing that a person is a political refugee,
a religious refugee, undocumented, or in the United States on one
kind of a visa or another helps the provider to assess other possible
stressors that the patient may not be talking about. It is critical that
the patient understand why this information is being sought and
that it will remain privileged.

*Degree of acculturation.* Patients do not want it to be assumed
that they are foreigners if they have a long history of living in the
United States. Therefore, what a provider has learned about another culture and found helpful in becoming culturally proficient
may become less relevant as he or she encounters patients who are
third- or fourth-generation Americans.

*Premigration history.* The fact that an individual may have spent
time in a refugee camp or traveled to many different countries
prior to arriving in the United States is crucial in understanding

that person's physical and mental health status. This knowledge, combined with the patient's experience of migration, helps to put the patient's worldview as it was colored by more recent experiences into perspective.

*Degree of loss.* Often patients have experienced multiple traumas in their country of origin, their transition to the United States, or their experiences when they first arrived. Americans tend to take the loss of family members, friends, and other important people for granted, because mainstream America does not have much recent history of traumatic losses of life on a large-scale basis. For example, the experiences of immigrants from Lebanon and what was formerly Yugoslavia, Rwanda, and Cambodia must be handled delicately and sensitively but should be acknowledged.

*Work and financial history.* It is not sufficient to assume that a person who is a laborer in the United States was a laborer in his or her native country. People now holding blue-collar jobs may have been managers or even health care professionals in their countries of origin. In addition, a person's financial status in his or her native country might have been quite different from the current situation. This information also helps clinicians to understand that person's potential for a meaningful economic existence here or the consequences of a major loss of status.

*Support systems.* A person who lives alone may have had a completely different experience in his or her country of origin. Someone who attempts to be sociable here because that was the natural mode of existence in his or her own country may abruptly find that U.S. socialization patterns and mores are quite different from those of other settings.

These items, which form a cultural assessment paradigm, serve to establish rapport with a patient, get a better sense of who the person is and why he or she is seeking health care, and provide valuable pieces of information that can be useful in formulating treatment plans and establishing long-lasting therapeutic relationships.

## Conclusion

Health care practitioners who work with newcomers need to make a conceptual leap to understand the patient's health care–seeking behaviors, expectations, and symptoms in their appropriate context. Although the provider does not have to agree with patients' health beliefs in order to provide appropriate care, understanding and acknowledging them will make it easier to integrate Western medicine with other treatment modalities, and ensure adherence and patient and provider satisfaction with the relationship. For example, many Chinese patients believe that once blood is drawn, it never will be replaced. If phlebotomy is kept to a minimum, the need for it explained to the Chinese patient, and herbal remedies or teas that are believed to enhance blood production are prescribed, there is a greater chance the patient will return (Gany and Thiel-deBocanegra, 1996). Kleinman's questions to determine a patient's explanatory model of disease are useful regardless of his or her cultural or personal belief system. Cultural understanding at this level can bring about satisfying provider-patient relationships and lead to more accurate diagnoses and treatments.

Chapter Three

# Linguistic Issues

*Sherry Riddick*

Given reports that show that language gaps and cultural differences play an important role in underutilization of health services by some subgroups of the population (Association of State and Territorial Health Officials, 1992; National Coalition of Hispanic Health and Human Services Organizations, 1990), health care institutions have begun to examine more carefully how they serve their limited-English-proficient (LEP) clients. This action was precipitated by increased concern about malpractice liability, the need to comply with civil rights laws, and advocacy by ethnic and other community-based organizations.

This chapter describes concepts, strategies, and models currently being used to improve quality and access to health care for LEP individuals in various health care settings around the country.

Research for this chapter was supported in part by the Henry J. Kaiser Family Foundation and was prepared for the Kaiser Family Foundation Forum on Responding to Language Barriers to Health Care, Washington, D.C., September 18–19, 1995. Major portions of this chapter appear in the *Journal of Health Care for the Poor and Underserved*, 1998, *9*(2). I am grateful to Julia Puebla Fortier, health policy consultant and director, Resources for Cross Cultural Health, and Francis S. Chang, program officer, Henry J. Kaiser Family Foundation, for insightful comments and critical review of drafts of this chapter.

## Bilingual and Bicultural Providers

Hiring bilingual staff who can communicate directly with patients without need of an interpreter is the ideal approach for dealing with language barriers; some also think that it is the most efficient method of communication. If providers speak the same language as their patients and have similar cultural backgrounds, they will avoid many of the problems encountered by their colleagues whose linguistic and cultural backgrounds are different. An overriding problem with this approach is the lack of trained health care professionals at all levels who are bilingual and bicultural. The demographics of the health care professions do not match the demographics of the population at large, and recruitment for bilingual positions can be problematic, even for widely spoken languages such as Spanish (National Coalition of Hispanic Health and Human Services Organizations, 1995). Some health care organizations have implemented creative approaches to fill this gap. One approach is the use of foreign-trained health care professionals and nontraditional health care workers such as shaman and herbalists from the community. Another approach is to encourage health care providers to study another language while in college or medical school, especially if they expect to practice in an area with many non-English-speaking people.

A second area of concern with this strategy is that most bilingual staff have not been formally assessed for their language skills or their cultural awareness. Few sites that make concerted efforts to hire bilingual staff actually assess language abilities, leaving to chance the quality of bilingual services that are provided (National Coalition of Hispanic Health and Human Services Organizations, 1995). Although the need to assess a nonnative speaker's linguistic skills is clear, whether native-speaking health care providers should be evaluated is less obvious. Although we can assume that native speakers generally are more proficient in the target language and more aware of cultural nuances than nonnative speakers, problems can arise nonetheless. The dialect may be inappropriate to the specific patient population, sociocultural differences (such as class or gender) may interfere with effective communication, and medical terminology in the target language may be lacking, especially if the provider received medical training in the United States.

Although these problems may not arise often, there is a need to develop standardized evaluation tools for a provider's linguistic skills.

## Community Health Workers

Access to health care can be much improved for the LEP population through the development of programs that reach out to the community. Programs that use community health workers have been especially successful. The generic term *community health worker* defines "community members who work almost exclusively in community settings and who serve as connectors between health care consumers and providers to promote health among groups that traditionally have lacked access to adequate care" (Witmer and others, 1995, p. 1055). By hiring staff who reflect the linguistic and cultural diversity of the community, community health worker programs improve the quality of health care services in several ways. They facilitate access through outreach and health promotion activities, encourage community participation in the health care system, and educate providers about cultural relevance. Equally important, as members of a comprehensive health care team, they contribute to the continuity, coordination, and overall quality of care.

## Language Bank Interpreters

The in-house language bank is one of the oldest strategies for dealing with language barriers in health institutions. Commonly used by hospitals, this approach recruits employees who speak other languages to volunteer for the language bank, which calls individuals as needed to interpret for patients who speak their language. One advantage of this strategy is its apparent low cost, since no extra staff need be hired. In addition, the language bank interpreter may be readily available for emergency or immediate requests, provided they occur on his or her shift.

Language banks nevertheless have multiple problems. Employees usually have not been evaluated for language skills and have simply filled out forms on which they self-rate their own degree of fluency. Further, few have received any training in medical interpreting skills, ethics, or vocabulary. This may lead to inappropriate situations: for example, a hospital housekeeper, newly arrived in the United States and barely speaking English, may be called on to interpret for a patient being prepared for surgery; or a U.S.-born nurse with two years of college French may be asked to interpret for a Creole-speaking Haitian refugee with a grade school education. In these two situations, neither "interpreter" will be able to do a good job. Finally, job conflict can result from lack of inclusion of interpreting duties in employees' job descriptions. Supervisors and co-workers may blame the bilingual employee for time spent away from formally assigned duties while interpreting, a situation that can lead to a negative work environment and resentment by the employee as well as colleagues and supervisors.

The quality of language banks can be improved by assigning a coordinator to be responsible for assessing the language and interpretation skills of employees, maintaining updated lists of participant employees, providing at least a minimal level of interpreter training, and continuously assessing the quality of the service provided. It also is helpful to include interpretation as a listed job duty and to enlist the support and cooperation of supervisors and co-workers. Finally, compensation for bilingual skills as a bonus or differential should be provided, especially when the time spent interpreting is significant. When managed properly, language banks can be an effective backup to other strategies.

## Professional Interpreters

When bilingual providers are not available to care for monolingual patients, well-trained professional interpreters can do much to bridge the language and culture gaps. A variety of hiring approaches is used to obtain the services of professional interpreters. Hiring interpreters as full-time or part-time regular employees is most commonly practiced when a particular language is prevalent and the expense of maintaining the employee can be justified. Hiring interpreters as hourly, on-call employees or as independent contractors is most useful when demand for a particular language is intermittent. It works best when most of the demand is for prescheduled appointments, although emergency needs can be met when interpreters are willing (or paid) to carry pagers and be accessible night and day. Finally, in some communities, interpreter services are obtained through outside agencies that specialize in medical interpretation. This works well when need is intermittent and diverse; it also can supplement an organization's regular interpretation staff.

Professionally trained interpreters are relatively rare in the medical arena, and there is a lack of clearly defined standards and training for them. Some medical institutions and agencies have developed their own role definitions, assessment tools, and training programs for interpreters, but a nationally accepted model has not been developed, and most health care programs have neither assessed nor trained their "professional" interpreters. In Washington and Massachusetts, recently formed medical interpreter associations are working to develop statewide, and even national, professional standards and training programs for interpreters. Other organizations responsible for ensuring quality health care could work with groups such as these to establish standards of training and competency.

The extra cost of hiring interpreters often is cited as a barrier to using paid, dedicated personnel. However, the cost of using untrained or ad hoc interpreters (family, friends, other patients) rarely is examined. Potential liability costs, the cost of lower-quality health care, and adverse health outcomes that result from inadequate communication may be more expensive than providing well-trained interpreters.

## Remote Consecutive Interpretation

This is the method used in most telephone interpretation services. Many hospitals use such services for emergencies when it will take too long to get an interpreter in person. They also may use telephone interpretation for simple communications and many routine functions such as setting up appointments, giving lab results, and doing follow-up with patients. It may be more affordable for health care facilities to purchase this type of service for languages that are infrequently encountered than to try to provide them in-house.

When the patient is at home, it is most helpful to have conference calling capability for a three-way conversation. When the patient is present in the health facility, having a speaker telephone available avoids the necessity of passing the telephone back and forth from patient to provider. However, this can breach confidentiality if the conversation is overheard by others.

Another problem with this method is the lack of visual input. The absence of facial expression, gestures, and other nonverbal cues may have an impact on the accuracy of the interpretation. Also, providers and patients may feel uncomfortable or insecure about the quality of the interpretation. Because the interpreters and their qualifications often are unknown to the health care facility staff, it would be wise for the staff to ascertain the interpreter's level of experience and knowledge before beginning the interpreted conversation, especially when important medical information needs to be imparted.

## Nonprofessional Interpreters: Volunteers and Family and Friends

Formal volunteer programs sometimes recruit volunteers from the community to function as interpreters. Hospitals often have volunteer departments that may be responsible for recruiting interpreters. Occasionally these volunteers may be trained, professional interpreters, but more often they are not. A survey of teaching hospitals found that only 14 percent of those that use volunteer interpreters provide any training, and of these, only half required it (Ginsberg and others, 1995, p. 28). The issues surrounding the use of unassessed, untrained volunteers as interpreters are the same as those for language banks and professional interpreters. Therefore, the apparent cost advantage of using volunteers may be overridden by their lack of effectiveness in providing this type of service.

The use of family and friends of patients as interpreters has long been a fallback for health institutions; unfortunately, it is the primary strategy used for serving LEP populations in some areas. Although there are times when it may be necessary to use a relative or friend, this never should be the method of choice. Family, friends, and other individuals who are called on as interpreters may lack appropriate language skills and knowledge of medical terminology, and gross errors in communication can occur. Use of family members is especially problematic. Confidentiality is compromised, vital information may be censored, and internal family dynamics may be jeopardized, especially when children are used to interpret (Woloshin and others, 1995).

## Written Translation Materials

Translation materials that place English alongside the target language, such as health education pamphlets that allow each party to find and point to the appropriate phrase in their language, sometimes are used to communicate with patients. This method, which is used most often in emergencies in the absence of a readily available interpreter or for simple needs an inpatient might have, such as indicating the need for a bedpan or a drink of water, is inherently limited in usefulness and obviously requires the patient to be literate in the native language. However, it also may be useful for a receptionist who needs to identify the language of a patient before requesting an interpreter or using a telephone interpretation service.

Translated forms, documents, and health education materials such as discharge instructions also play a role in increasing access to service and assuring adherence. Many agencies have developed a variety of translated materials, and these can be useful with some populations if they are tailored to the reading level of the audience and adapted and tested for cultural appropriateness. Protocols for translated materials must be standardized, and clearinghouses developed to aid in the dissemination of appropriate and effective materials. Policies that govern the use of such materials should make clear that translated handouts do not take the place of verbal communication with a patient.

## Conclusion

In a survey of public and private hospitals, Ginsberg and others (1995, p. 1) found that hospitals and other health care organizations "have developed numerous responses designed to address the growing need for interpretation in the medical setting. The diversity of these responses has increased without overarching guidance from a regulatory body delineating standards for medical interpretation or guidelines for training, compensation, and evaluation." Despite the creativity and diligence applied by many organizations to improve their access and services for the LEP population, much remains to be done. The list of recommendations that follows, summarized from several reports and surveys, could be useful to individual health care organizations, state and local government, advocacy groups, and others striving to serve their diverse communities better (Association of State and Territorial Health Officials, 1992; National Coalition of Hispanic Health and Human Services Organizations, 1995; Ginsberg and others, 1995; National Association of County Health Officials, 1992; U.S. Conference of Mayors and U.S. Conference of Local Health Officers, 1993).

## *Recruiting and Training Bilingual and Bicultural Staff*

- Make greater efforts to recruit and retain bilingual and bicultural staff at all levels of organizations.
- Work with universities and colleges to recruit more minorities into health professions.
- Train health professionals within the multicultural and underserved communities where they will work.
- Train health professionals in cultural competency, including the cultural histories, norms, and values of those served.
- Provide in-depth language training to health professionals planning to work in areas with LEP populations.
- Use the skills of nontraditional health care workers where possible.
- Train and hire members of the community as community health workers, outreach workers, and advocates.

## *Interpreter Standards, Testing, and Training and Service Models*

- Define the role of interpreters and situations in which interpreters should be used.
- Develop models for training interpreters, and ensure that all interpreters are trained.
- Develop minimal standards and qualifications for medical interpreters, ensuring that all interpreters are assessed for language, cultural, and interpreting skills.
- Develop guidelines for using bilingual staff as interpreters,

and ensure that minimal standards, qualifications, and training needs are met.

- Develop models appropriate to the needs of various types of facilities, for example, by size, language mix, and need for emergency service.
- Develop mechanisms for sharing interpretation models, testing, and training on a national basis.

## Translation of Materials

- Develop protocols for accurate and appropriate translation of patient materials, such as consent forms and health promotion materials.
- Develop clearinghouses or other mechanisms to promote sharing of bilingual written materials.

## Funding

- Encourage public institutions, such as state health agencies, to allocate resources to ensure the access of linguistic minorities to their health care services.
- Encourage coverage of interpreter services by third-party payers.

## Quality Assurance

- Develop formal quality assurance standards to monitor and evaluate multilingual and multicultural program effectiveness, including interpreter services.

# Chapter Four

# Health Services Utilization and Access to Care

*Susan L. Ivey*

Understanding the daily lives of immigrant women and the barriers they face in their efforts to access health care may be especially important to understanding their utilization of health services (Juarbe, 1995). A number of authors have defined *utilization* as a function of access and developed frameworks within which it can be examined (Aday and Andersen, 1981). Several studies have concluded that for low-income minorities, particularly Hispanics, financial variables (affordability) and structural variables (including availability and accessibility of services, plus language and translation difficulty) account for most of the difference in health services utilization between and among ethnic groups (Institute of Medicine, 1993; Solis, Marks, Garcia, and Shelton, 1990). Insurance status, including Medicaid coverage, is known to have a significant impact on medical care utilization (Freeman and Corey, 1993; Guendelman and Schwalbe, 1986; Trevino and Moss, 1983). In a study that compared documented and undocumented Latinos with non-Hispanic whites in southern California, Hubbell and others (1991) found that health insurance status, not ethnicity, was the most important predictor of access to medical care, although having insurance does not guarantee women access.

In addition to financial and structural barriers, number of years of U.S. residence is correlated with increased utilization. Using the 1990 National Health Interview Survey supplement and after adjusting for socioeconomic and insurance status, LeClere,

Jensen, and Biddlecom (1994) concluded that duration of residence in the United States had a major effect on health services utilization by immigrants. However, after including measures of adaptation, such as age at immigration and language in which the survey interview was conducted, immigrants who had resided in the United States more than ten years used health services similarly to native-born Americans.

Recent immigrants tend to use fewer preventive services, a pattern that for Hispanic adults has been noted to be a function of insurance status and not acculturation per se (Solis, Marks, Garcia, and Shelton, 1990). Although immigrants may obtain health care from many sources, they often get services from safety net providers, such as public hospitals, federally qualified and other types of neighborhood health centers, emergency departments of hospitals, and traditional practitioners. Clinics and providers with a tradition of caring for underserved groups including immigrant women are another common source of care.

## Limitations of Current Studies

Because of limitations of available studies, a variety of sources must be used to arrive at a description of utilization by immigrant women. The 1990 National Health Interview Survey supplement examined the impact of length of U.S. residence and language of the survey interview (as proxies for adaptation) on overall utilization of health services (LeClere, Jensen, and Biddlecom, 1994). The National Hospital Ambulatory Medical Care Survey (NHAMCS) and National Ambulatory Medical Care Survey (NAMCS) examine utilization by racial group or Hispanic ethnic group but not by immigration status. Case studies in cities with large immigrant populations have explored utilization, including that by undocumented persons (Hubbell and others, 1991). However, case studies may lack generalizability outside the specific location in which they were conducted. Data from NAMCS demonstrate that women tend to have more overall visits to physicians than men, with visit rates increasing after age twenty-four. The office visit rate is higher for white than for nonwhite persons. Of all ambulatory visits, white persons made 85.2 percent; blacks, 11.1 percent; and Asian–Pacific Islanders (APIs), 3.3 percent

(Woodwell, 1997). This compares to data showing that 69.4 percent of all hospital-based outpatient visits in the NHAMCS were made by whites, 27.4 percent by blacks, and 3.0 percent by APIs (McCaig and Stussman, 1997). Although Hispanic heritage was not analyzed, it would appear that whites use the private ambulatory sector more, and blacks use the hospital outpatient department more, with APIs using both public and private sectors at similar rates.

## Sources of Care

Because of limited access to care within the formal U.S. health system, immigrants may depend disproportionately on safety net providers, including federally qualified health centers, public hospitals, and emergency departments. Given options, patients' choices of site also may reflect the types of health care delivery systems in their countries of origin. For example, Europeans and Canadians tend to use the emergency departments (EDs) in their native countries at higher rates than people use the ED in the United States (Fulton, 1993; Kooiman, Van de Wetering, and Van der Mast, 1989). Conversely, rates of hospital use might be expected to be much lower among people from countries with few large hospitals, and those from rural regions where the hospital is less likely to be viewed as a primary source of medical care. For instance, in Vietnam, there are very few large hospitals or organized emergency services (Richards, 1997). In other countries, gatekeepers may have been necessary, as in Bosnia, where a patient would need a written and stamped note from an *ambulanta,* or primary care clinic, in order to be seen at the hospital (Lasseter, Pyles, and Galijasevic, 1997).

### Federally Qualified Health Centers

The term *federally qualified health center* (FQHC) covers health centers that were consolidated under section 330 of the Public Health Service Act. These include migrant health centers, which provide services to migrant and seasonal farmworkers and their families; community health centers, which provide services to medically underserved populations living in both rural and urban underserved communities; health care for the homeless programs, which provide services to homeless individuals and children at locations that are accessible to them; and health services for residents of public housing. Most funding for these programs comes from the Bureau of Primary Health Care (BPHC), a federal agency within the U.S. Public Health Service. Services are offered to all who seek them, and, historically, they have been provided on a sliding-scale fee basis or at no cost to the patient where necessary. Required primary care services include enabling assistance such as outreach, transportation, translation, and patient education.

More than eight million individuals are served by this network of clinics (Bureau of Primary Health Care, 1998). Health services are provided to approximately 600,000 migrants and seasonal farmworkers at more than 390 delivery sites that belong to a network of 122 migrant health centers. Community health centers currently serve medically underserved people at 1,650 delivery sites. Approximately 124 organizations, including community health centers, public health departments, and other community-based health service providers, offer services to the homeless at nearly 200 sites in both rural and urban areas (Bureau of Primary Health Care, 1998). An additional ten grantees provide services to homeless children. The proportion of immigrants served by FQHCs is not known. Statistics from BPHC show that women use over 60 percent of the services in these clinics. Utilization of services by race is as follows: 38.0 percent whites, 28.5 percent African Americans, 27.6 percent Hispanics, and 2.3 percent Asians. These percentages vary widely by state. In Texas, 84.2 percent of users are Hispanic; in California, 57.7 percent are Hispanic, and 7.2 percent are Asian (Bureau of Primary Health Care, 1998).

## Public Hospitals

The nation's public general hospitals are the major providers of inpatient hospital care, and significant providers of outpatient care, to the uninsured and underinsured, many of whom are immigrants. Mandates from all levels of government in the past required these hospitals to care for all who sought their services. In its most recent member survey, the National Association of Public Hospitals (NAPH) reported that ninety of its member institutions had 1.4 million admissions, with 10.9 million inpatient-days (National Association of Public Hospitals, 1997, p. 10).

Safety net hospitals often serve as the primary care provider for people in medically underserved areas. In 1995, sixty-seven NAPH member hospitals provided 22.2 million outpatient visits. Since 1988, the average number of outpatient visits provided by twenty-four NAPH members has increased 17.6 percent. Further, fewer than 20 percent of the 22 million reported outpatient visits were to EDs, and ED visits at NAPH member hospitals declined 4.7 percent from 1993 to 1995 (National Association of Public Hospitals, 1997, p. 11). These figures suggest that patients use appropriate outpatient sites when they are available in the safety net.

Key informant interviews conducted in 1997 with a group of safety net hospitals that are members of the NAPH gave ranges of the immigrant population served by the hospitals as between 30 and 60 percent of patients at the facilities interviewed (National Association of Public Hospitals, personal communication).

## Emergency Departments

Lack of entitlement to health care has its own impact on utilization patterns of immigrant women. Preventive care is discouraged and medical care often deferred until needs are more acute (Rask, Williams, Parker, and McNagny, 1994). Patients may then present to EDs. Many low-income and self-pay patients use the ED as their main source of medical care (Pane, Farner, and Salness, 1991).

The total number of ED visits per 100 persons varies by age, gender, and race (McCaig and Stussman, 1997). ED utilization patterns appear to differ for various ethnic groups, as well as by generation of migration (Baker, Stevens, and Brook, 1994; Markides, Levin, and Ray, 1985). In 1996, ED visit rates per 100 persons per year were 31.5 for whites, 58.0 for blacks, and 16.6 for APIs (McCaig and Stussman, 1997). Less is known about ED use based on immigrant versus nonimmigrant status. However, examination of the few existing articles on immigrant utilization of ED services suggests that the pattern for Mexican immigrants may be similar to patterns of use for other low-income populations (Chan, Krishel, Bramwell, and Clark, 1996; Chavez, Cornelius, and Jones, 1985; Zambrana and others, 1994). Examination of patterns of utilization of Samoans living in Hawaii also has shown a preference for use of the ED or drop-in visits over scheduled clinic visits (Forbes and Wegner, 1987).

Average ranges of 45 to 55 percent of all ED visits being non-urgent are common (Health Care Advisory Board, 1993; Jones, Jones, and Yoder, 1982). Although nonemergency care frequently is viewed as inappropriate utilization of the ED, it should be deemed inappropriate only if a more appropriate source of care for immigrant women exists. This means they would need to have access to care that is available, geographically and temporally accessible, acceptable according to the patient's cultural perspective, and affordable. It is exceedingly unlikely that all of these conditions for ensuring access will be met for many recent immigrants.

Of the groups most likely to contain recent immigrants, Hispanic ED utilization has been best studied. Cunningham, Clancy, Cohen, and Wilets (1995) used the National Medical Expenditure Survey to examine nonurgent ED utilization for white, black, and Hispanic racial and ethnic categories and found that the probability of nonurgent ED utilization was lowest for Hispanic Americans. The proportion of all physician visits that were nonurgent ED visits was similar for Hispanics and African Americans, who had the highest probability of nonurgent ED visits. Although overall health services utilization by Hispanics is the lowest of all the groups examined, a not-unexpected finding given that they appear to be the ethnic group who are least likely to have health insurance (Cornelius, 1993; Berk, Albers, and Schur, 1996), the higher percentage of all physician visits made by Hispanics that are nonurgent ED visits indicates that they often depend on the ED as a source for nonurgent care.

One study found that Hispanic immigrants sought care in the ED due to lack of health insurance, and an additional 19 percent said that their restricted Medicaid benefits required them to seek care at an ED in order to be covered. More than a third of the respondents said they could not obtain care at other sites because of their undocumented status (Chan, Krishel, Bramwell, and Clark, 1996).

Nonurgent use of the ED also varies by type of insurance coverage: Medicaid, other third-party coverage, or no insurance (Ahern and McCoy, 1992; Gooding, Smith, and Peyrot, 1996).

Uninsured patients use fewer total health services than insured individuals (U.S. Congress, 1992). However, in Gooding, Smith, and Peyrot's (1996) analysis of data from the 1992 NAMCS, Medicaid patients had a higher rate of nonurgent ED utilization than either other insured or uninsured groups. Thus, it would appear that uninsured and Medicaid-insured individuals use the ED for nonurgent care, as a proportion of all care, more frequently than privately insured individuals, a finding that likely translates into an overdependence on EDs by immigrants who are seeking nonurgent care. In addition, case studies have shown that immigrants use the ED when they face truncated access to other segments of the health care system (Chavez, Cornelius, and Jones, 1985). Emergency medical transfer law mandates medical screening examinations prior to gatekeeping but has no provision for providing treatment that is deemed nonurgent.

There are a number of pitfalls to reliance on the hospital as the safety net. One concern has been that public hospitals will receive the bulk of the burden of indigent care. However, the federal emergency medical transfer law applies to hospitals of all types, not just public hospitals (Cross, 1992). Urban sites are not the only areas affected. Although immigrants often settle in cities initially, they migrate to other areas. As part of their resettlement terms, refugees may be settled in specific areas of the country outside major entry ports. Undocumented immigrants may settle in rural areas as seasonal farmworkers.

In general, EDs were not meant to function as sites for delivery of primary care services. However, when framed in the context of current policies, it is not unexpected that immigrants will use the ED for medical care, particularly if it is the only available or accessible source of care in the community. Further, the ED may be seen as a relatively anonymous place, a perception with appeal to undocumented individuals, who may fear being discovered.

## Costs of Acute Care

There are no valid statistics on the costs of care incurred specifically by unqualified immigrants, who may generate higher costs than they are capable of paying. This produces externalized costs, which society must subsidize. The savings promised by denial of medical benefits to nonqualifying immigrants could potentially translate into additional costs incurred by safety net facilities, particularly EDs and hospitals. Although costs for emergency care alone represent a small portion of national health expenditures (Tyrance, Himmelstein, and Woolhandler, 1997), a large proportion of hospitalizations result from admissions from the ED.

## The Access Gap

Access to care is a key determinant of utilization. Bindman and others (1995) found that self-reported lack of access to care correlates well with an aggregate measure of preventable hospitalizations. Similar findings on obstacles to care suggest that those who lack access, including financial access, may delay seeking early diagnosis and treatment of illnesses (Rask, Williams, Parker, and McNagny, 1994). Persons with lower access to care or no regular provider are less likely to receive preventive services (Lambrew and others, 1996; Bindman and others, 1996). Finally, persons with no regular source of care (defined as a regular provider or site) report lower access to services of all types in the Behavioral Risk Factor Surveillance System. Although women were at less risk than men, Hispanics were more likely to report this barrier to access (Centers for Disease Control, 1998a).

## Preservation of Access to Health Care

Although the concept of universal access to care has lost popularity since the ungracious demise of the Clinton health care reform plan, there is a movement toward examining barriers to care that specific subpopulations face and finding methods to reduce those barriers. One successful model uses volunteer or paid lay health outreach workers who are trained to provide basic health education to specific target populations, such as recent immigrant groups. The workers typically are recruited from a specific ethnic and language group to serve as liaisons between the patient and the health system and, in many cases, the social services agencies. In some areas, they also enroll individuals who are eligible for specific services (such as pregnant women in prenatal care). A good summary of existing programs can be found in the Centers for Disease Control's two-volume set: *Community Health Advisors: Models, Research, and Practice,* and *Community Health Advisors: Health Promotion and Disease Prevention* (1994).

Historically, the public sector has funded certain essential community medical services, including emergency services, trauma centers, burn centers, neonatal intensive care services, immunization and disease surveillance, and community health clinics for ambulatory care to indigent individuals. The public sector never has fit the market economy model because there is little competition to deliver services that have a high risk for not being reimbursed. Some populations, including recent immigrants, migrant farmworkers, and the homeless, remain unattractive to service providers. The market model has provided little in the way of relief for uninsured individuals.

In the past, public hospitals and community clinics were able to subsidize care to the uninsured, including immigrants, with revenues from federal sources (Medicare, Medicaid, and Disproportionate Share to Hospital funds, which also come from Medicaid). More recently, they have sometimes lost Medicare and Medicaid patients to private managed care entities that are able to offer more attractive packages to beneficiaries (Andrulis, 1997). These providers now see themselves as being left with disproportionate numbers of indigent patients, including recent immigrants, and unable to engage in any cost shifting due to fewer insured patients (including Medicaid insured). Closures of some public hospitals and the financial crises of others show that concerns about the survival of the safety net are not unfounded (Andrulis, 1997). Even well-established clinics that serve large immigrant populations have faced significant decreases in revenue and have been forced to reexamine their capacity to treat all categories of patients (K. Hendry, personal communication, 1998).

Nationally, a review of gross patient revenues from one hundred public hospitals by the National Public Health and Hospital Institute showed a reduction in government support from 15.9 percent of total revenues in 1980 to 8.9 percent in 1993 (National Public Health and Hospital Institute, 1995a). Some institutions have been able to survive these changes by engaging as full partners with managed care companies and presumably having a higher ratio of paying to indigent patients. But what about cities, such as Los Angeles and New York, where the number of immigrants is high and resources for those individuals to receive insurance of any kind are becoming increasingly scarce? Will clinics and hospitals in these areas need the types of federal bailouts that Los Angeles County Hospital needed in 1996?

Future crises may arise as immigrants who previously were eligible for subsidized programs shift from federal funding, to county funding, to uninsured status. California already has stated its intention to deny prenatal coverage to undocumented women. A similar dilemma confronts federally qualified health centers and clinics, which historically have cared for immigrants. One clinic's strategic plan to preserve its mission is detailed in Chapter Eighteen.

Concern remains that by curtailing access to nonemergency services, including preventive care, immunizations, early detection and treatment of infectious diseases, and prenatal care, we risk overburdening safety net facilities, which already face staffing shortages and financial crises. Appropriate utilization of the health care delivery system and each of its sectors hinges on federal financing of all necessary services: preventive, primary care, and acute care.

# Chapter Five

# Utilization of Mental Health Services

*Kevin M. Chun and*
*Phillip D. Akutsu*

API women and Latina Americans may be considered unique client populations with special mental health needs. However, their service needs and utilization patterns remain largely a matter of conjecture due to the paucity of data for immigrant and refugee women on utilization rates, types of services received, and treatment outcomes. Nonetheless, study findings for the overall API and Latino and Latina populations consistently show that proportionally fewer individuals utilize mental health services compared to European Americans (Sue, Zane, and Young, 1994). One investigation, which used the 1986 National Institute of Mental Health national survey data of patient populations, found that APIs were three times less likely to utilize mental health services compared to European Americans (Matsuoka, Breaux, and Ryujin, 1997). Another study analyzed utilization patterns of five different Asian American groups who were treated in the Los Angeles County mental health system from 1983 to 1988 (Ying and Hu, 1994). Results showed variable utilization patterns and treatment outcomes across Asian American groups: Filipinos were underrepresented in this public mental health system relative to their overall county population, while Southeast Asians were overrepresented and reported the least improvement following therapy. In an earlier study using the same Los Angeles County data set, Sue, Fujino, Hu, and Takeuchi (1991) found that Mexican Americans also underutilized public mental health services; these findings were in contrast to African Americans, who overutilized services.

Significant ethnic differences in the types of services received in public mental health systems also have been highlighted. For instance, Asian and Latino American clients used fewer emergency and inpatient services but more outpatient care compared to European American clients served in San Francisco and Santa Clara counties (Hu, Snowden, Jerrell, and Nguyen, 1991). Similar ethnic differences were found for clients who were being treated for severe mental illness at public mental health clinics. In examining mental health records for two large West Coast counties, researchers found that in one county, Asian and Latino American clients suffering from severe psychopathology and psychosocial dysfunction utilized more outpatient and supportive services, but fewer inpatient services compared to European Americans (Snowden and Hu, 1997). Asian and Latino American clients in the second county exhibited an opposite service pattern: they were more likely to be hospitalized compared to European American clients.

A broad range of variables have been identified to account for ethnic differences in utilization rates, treatment outcomes, and types of services: clients' demographic backgrounds, cultural values and norms, illness beliefs, help-seeking strategies, therapist characteristics, assessment and treatment techniques, and organizational and structural characteristics of the mental health agency (Echeverry, 1997; Uba, 1994). However, discussion of these variables often is devoid of a conceptual framework to understand their significance to the *process* of service utilization among immigrant and refugee populations. To this end, mental health service issues for these special client populations may be analyzed using a stage model of utilization that extends past discussions of utilization pathways (Howard and others, 1996; Saunders, 1993) and change processes (Prochaska, DiClemente, and Norcross, 1992).

The proposed stage model of utilization assumes that clients will progress through a series of identifiable and interrelated stages that characterize service utilization as a multilevel process involving numerous individual, organizational and structural, and treatment variables: problem recognition, coping response, agency contact, and service engagement. The following discussion outlines the various issues in each stage for immigrant and refugee populations, with particular attention to sociocultural and structural barriers that may prevent API women and Latinas from accessing mental health care systems.

## Problem Recognition

In this stage, individuals first become aware of their psychological distress and related symptomatology. They form initial illness attributions, which are contingent on their level of acculturation. API women and Latinas may view their presenting problems in culturally distinct ways that ultimately inform their coping strategies, including their decision on whether to utilize mental health services.

API women and Latinas may hold culturally embedded views of mental health that focus on a dynamic interaction between the mind and body (Chun, Eastman, Wang, and Sue, 1998). This, of course, is different from Western psychological perspectives, which primarily attend to mental processes. This was poignantly illustrated in the traditional health beliefs found in a community sample of immigrant Chinese women in San Francisco's Chinatown, who attributed major depression to both psychological (for example, "low/unstable mood") and physiological (for example, "heart problems") causes (Ying, 1990).

Latinas also may hold culturally distinct conceptualizations of psychological distress that may involve physical symptoms. For example, it has been suggested that *ataques de nervios* in immigrant Puerto Rican women is a permissible way for Puerto Rican women to express anger within their cultural milieu (Oquendo, 1994).

## Coping Response

Individuals in this stage initiate coping strategies aimed at alleviating their psychological distress. They may attempt to resolve their problems individually or with the aid of resources in their sociocultural environment. API women and Latinas may initiate multiple coping responses before considering mental health services due to cultural conceptualizations of illness, availability of informal social support networks, cultural norms and values, gender role expectations, lack of awareness of the availability and nature of mental health services, and cultural distrust of agencies.

Initially they may seek help from medical rather than mental health professionals (Canino, 1982; Lin, Carter, and Kleinman, 1985; Lin, Ihle, and Tazuma, 1985). They also may be more comfortable accessing coping resources that are more compatible with their cultural belief systems (Dworkin and Adams, 1987; Lee, 1997; Reeves, 1986; Uba, 1994). Within the Asian and Latin American cultures, this may include seeking help from indigenous folk healers or the church and clergy (Akutsu, Snowden, and Organista, 1996; Flaskerud, 1986; Garcia and Zea, 1997; Lee, 1997; Leong, Wagner, and Tata, 1995; Uba, 1994). For example, many Hmong and Mien refugees who have relocated to the United States continue to seek shamans and use traditional herbal remedies to treat their psychological problems (Westermeyer, 1988).

Historically, API women and Latinas have turned to informal social supports, such as immediate and extended family and close friends, when personal remedies for psychological distress are inadequate (Cheung, 1987; Lin, Inui, Kleinman, and Womack, 1982). Cultural norms that ascribe shame and stigma to mental illness may also contribute to underutilization of mental health services (Jayakar, 1994; Vargas-Willis and Cervantes, 1987). Personal disclosures of mental health problems to individuals outside the immediate and extended family often are seen as cultural taboos that bring shame and dishonor to the entire family. Similarly, mental health problems often are viewed as a sign of moral weakness or a lack of moral character (Echeverry, 1997). As such, API women and Latinas are more likely to strengthen their willpower and suffer in silence instead of seeking professional help (Bradshaw, 1994). Korean immigrants, for example, have taken great pride in their silent endurance and resiliency under the most adverse conditions in immigrating to the United States (Kim, 1994).

Cultural values of harmony and group cohesion may further discourage these women from disclosing their problems even to their own families. For example, one study found that Spanish-speaking Latinas infected with the human immunodeficiency virus (HIV) were less likely to disclose their seropositivity or HIV-related worries with their family and friends, compared to African and European Americans and English-speaking Latinas (Simoni and others, 1995). Cultural norms such as *simpatica* (emphasizing harmonious social relationships) and "familism" (promoting family solidarity) may have inhibited these Latinas from disclosing to family and friends in order to avoid disruption of interpersonal relations.

Puerto Rican American women may adhere to *marianismo*, which incorporates Catholic beliefs surrounding the Virgin Mary. This gender role prescription maintains that women are spiritually superior to men, thereby allowing them to endure the suffering caused by men (Comas-Diaz, 1988). This notion of self-sacrifice may reinforce Latinas to cope with their problems on an individual basis. Such gender role expectations are seen in Asian American cultures as well. In the Japanese culture, the expression *shi-ka-ta-ga-nai* or ("it cannot be helped") encourages women to tolerate life's suffering without complaint or help from others.

Lack of awareness of available services and lack of familiarity with the nature of therapy further mitigate API women and Latinas' seeking professional help (Starrett and others, 1990; Uba, 1994). For example, a lack of awareness of community mental health resources has been found to contribute to lower utilization rates (Loo, Tong, and True, 1989). Researchers also have noted that many immigrant and refugee groups may be reluctant to seek psychotherapy because they are unfamiliar with the nature and benefits of this treatment modality (Uba, 1994).

Cultural distrust may inhibit Asian American–Pacific Islander women and Latinas from using mental health services even if they are aware of their availability. Invariably, there is a recurrent fear that services or information disclosed in therapy may not be confidential and may become a part of public record where families, neighbors, or the community at large are privy to highly personal information (Echeverry, 1997; Ishisaka, Nguyen, and Okimoto, 1985). This fear is particularly important for undocumented women, who may not seek services in a government-sponsored clinic because they assume it is affiliated with the Immigration and Naturalization Service (INS) and that they will be deported if their illegal status is disclosed (Echeverry, 1997).

Given these reasons, it is not uncommon for immigrant and refugee women initially to attempt to resolve their personal difficulties alone or within their immediate and extended families, including trusted friends. Next, they may seek consultation with an indigenous folk healer, spiritualist, clergy, or medical professional (Koss-Chioino, 1995), and if these resources fail to alleviate the problem, they may finally go to an emergency room or a mental health clinic when the situation reaches crisis proportion (Wallen, 1992).

## Agency Contact

Individuals in this stage make the initial step of contacting mental health agencies to determine the feasibility and relative merits of utilizing professional services. API women and Latinas may still harbor reservations about mental health care. Consequently, they may spend considerable time inquiring about agency services, structure, and policy, without making a commitment to utilization.

In order to improve mental health service use within Asian and Latina American communities, clinicians and researchers have emphasized the importance of hiring culturally competent and bilingual staff, improving accessibility to agencies, increasing availability of agency services, improving affordability of services and fees, and providing additional services targeting immigrant and refugee populations. Marin (1993) advises that culturally appropriate strategies must address some basic criteria for Asian and Latin American populations:

1. The intervention is based on the cultural values of the targeted group.
2. Intervention strategies reflect the subjective culture (attitudes, expectancies, norms) of the group.
3. The components comprising these strategies incorporate the behavioral preferences and expectations of the group's members.

Because Latinas and API women may be unfamiliar with mental health services, agencies should be staffed with culturally competent individuals who are sensitive to their unique concerns and needs. This includes orienting staff to cultural expectations for psychological treatment among refugee and immigrant women (Acosta, Yamamoto, and Evans, 1982; Tien, 1994; Vargas-Willis and Cervantes, 1987). It is likely that these women will be contacting the agency after exhausting other culturally sanctioned coping responses, so it is critical to address possible feelings of guilt and shame immediately that may accompany their decision to seek services. This may require pretreatment client education on the nature and course of therapy, as well as the roles of the client and therapist. The provision of such information prior to treatment is associated with increased knowledge about psychotherapy and more positive attitudes toward treatment for API women and Latinas (Acosta, Yamamoto, Evans, and Skilbeck, 1983; Uba, 1994).

The availability of bilingual staff affects service utilization for APIs and Latinas as well (Echeverry, 1997; Uba, 1994). Most immigrant and refugee women clients who are primarily monolingual tend to prefer services offered in their native tongue or dialect. The inability of most therapists and staff to communicate effectively with clients who have limited English-language skills seriously compromises the quality of services (Bamford, 1991; Malgady, Rogler, and Constantino, 1987). This is especially evident during initial contact, where speaking to the agency receptionist in one's native tongue may be decisive in forgoing or pursuing professional help. Although children may act as translators for the family, this is not necessarily an effective method of communication (Chung and Lin, 1994), and the use of bilingual professionals in the field is preferred (Comas-Diaz and Greene, 1994).

Accessibility and geographic location of mental health agencies also influence service (Echeverry, 1997; Uba, 1994). Since many immigrant and refugee clients come from impoverished backgrounds, it is likely that they have to rely on public transportation, which means spending considerable time and effort traveling to seek professional help. A family also must have enough funds to pay transportation fares for several people. Reliance on public transportation can be a potential source of embarrassment for those traveling with a family member who may be visibly disturbed or difficult to manage (Echeverry, 1997).

Agency hours of operation or availability play a critical role in determining whether greater service use will occur. Work schedules for immigrant and refugee women may conflict with regular business hours, a significant obstacle for those who are primary caretakers of their children and other family members. In addition, many employed women of color are unable to take sick leave for mental health treatment (Echeverry, 1997; Uba, 1994). In response to these challenges, many culturally sensitive programs have increased their hours of operation to include evening and weekend hours.

High costs and service fees and lack of health insurance or benefits may further restrict access to mental health care (Ruiz, 1993; Wells and others, 1987). Many immigrant and refugee women and their families live below the poverty level and tend to have low-wage jobs that prevent them from utilizing mental health services (O'Hare, 1992). Newly arrived immigrants and refugees are particularly intimidated by the cost of mental health services, either because they lack health insurance or their health insurance is inadequate (Wong, 1985).

Service utilization may increase with the incorporation of mental health services into multiservice centers that provide legal and social services, as well as language programs that meet the unique needs of immigrant and refugee populations (Sue and Zane, 1987). This multiservice center option can diminish the stigma associated with mental health care by presenting psychotherapy as just one of many service options available to prospective clients (Uba, 1982).

## Service Engagement

Once individuals have made an initial commitment to enter therapy, whether they will remain engaged in the treatment process depends on the client-therapist ethnic and gender match, culturally sensitive therapy techniques, and therapist credibility.

Attention to gender issues is a key factor in service engagement for API women and Latinas. In the previously discussed study of psychiatric outpatients in the Los Angeles County mental health system, ethnic match between client and therapist was positively related to the number of therapy sessions for Asian and Mexican Americans (Sue and others, 1991). Moreover, it contributed both to fewer premature terminations and positive treatment outcome for those who did not have English as a primary language. Another study, which used the same data, found that Asian American women who were matched with their therapist on both ethnicity and gender were twenty times less likely to drop out of treatment after one session compared to women who were not matched on either ethnicity or gender (Fujino, Okazaki, and Young, 1994).

Treatment benefits associated with client-therapist ethnic and gender match may be related to heightened sensitivity to cultural and gender issues in the therapy session. Although studies have yet to investigate the relationship of specific treatment variables to outcome for API women and Latina clients, culturally sensitive therapy techniques have been recommended. These have included a directive and active counseling style and attention to nonverbal communication and implicit social cues reflected in body language, eye contact, and tone of voice. For Mexican American women clients, in particular, *dichos,* or cultural proverbs, may be used to overcome discomfort with the psychotherapy process and promote change. Examples of such proverbs include *"Lo que pasó voló,"* or let bygones be bygones, and *"Al que le duela la muela que se la saque,"* which literally means that the person with tooth pain should pull it out, or "God helps those who help themselves" (Zuniga, 1991).

Culturally diverse immigrant and refugee women may be more likely to remain engaged in treatment if gender issues are addressed as well. In addition to exploring grief and loneliness stemming from the immigration and refugee experience, therapists should be aware that some women may feel guilt and shame if they fail to meet gender role expectations. This may represent a salient treatment issue for those who come to the United States alone, leaving family and children behind in their home countries (Espin, 1987). Therapy may incorporate feminist approaches of self-empowerment that allow immigrant and refugee women to redefine their social and family roles and develop self-acceptance and autonomy (Vargas-Willis and Cervantes, 1987). However, feminist approaches should be adapted to meet the sociocultural experiences of ethnically diverse groups (Comas-Diaz, 1988; Sieng and Thompson, 1992). For instance, awareness, education, openness, and confrontation of sexual and cultural stereotypes may be an integral component of treatment (Chan, 1988). In addition, analysis of power relationships that are affecting the client's situation and identification of potential power may prove beneficial to ethnic minority women (Gutierrez, 1990). This may encompass identifying positive role models of adaptation in the community or in traditional folk legends, and developing support groups for women (True, 1990). The ultimate goal of these treatment considerations is to help immigrant and refugee women to integrate ethnic, gender, and racial components into their identity (Comas-Diaz, 1988).

Finally, therapist credibility may be considered more proximal to the goal of positive treatment outcome than ethnic match, gender match, culturally sensitive techniques, and attention to gender issues alone. According to Sue and Zane (1987), ascribed and achieved credibility is fundamental to treatment success. Ascribed credibility relates to the status that is assigned to the therapist prior to the therapy session, whereas achieved credibility refers to the therapist's actual skills and actions. In this context, API women and Latinas may ascribe high credibility to their therapists if they are women who share similar cultural backgrounds. Moreover, therapists can achieve credibility if they develop culturally appropriate conceptualizations of problems, problem resolution strategies, and treatment goals. Therapists who have low ascribed credibility initially may thus achieve credibility over time.

## Conclusion

The stage model of utilization is intended to broaden past discussions that typically have been confined to one aspect of a multilevel process. Delineation of stages toward utilization allows for the systematic analysis of individual, organizational and structural, and treatment process variables and their relationship to the service needs and utilization patterns of immigrant and refugee women. A number of recommendations aimed at improving service utilization can thus be formulated for the different stages in this model.

First, in terms of problem recognition, it is important to gain a better understanding of emic constructions of illness in order to estimate the prevalence of psychological distress within immigrant and refugee communities. This will allow practitioners to understand the mental health service needs of specific cultural groups better. With regard to coping responses, it is imperative that mental health agencies implement culturally appropriate interventions that increase community awareness of available mental health care. To this end, mental health agencies may enlist the help of community leaders to serve as educators or lay counselors, who can provide information about services to fellow immigrant and refugee women. In relation to agency contact, the hiring of culturally competent, bilingual staff should remain a priority in light of the growing size of immigrant and refugee populations who require mental health care. Furthermore, agencies should continue to offer additional services, such as parenting support groups and public seminars on women's health care, to diminish the stigma associated with mental health service use. For the last stage of service engagement, continued research on specific process variables associated with therapist credibility will lead to improved treatment approaches for culturally diverse groups. The efficacy of modified feminist treatment approaches also should be examined to develop strategies for empowerment that incorporate the sociocultural realities of immigrant and refugee women.

*Chapter Six*

# The Impact of Recent Legislation on the Delivery of Health Care to Immigrants

# Welfare and Immigration Reforms in 1996 and 1997

*Susan L. Ivey*

Health care facilities of all types are faced with the possibility of increasing numbers of immigrants who seek care but lack the resources to pay for it. Two recent laws, the Personal Responsibility and Work Opportunity Reconciliation Act (PRWORA, Public Law [PL] 104–193, 1996) and the Illegal Immigration Reform and Immigrant Responsibility Act of 1996, hereafter referred to as the immigration reform act (IIRIRA, PL 104–208, sec. 803, div. C), would restrict benefits for Social Security, Medicaid, and Medicare to immigrants deemed "qualified" by virtue of having worked forty quarters (at least ten years) during which they paid into the Social Security system.

Some immigrants may have arrived in the United States late in their working years; others may have come to join relatives here upon retirement. Some immigrants have been receiving various forms of assistance (Supplemental Security Income, Medicare, Medicaid) for a number of years. The possibility exists that legal immigrants who were receiving assistance prior to 1997 will lose their benefits, and their families will not be able to support them. Bills have been proposed in both the House and the Senate to repeal that portion of the law that relates to individuals who are over age sixty-five, disabled, or blind (U.S. Congress, 1997b). Immediate implementation of the changes for these groups has been stayed by presidential order, allowing recipients a brief reprieve (*Washington Post*, 1997, p. A3). Nevertheless, the effects of implementation of other portions of the laws have begun to unfold.

# Federal Funding for Health Care

As funding for financing health care for immigrants is reduced (as was threatened under California's Proposition 187 and implemented as part of federal immigration reform in 1996), traditional settings in the community no longer are financially able to care for large numbers of uninsured immigrants. The burden of providing such care may shift to hospitals and emergency departments (National Association of Public Hospitals and Health Systems, 1997). The welfare reform act contains explicit exceptions for provision of emergency services necessary to preserve life or safety (PRWORA, sec. 401(b)(1)). They are in keeping with the federal Emergency Medical Treatment and Active Labor Act (EMTALA), and services covered under EMTALA must be provided without regard to insurance or immigration status. Sanctions and financial penalties can be levied against providers and hospitals for violating this law.

The language in the welfare reform act allows the use of state and federal funds for emergency care and care related to symptoms of infectious diseases regardless of whether the final diagnosis is a communicable disease (PRWORA, sec. 401(b)(1)(A,B,C)). However, the immigration reform act stipulates that in order to apply for those specific funds, information ascertaining illegal immigrant status must be collected by providers and reported to the federal government (IIRIRA, subtitle D, sec. 562). In the past, hospitals have applied for disproportionate share (DSH) payments from Medicaid to offset the cost of indigent care. This portion of the Medicaid budget had been one of the most rapidly growing uses of Medicaid funds prior to the 1996 changes (Kaiser Family Foundation, 1995). DSH funds also are targeted for cutbacks under federal Medicaid reform. It is not clear whether the funds for provision of emergency medical services to uncovered immigrants will come from the Medicaid budget or other sources. And it is similarly unclear whether hospitals that are unable or unwilling to report specific information regarding the legal status of their patients will be able to apply for such funds.

The fallout from the recent federal changes in eligibility could result in longer waits for care, an increasing number of preventable hospitalizations among immigrants who delay seeking care, and a shift in site of care from federally qualified health clinics and traditional community structures to the emergency department as site of last resort. Although welfare reform has been in place for only a few months at the time of this writing, San Francisco area hospitals have reported increases of 5 to 25 percent in emergency department utilization compared to the same period one year earlier (*San Francisco Examiner,* 1997). Whether these are one-time increases or part of a pattern of sustained change in the site of care delivery remains to be seen.

## Other Affected Programs

Changes to Medicaid included the unlinking of eligibility from eligibility for the program now known as Temporary Assistance to Needy Families (TANF), formerly Aid to Families with Dependent Children. Other restrictions of the welfare reform act, such as decreased eligibility for subsidized housing and food stamp programs, were implemented in 1997. Although states have the option of continuing to provide assistance to immigrants with their own funds, immigrants who formerly qualified for assistance may find only safety net services available in many states (Andrulis, 1997; National Association of Public Hospitals, 1997b).

The welfare reform act also eliminated food stamp benefits for "nonqualified aliens." The immigration reform act extended food stamp eligibility for "qualified immigrants currently receiving benefits" to April 1, 1997. Immigrants who lose access to food stamps and housing assistance are likely to contribute to the increase in applications for food and emergency general assistance predicted by many big city mayors in 1996 (U.S. Conference of Mayors, 1996). Repeal of the changes in the food stamp program has been discussed in the 105th Congress.

Elderly persons, already at risk for poor nutrition, and those with mental illness are especially likely to be affected by food and housing restrictions. One solution to less available housing would be for extended families to live together in order to conserve resources. This might result in increases in household density (the number of persons occupying a household). Overcrowding can lead to easier spread of infectious diseases and increased levels of family stress. Reduced access to food stamps and Women, Infants, and Children (WIC) food programs might result in poorer nutrition for pregnant women, thereby leading to diminished birth outcomes.

## Special Protections for Women

The welfare reform act of 1996 also allows for temporary treatment of battered "aliens" as "qualified aliens" (PRWORA, sec. 431(b)). This was further defined in the immigration reform act (PL 104–208, sec. 803, div. C, title IV, subtitle A, sec. 501, 552). Similar attention was given to the mail-order bride trade (sec. 652). However, many immigrant women are reluctant to report domestic violence (see Chapter Ten). The potential impact of these protections under federal law is unclear. Similarly, female genital mutilation is recognized as a crime under the immigration reform act (sec. 645), amending U.S. Code Title 18, section 116.

## Access to Emergency and Labor Services

The welfare reform act and the immigration reform act reaffirm the intent of EMTALA to maintain access to care for life-threatening emergencies for all who present regardless of ability to pay. Although the intent of both laws is to preserve the availability of safety net services, no funding was mandated under EMTALA. The welfare reform act states only that emergency funds will be available under Title XIX of the Social Security Act (sec. 1903 (v)(3)) without specifying a mechanism for funding or whether the funds will be in addition to or in place of the previous DSH payments that enable many hospitals to provide uncompensated care to indigent patients (PRWORA, sec. 401(b)).

Eligibility for services hinges on meeting eligibility requirements for medical assistance under each state's plan. The immigration reform act, section 562(b), states that no payments for treatment of emergency medical conditions will be made to public hospitals, public facilities, or eligible nonprofit hospitals without verification of immigration status, and that payment under this mechanism will be made only to the extent that costs cannot be recovered from other programs and the "alien or another person." This means that sponsors will likely be held responsible for payment as well.

## Immigrant Versus Immigration Policy

The goals of immigration policy reform (such as border control and allocation of temporary work visas for seasonal farmworkers) can be separated from U.S. immigrant policy (provision of health care and food benefits while workers and families are here). This is the case in many other countries, which have universal or near-universal health care coverage. It is unlikely that the United States will see shrinking numbers of recent immigrants requiring medical care in the near future. Immigration to the United States is at the highest level since the early part of the century. Once immigrants are here, there must be a rational allocation of resources for preventive and safety net services. The 1996 immigration reforms evidenced little concern for the people who immigrate for reasons of severe economic deprivation in their own countries, focusing instead on specific groups who might seek asylum.

## The Potential for Shifting Sites of Health Care

Community-based providers of care to immigrants have expressed great concern about their ability to sustain services to immigrants in the face of proposed funding cuts to Medicaid. Federally qualified health centers provide preventive services, immunizations, and acute care for nonemergent problems. Problems such as children with fevers and otitis media, adults with respiratory ailments (such as cough with fever), and minor injuries such as strains or sprains might be better thought of as requiring care within twenty-four hours rather than as emergencies.

Increasing numbers of preventable hospitalizations could occur if access to outpatient clinics and community health centers is curtailed, and people delay seeking care earlier in the course of illness (Bindman and others, 1995; Rask, Williams, Parker, and McNagny, 1994). Although this may not increase emergency department visits or hospitalizations overall (since individuals may seek care only if they are truly ill), it could result in increased acuity of visits and a shift in site of care from federally qualified health clinics and traditional community structures to emergency departments or hospitals as sites of last resort (Ivey and Kramer, 1998).

Attempts in California to exclude undocumented immigrants from both the education and health systems (Proposition 187, which was passed in 1995) have been enjoined while the courts examine the tensions between federal and state obligations. The appellate court has ordered California to provide certain emergency and prenatal benefits (Richman, 1998). Although the changes seen following passage of Proposition 187 appeared to be transient, given that a law was passed but never implemented, much larger sustained alterations in site of service delivery could be expected to occur with the changes in federal law. There is an urgent need for research on the changes in utilization, costs, and health outcomes associated with this broad policy change.

# Proposition 187: California's Anti-Immigrant Statute

*Nobuko Mizoguchi*

In 1994, 58.5 percent of California voters passed Proposition 187, a ballot initiative that made undocumented residents ineligible for nonemergency publicly funded health care services, public social services, and public education. In addition, Proposition 187 required service providers, school districts, and educational institutions to report any person who is determined to be or reasonably suspected of being undocumented to the U.S. Immigration and Naturalization Service. The measure also contained a provision that created new state crimes involving manufacture, distribution, sale, or use of false citizenship or resident alien documents (California, 1994).

Proposition 187 passed in the context of a larger anti-immigrant backlash, spurred by the economic recession that hit California in the early 1990s and the increasing racial diversification of the state population, which was perceived by some as a threat. Throughout history, immigrants have been targets of hostility during times of economic recession. Proposition 187 passed in a year of economical difficulties for Californians. The state was just beginning to recover from a deep recession through which it had been suffering since 1990. The state unemployment rate was at 8.6 percent, the number of wage and salary workers in nonfarm establishments had decreased 2.7 percent since 1990, and the per capita personal income of Californians had increased only 1.9 percent since the previous year (California, 1997).

In addition, the demographic landscape of California had changed rapidly during the 1980s. By 1990, ethnic minorities composed 43 percent of the population. Growth was particularly great among Asian and Latino populations. Between 1980 and 1990, the Asian population more than doubled, from 1.2 million to 2.7 million, and the Latino population increased by approximately 70 percent, to 7.7 million in 1990. In comparison, the African American and white populations grew at a slower rate. The African American population (excluding Latinos) increased by 17 percent, to 2.1 million, and the non-Latino white population rose by 7.4 percent, to 17 million (California, 1991).

Proposition 187 became largely a symbolic measure aimed at sending a message to policymakers, immigrants, and potential immigrants. Arguments in favor of it included a call to stop the flow of "illegal aliens," asserting that undocumented residents are a social and economic burden to taxpayers, that Californians suffer from crimes committed by undocumented residents, and that public health and social services draw immigrants to the United States. Arguments against the measure claimed that Proposition 187 would result in additional costs to the taxpayers, it conflicted with federal laws, it was racist, it threatened the health of all Californians, and it would not stop the flow of immigrants (California, 1994). The symbolic nature of the proposition was propelled when Pete Wilson made Proposition 187 the cornerstone of his gubernatorial campaign.

Proposition 187 created a great deal of concern among health care professionals regarding the impact of such a measure on the health of undocumented residents and the public. Although the courts have prohibited implementation of Proposition 187, health care providers have argued that the fear generated by its passage has had a detrimental effect on the health of immigrants and the public.

Many medical groups and public health organizations, including the American Medical Association, the California Medical Association, the California Nurses Association, and the American Public Health Association, have spoken out against Proposition 187. Health care professionals argued that infectious diseases, such as tuberculosis and measles, may spread if undocumented residents do not seek care (Ziv and Lo, 1995; Levy, 1994). One study conducted prior to the passage of Proposition 187 showed that fear of immigration authorities was closely associated with delay in care of patients with symptomatic tuberculosis (Asch, Leake, and Gelberg, 1994). Although only 6 percent stated that they feared that going to a physician might lead to problems with immigration authorities, those who did were about four times as likely to delay care for more than two months. The authors of the report expressed apprehension that policies that increase undocumented residents' fear of being reported to immigration authorities by health care professionals may exacerbate the tuberculosis epidemic. In addition to infectious diseases, many health care providers claimed that denial of prenatal care to undocumented women would hurt children born in California who are U.S. citizens.

Anecdotal reports indicate that there have been deaths as a result of immigrants' not seeking health care services due to fear of Proposition 187, as well as a general decrease in the number of immigrants seeking care (Burdman, 1994a, 1994b; Salladay, 1994).

A handful of studies that measured the impact of the passage of Proposition 187 support the anecdotal reports that the number of immigrants seeking health care services declined. One study examined the effect of Proposition 187 on mental health service use in San Francisco by Latinos aged eighteen to forty-five. Fenton, Catalano, and Hargreaves (1996) analyzed services and demographic data from the San Francisco County Division of Mental Health and Substance Abuse Services (DMS) system covering the time period sixty-seven weeks before and twenty-three weeks after the passage of Proposition 187. Results of their time-series analyses showed a 26 percent decrease in initiation of outpatient services after the passage of Proposition 187 at sites with large numbers of Latino immigrant clients. No similar decrease was observed among young non-Latino whites. Furthermore, this decrease was sustained nearly six months after the election, until the end of the study period. In addition, the decrease in outpatient services by young Latinos was accompanied by an increase in crisis services. The authors suggest that this trend may have cost implications since crisis visits may be nearly five times more expensive than outpatient visits.

Spetz and others (1997) analyzed data from California's Birth Public Use files to determine the effects of the passage of Proposition 187 on prenatal care utilization and birth outcomes. The study focused on 147,886 foreign-born women with less than twelve years of education who gave birth in California between 1993 and 1995. Those without private insurance, Latino women, and women who gave birth in Los Angeles County were examined separately to obtain a more accurate picture of the effect of Proposition 187 on undocumented women. The authors considered these characteristics to be associated with a higher proportion of undocumented residents. The results showed a decrease in the use of prenatal care among foreign-born women with low educational levels giving birth in Los Angeles County after the passage of Proposition 187. No significant change in prenatal care use was observed on the statewide level. Despite the decline in prenatal care use in Los Angeles County, no change in average birth outcomes was observed in Los Angeles County or statewide.

Finally, a study surveyed a sample of 121 primary care clinics in California that serve low-income groups about the impact of Proposition 187 on the use of the clinics (Fenton, Moss, Khalil, and Asch, 1997). The authors reported no significant decline in total monthly visits from October 1994 to March 1995, compared to the previous year. However, when clinic directors were asked whether they noticed any change, 51 percent indicated that they were aware of a patient who delayed seeking care at their clinic due to fears related to Proposition 187. Sixty-five percent of clinic directors indicated that they either perceived a decrease in patient visits or were aware of a patient who delayed seeking care.

A study that measured the effect of Proposition 187 on ophthalmology clinic utilization at a major inner-city public hospital reported that the number of new walk-in patients significantly decreased for a two-month period around the election when Proposition 187 was being debated and there was confusion about its implementation (Marx and others, 1996). The authors attributed this decrease to Proposition 187. By December 1994, the number of walk-in patients returned to baseline levels. The authors concluded that the no-effect finding in December 1994 was due to alleviation of the confusion around implementation of Proposition 187, which was attributable to adequate publicity concerning court-ordered temporary injunctions. No statistically significant change in utilization was observed for cancellations and no-shows for the same period for new patients. In addition, no change in utilization was seen among return patients. However, the authors argued that walk-ins reflect a patient's spontaneous decision to seek medical care. Hence, the number of walk-ins is believed to be the best indicator of new patients' decisions over the risks and benefits involved in seeking care.

In addition to the studies that measured the impact of Proposition 187 on health care service use, one study examined how Proposition 187 was perceived by immigrant Latina women and how their perception might affect their use of clinical services (Moss, Baumeister, and Biewener, 1996). The study revealed that the women who were interviewed saw Proposition 187 as discriminatory and targeting primarily Latinos. In addition, many expressed fears about denial of services, payment, and threats of deportation. Some also were concerned about the spread of infectious disease. According to the study, the initiative intensified the general fears, common among immigrant Latina women, about being economically and socially marginalized in society.

The effect that Proposition 187 has had on health status is difficult to assess. Very few studies of this issue have been conducted. Despite the paucity of evidence, it seems apparent that Proposition 187 has had some harmful effects, and they could extend beyond undocumented residents. In addition to being a potential threat to the public's health, one study has suggested that it also may result in increased costs associated with decreased utilization of less expensive preventive services and increased use of higher-cost acute care services (Fenton, Catalano, and Hargreaves, 1996). As of September 1998, Proposition 187 is still enjoined. The appellate court has ruled that emergency and prenatal services cannot be denied to women "who otherwise qualify" just because they have border-crossing cards.

## Conclusion

The federal welfare and illegal immigration reform legislation that passed in 1996 is being implemented in many states. Whether this legislation will produce the types of changes seen following California's attempt to restrict access to public services for immigrants is unknown. The 105th Congress and the Clinton administration have moved to stay certain provisions of the laws that would have affected the most vulnerable: the elderly, disabled, and mentally ill. However, many states have proceeded with restrictions that affect women and children. It is imperative that providers be aware of policy changes that may affect the ability of women to obtain timely primary care, prenatal, and preventive services.

# Health Problems
# and Concerns

*Chapter Seven*

# Screening, Infectious Diseases, and Nutritional Concerns

# Initial Assessment, Screening, and Immunizations

*Susan L. Ivey*
*and Shotsy Faust*

The medical care of recent immigrant women must reach beyond the Western focus on identification of pathophysiologic processes that cause a symptom or might lead to disease. Clinicians are confronted with a variety of different backgrounds and experiences, all of which may have health consequences as well as an impact on communication, modesty, and use of health services. The goals of the primary care practitioner in the initial encounter with a new immigrant are to understand the impact of migration on health, incorporate the patient's health belief system into the therapeutic relationship, use screening tests only where indicated, and render necessary care and wraparound services in a culturally competent manner.

Whether the newcomer is an immigrant or a refugee, the length of time she has been in this country and whether she has had prior screening should be determined at the first visit. Although immigrants generally have time to plan their move, refugees often have to flee their country of origin with little planning or choice. The flight itself can have health consequences, and there may have been interim stays in refugee camps under

---

The anemia and hepatitis protocols were provided courtesy of Lori Kohler, medical director of the San Francisco General Hospital Refugee Clinic.

less-than-optimal conditions (DeLay and Faust, 1987). On the other hand, both groups have sustained the stress of a move and are newcomers to our society, with similar barriers in terms of language and understanding of a new culture and health system. Some legal immigrants from Central America, for example, may not technically be designated as refugees but have nevertheless undergone the same trauma of war and survivorship. Sluzki's migration history model (see Chapter One) presents the stages through which migrant women move.

In general, refugee patients are at higher risk for physical and emotional crises after arrival (Faust, 1996). Details of their migration experience may elicit emotional pain and should be pursued in a later visit if they are not directly related to making a diagnosis. It is important that the provider also establish trust with the patient by ensuring, as much as possible, that determination of immigration status will not affect the care delivered. Sluzki's model (1979) identifies five stages of migration: (1) planning stage, (2) act of migration, (3) period of overcompensation, (4) period of decompensation, and (5) resolution stage or stage of intergenerational support. Many refugees will have the assistance of the social service agency or sponsor in finding these essentials. There may be less social service support for immigrants, particularly for undocumented persons. During the period of decompensation, refugees who have obtained only initial screening services may now return for symptoms that may be either somatic manifestations of stress or exacerbations of chronic conditions for which they have delayed seeking care due to other concerns.

## First Clinic Visit

The initial clinic visit follows the format of a typical history and physical examination. It includes, however, initiation of a migration history and attention to any severe, acute problems.

### Taking the History

The migration history is generally ascertained over several clinic visits. At the first visit, simply eliciting when the patient arrived in the United States, her current living situation, and whether she resides with family, friends, or alone may be sufficient. After the initiation of a migration history, the provider should explore any medical symptoms. It is important not to define for the patient that symptoms are either physical or emotional, a paradigm unique to Western culture. Rather, a more comprehensive review of systems focusing on symptom elicitation should be used. The provider also should explore the patient's belief about the origin of her symptoms. Kleinman's explanatory belief model, discussed in Chapter Two, suits this purpose well. The most useful initial questions are those that elicit what the patient calls her problem, the kind of treatment she thinks she should receive, and the most important results she hopes to get from treatment.

In addition to determining her living situation, the social history should include whether the patient has a means of income or assistance and information on occupation. Smoking and substance use history should be taken as well. Tobacco use by household members should be ascertained; in many cultures, women who do not smoke (and they are less likely to) and their children may have high exposure to secondhand smoke, because immigrant male smoking rates are similar to or higher than those of U.S. men. The medication history should be elicited nonjudgmentally and should include use of herbs, alcohol, certain foods, and preparations from animal parts, since in many cultures all of these play a role in treating illness or promoting health and strength. Many of the preparations have pharmacologic properties and can cause symptoms or cross-react with medications the provider may want to prescribe. The patient also should be asked about traditional healing modalities.

Immunization records may be available for immigrants who had screening in their country of origin. Because immunization is a critical component of prevention, when records are missing, the provider should attempt to ascertain if the patient had any immunizations as a child, whether she received a set of immunizations prior to coming to the United States, and when the last set was given. It is important to ask whether the patient has received Bacillus of Calmette-Guérin (BCG), a vaccine frequently used in Mexico and Southeast Asia to prevent serious forms of tuberculosis when infection occurs.

When available, the overseas screening examination should be thoroughly reviewed, during the first clinic visit if at all possible. An initial screening assessment on arrival in the United States is important to detect other health problems that are not part of the overseas assessment, as well as problems that have developed since the overseas examination was performed. Many immigrants have no medical records for the provider to review. Asking whether the patient has had any screening prior to arrival can sometimes be a proxy for legal versus illegal immigration. It is important to try to build a history of previously received medical care and immunizations.

Women should be asked when their last period occurred and whether they think they are pregnant. These questions should be asked through an interpreter without family members present. The patient should be asked if she has had previous gynecologic examinations (including Pap screening). Because refugee women may have lost children, it might be more appropriate to defer a more extensive obstetrical history to another time unless it is needed for prenatal care. At the time that history is obtained, a detailed sexual history also should be elicited.

## Doing the Physical Examination

The initial history should direct the provider to an appropriate physical examination with attention to all major organ systems. The examination should include assessment of vital signs (including blood pressure), skin, breasts, nutritional status, dental status, and general emotional status. Unless the patient is presenting for a gynecologic complaint or prenatal care, one may defer genitourinary and rectal examination to a later date. This can be particularly important for immigrant women who come from cultures, such as Islamic ones, where modesty and chastity are considered obligatory. Honoring their belief can help to build a trusting relationship. On the other hand, the use of touch during the physical examination allows providers to reassure patients that they care about them and to reach beyond the bounds that a language mismatch may place on establishing a therapeutic relationship (Faust, 1996).

The physical examination also offers the provider a chance to look for stigmata of folk health practices, such as moxibustion, cupping, coin rubbing, use of special oils, and ritual scarification (see Chapter Two). At a later time, the provider may want to elicit specific information on female genital mutilation in a nonjudgmental manner. When viewing stigmata of any folk practices, it is important for the provider to ask for the patient's interpretation of those cultural practices and to inquire whether they are for treatment, protection, or beauty. Where possible, the provider can accept and promote those traditional practices that are safe. This will facilitate his or her ability to gradually introduce new concepts of health promotion and treatment that are more Western in origin or orientation (Faust, 1996).

## Doing Laboratory Assessments

Many patients equate blood with life's essence and may have a great deal of anxiety about having blood drawn. The provider should explain that the body makes new blood to replace the old blood. It can be helpful to give fluids orally to symbolize replacement of the fluid that has been taken from the patient. All necessary laboratory testing procedures should be explained to the patient. It is essential to demonstrate the importance of the laboratory portion of the examination by ensuring an in-person follow-up visit in which test results are reviewed with the patient through an interpreter. The screening protocol used by the San Francisco General Hospital (SFGH) Refugee Clinic, which was revised in June 1997, appears in Exhibit 7.1. Special protocols also were written for assessment of hepatitis B and anemia (see Exhibit 7.2). Although specific laboratory protocols vary, hepatitis B screening has been shown to be a cost-effective method for determining which immigrants need immunization (Gjerdingen and Lor, 1997).

## Second and Third Clinic Visits

Second and third clinic visits focus on reviewing the patient's health status, laboratory work, and recommended interventions. The practitioner continues the migration history, including time

**Exhibit 7.1. Screening Protocol for Refugee Women at San Francisco General Hospital's Refugee Clinic.**

CBC, urinalysis, stool ova and parasites times three, HBsAg if from high-prevalence group, RPR if clinically indicated (patient has symptoms, risk factors), pregnancy test if indicated.

In addition, both these groups receive a PPD, updating of indicated immunizations, and Snellen visual testing and audiology.

Note: Many patients will have had a VDRL as part of the overseas exam for the visa; however, for those patients who do not have a record, an RPR is used at SFGH for screening. HIV testing has often been done prior to arrival but might be considered in patients from East Africa and Haiti, or who have other risk factors, if none has been documented in the past.

Courtesy of the San Francisco General Hospital's Refugee Clinic.

of arrival and the recent past, temporally continuing from the history obtained during the first visit. The history should use the patient's words as much as possible. Refugee patients should be engaged in a discussion of health status or events that occurred in the refugee camp.

During the third visit, the practitioner continues to evaluate symptoms and assess the efficacy of interventions. It is now appropriate to begin more probing questions about migration, such as reasons for leaving the country of origin, status of family and friends left behind, and details of the flight. Now the medical evaluation also is underway or may have been completed, and symptoms can be evaluated using a combination of traditional medical, psychological, and cultural approaches (Faust, 1996).

## Formulating a Treatment Plan

In discussing the differential diagnosis with the patient, the provider should use the words the patient has used for her symptom and illness and join this description to the Western terms for the problem. Providers also can explain that it is their belief that Western treatment with a particular agent will help this condition. In some cases, the diagnosis will be somatization of emotional

**Exhibit 7.2.   Screening Protocol for All Refugees from Countries with High Prevalence of Hepatitis B Carriers.**

Universal Hepatitis B vaccination for all children aged 11 years and less.

HbsAg on all refugees from high-prevalence countries who are aged 12 years and older. Immunization of all children aged 12–18 years old if HBsAg is negative.

If HBsAg is positive, order liver function studies and alpha-fetoprotein (AFP).

Vaccinate all household contacts with first hepatitis B immunization and draw HBcAb on the household contact. If HBcAb is positive, draw HBsAg and do not continue vaccine series.

If LFT and AFP are normal, no follow-up until age 40 or new symptoms.

If AFP > 20, order right upper quadrant abdominal ultrasound to assess liver.

If LFTs are high but AFP < 20, redraw labs in 6 mos.

## Prevalence of Hepatitis B Virus Carriers in Population by Country of Origin

| High Prevalence | Medium Prevalence | Low Prevalence |
|---|---|---|
| Africa: All countries | Afghanistan | Former Soviet |
| Southeast Asia: all countries | Iraq | Republics: |
| Former Soviet Republics: | Russia | Belarus |
|   Armenia | Haiti | Estonia |
|   Azerbaijan | Bosnia and | Latvia |
|   Georgia |   Herzegovina | Lithuania |
|   Kazakhstan | | Ukraine |
|   Kyrgyzstan | | Latin America |
|   Moldova | |   and Cuba |
|   Tajikistan | | Eastern Europe: |
|   Turkmenistan | |   Czech Republic |
|   Uzbekistan | |   Hungary |
| Eastern Europe: | |   Poland |
|   Albania | | |
|   Bulgaria | | |
|   Romania | | |

Courtesy of the San Francisco General Hospital's Refugee Clinic.

symptoms, although rarely will the provider label the patient's symptoms to the patient as somatization or depression. Interpretation of bodily sensations in different cultures is discussed in Chapter Thirteen.

Because of the central role of the family as the unit of care in most cultures, the provider should include the family in the treatment plan whenever possible, thereby demonstrating an understanding that an illness affects all members of a household. The provider also may inquire as to whether certain family members (such as the head of the household) should be present when the treatment plan is reviewed with the patient. This demonstrates the provider's respect for family and culture and improves the prospect of adherence to the therapeutic regimen.

Because dietary manipulation is a common treatment modality in most cultures, it is useful to discuss a healthy diet in relation to the patient's symptomatic complaint, in addition to prescribing medications.

## Prescribing Medications

Providers should not assume that recent immigrants have access to common remedies (such as over-the-counter medications) due to barriers such as language, literacy levels, and income. Prescription medications may be unaffordable if the patient has no insurance, or unusable if provided with instructions in English. At the SFGH Refugee Clinic, simple symptomatic over-the-counter remedies such as acetaminophen, cough syrup, and antacid commonly are given to the patients at the initial visit, when indicated. Medication cards or instructions can be provided to the patient at the clinic, with an illustration of how to take the medicine. At some locations, commercially available computer software can be used to prepare discharge and medication instructions in various languages and at various literacy levels.

## Giving Instructions at Discharge

Wherever possible, information related to diagnosis and treatment should be delivered through a trained interpreter who ensures that all questions are relayed to the provider and answered to the patient's satisfaction, and that the patient understands the discharge instructions.

## Visa-Mandated Medical Examinations

Individuals who enter the United States as legal immigrants for the purpose of establishing residence will have had a medical examination in their country of origin (or sometimes the initial country of asylum in the case of refugees). That examination, which is used to determine whether an individual should be excluded from the United States based on certain conditions, includes a medical examination, chest X ray, sputum smear for acid-fast bacilli, testing for human immunodeficiency virus (HIV), serologic testing for syphilis, screening for leprosy, and screening for mental disorders (Ackerman, 1997). Class A conditions, which warrant detainment, include cholera, diphtheria, infectious tuberculosis, plague, smallpox, yellow fever, viral hemorrhagic fevers, HIV, and leprosy. Class B conditions are serious ones that require follow-up but are not generally communicable (for example, diabetes, hypertension, and clinically active but not infectious tuberculosis).

## Screening Protocols

Any screening protocol for immigrants must be based on risk factors and epidemiology for that specific high-risk group. With the exception of a recommendation that immigrants be screened for tuberculosis, the U.S. Preventive Services Task Force guidelines (1996) say very little about screening immigrant women. Guidelines for screening immigrant women tend to be drawn from infectious disease profiles of local and state public health agencies and the Centers for Disease Control (CDC). The protocols presented in this chapter are those of the SFGH Refugee Clinic. In addition, studies done in other countries inform us about the prevalence of certain conditions in those populations (such as iron deficiency anemia). Screening recommendations that do not apply to the general population (such as screening for anemia), nevertheless could be appropriate in high-risk groups, including immigrant women.

# Anemia Screening

Every female patient at SFGH Refugee Clinic receives a complete blood count, because anemia is a common condition in immigrants. Usually, it is the hypochromic, microcytic type. The anemia may result from dietary iron deficiency or parasitic infestation that contributes to microscopic blood loss in the stool. It is difficult to distinguish this form of anemia from thalassemia, which is common in certain ethnic groups (Mediterranean, Asian). Women and girls over the age of twelve who have an initial hemoglobin (Hb) below 10 g/dl and hematocrit (hct) below 33 percent should be evaluated further, either by treating with iron and reevaluating or by ascertaining the cause of the anemia.

A conservative initial approach to treating anemia is to educate the patient about an iron-rich diet, and treat her with an oral iron preparation twice daily. The goal is to provide 3 mg/kg body weight of elemental iron divided into two daily doses for six to eight weeks. Any abnormalities identified on stool ova and parasite (O&P) preparation also are treated at the same time. The complete blood count (CBC) is then rechecked in six weeks. If the Hb/hct has returned to normal, no further evaluation is performed. If the Hb/hct remains low, the provider should exclude continuing blood loss (stool O&P, stool occult blood, menstruation history) and consider testing serum iron, total iron-binding capacity, serum ferritin, and lead level. Hemoglobin electrophoresis generally is reserved for children and pregnant women. Other nutritional deficiencies also may cause anemia.

# Tuberculosis Screening and Prophylaxis

Tuberculosis (TB) is both a very old and an emerging infection risk throughout the world. Old patterns of disease have changed with the advent of multiple-drug-resistant strains of *Mycobacterium species*. Countries that had lower rates in the past may have higher rates now due to less available medication (for example, former Soviet Union countries). HIV adds a significant comorbid condition that makes the treatment of TB more complex. It is important, therefore, that all newcomers be screened for TB using a purified protein derivative (PPD), regardless of BCG status. This includes those with Class B TB (positive PPD with evidence of past but not active disease on chest X ray) listed on screening forms that arrive with recent immigrants and refugees. The only exclusions should be patients with documentation of a positive PPD and those currently receiving TB medications. The appearance of 10 mm or more of induration within forty-eight to seventy-two hours after subcutaneous administration of PPD indicates a positive reaction in high-risk groups. The reading should be performed by a trained health care worker whenever possible. In recent contacts of persons known to have active TB, 5 mm of induration is considered positive (Pickwell, 1995). Boosting an immune response to PPD by repeating the test two weeks later might be considered in patients who are negative but for whom there is a high index of suspicion, such as the elderly.

Although previous BCG administration can make the interpretation of the PPD more complex, the CDC recommended in 1979 that the PPD test be interpreted as positive based on the size of induration, regardless of the patient's BCG vaccination status (Centers for Disease Control, 1988). Although BCG vaccination confers a variable degree of skin test positivity, which wanes with time, its effectiveness varies in different settings, and current recommendations are to treat positive PPD skin tests as positive reactions even if there is a history of BCG vaccination (Centers for Disease Control, 1991). Individuals with positive reactions but no active disease should be considered candidates for prophylaxis (Centers for Disease Control, 1991).

Most legal migrants will bring overseas chest X rays with them; they should be sent for formal reading by a radiologist if there is any suspicion of active disease. Films of poor technical quality should be repeated, with appropriate attention to the use of protective lead aprons. If a patient does not have a chest X ray and is PPD positive, a single posterior-anterior view X ray of the chest should be ordered, with additional views (lateral, apical lordotic) as indicated. If the chest X ray is abnormal, a sputum specimen should be collected.

HIV infection, diabetes mellitus, other chronic medical conditions, and use of immunocompromising or suppressive medications (including steroids) are considered to exacerbate TB risk.

In general, isoniazid remains the standard of prophylaxis for inactive disease, although practice varies when prophylaxis is being administered to patients from areas where multiple-drug-resistant TB is prevalent. Persons under age thirty-five with 10 mm or more of induration on PPD screening and persons over thirty-five with 15 mm or more of induration should be considered candidates for a six-month course of isoniazid chemoprophylaxis. Patients who are HIV-positive and those with abnormal chest X rays suggestive of previous TB should receive twelve months of combined therapy. Preventive therapy generally consists of six to twelve months of isoniazid (10 mg/kg for children, to a maximum dose of 300 mg per day for adults). Patients who are HIV-positive should receive twelve months of therapy. When therapy is directly observed, isoniazid can be given twice weekly in a dose of 15 mg/kg (up to 900 mg) (Centers for Disease Control, 1990b).

## Immunizations for Adults

A key part of the initial assessment of any immigrant patient is to ascertain immunization history and provide missing immunizations for vaccine-preventable diseases. Many patients will not have received a complete primary series by U.S. standards. The currently recommended U.S. primary series appears in Table 7.1. Adults who have not had the complete series should receive indicated immunizations (Centers for Disease Control, 1996–1997). As noted in Table 7.2, this would include an adult tetanus-diphtheria (Td) immunization (0.5 cc intramuscular [IM]) if none has been received in the past ten years, or two, six months apart, if one has never been given.

If the immunization history at the time of an injury to the skin reveals that a patient never has been immunized or has been inadequately immunized (fewer than three immunizations), tetanus immunoglobulin (TIG) injection (250 mg IM of TIG) may also be administered. The decision to use TIG should be predicated on whether there is a high likelihood of contamination of the wound (bites, soil contamination, puncture wounds, burns, or crush injuries). TIG provides passive immunity only, affording protection against tetanus for the immediate event. The inadequately immunized patient also should receive Td (0.5 cc IM) in addition to TIG

**Table 7.1. Recommended Primary Immunization Schedule in the United States, 1998.**

| | Birth | 1 Month | 2 Months | 4 Months | 6 Months | 12 Months | 15 Months | 18 Months | 4–6 Years | 11–12 Years | 14–16 Years |
|---|---|---|---|---|---|---|---|---|---|---|---|
| Hepatitis B | X | X | | | X | | | | | X (if not given in past) | |
| Diphtheria, tetanus, pertussis | | | DTaP or DTP | DTaP or DTP | DTaP or DTP | | DTaP or DTP | | DTaP or DTP | X (tetanus and diphtheria every 10 years) | |
| H. Influenzae B | | | X | X | X | X | | | | | |
| Polio | | | IPV or OPV | IPV or OPV | | X | | | X | | |
| Measles, mumps, rubella | | | | | | X | | | X or | X | |
| Varicella | | | | | | X | | | | X (if not given in past) | |

*Note:* Vaccines are listed at routinely recommended ages. Catch-up immunization should be done during any visit if feasible. Hepatitis B; measles, mumps, and rubella (MMR); and varicella immunization status should be reassessed at adolescent visit and at initial assessment. Injectable polio vaccine (IPV) or oral polio vaccine (OPV) can be given to persons under the age of 18 years for primary polio immunization. DTaP = Diphtheria, Tetanus, acellular Pertussis toxoids. DTP = Diphtheria, Tetanus, Pertussis toxoids (pediatric).

*Source:* Advisory Committee on Immunization Practices and American Academy of Family Practice, 1998.

**Table 7.2.  Recommended Adult Immunization Schedule in the United States, 1998.**

| | 11–12 Years | 14–18 Years | Adults (18–64 Years) | Over Age 65 |
|---|---|---|---|---|
| Hepatitis B | If not given in past | | | |
| Tetanus/diphtheria | Every 10 years | | | |
| S. pneumoniae | High-risk groups | | | Once |
| Polio | If not given in past | | | |
| Measles, mumps, rubella | Assess MMR status and give if not immune | | | |
| Influenza (Type B) | Annually for all high risk and over 65 years old | | | |

*Note:* Vaccines are listed as routinely recommended. Catch-up immunization should be done during any visit if feasible. High-risk groups include asplenia, sickle cell disease, chronic lung and cardiac conditions, and impaired immunity. Hepatitis B and measles, mumps, and rubella (MMR) immunization status should be assessed at the time of initial assessment and provided if indicated. MMR is contraindicated in pregnancy.

*Source:* Advisory Committee on Immunization Practices and American Academy of Family Practice, 1998.

in order to trigger active immunity. Patients should then receive a tetanus booster within six months.

Measles, mumps, and rubella (MMR) immunization should be given to all persons born after 1956, especially adolescents, women who are not currently pregnant who have negative rubella titers, day care providers, and health care workers. Rubella vaccine is not commonly given in the countries that constitute the former Soviet Union. Recent immigrants from that region born after 1957 should receive an MMR if it is not contraindicated (Ackerman, 1997). MMR vaccination is contraindicated in pregnant women. Hepatitis B vaccination should be considered for all adolescents who were not previously immunized and are negative on hepatitis B surface antigen (HBsAg) screening, the marker of a chronic carrier, and adults with exposure risks: household members or partners who are infected with hepatitis B, bisexual and gay men, heterosexual patients with multiple sex partners, and health care workers.

Pneumococcal vaccination should be given to patients over sixty-five years of age and to those persons with risk factors such as asthma, chronic obstructive pulmonary disease, asplenia, cardiac disease, and renal disease. Influenza vaccination should be given annually to individuals over sixty-five years of age and those with chronic cardiac, respiratory, renal, or metabolic diseases (Advisory Committee on Immunization Practices, 1998).

In addition to the pneumococcal vaccination, all patients with asplenia (whether functional or surgical) should receive meningococcal vaccine, *Haemophilus influenzae* (HIB) vaccine, and annual influenza vaccination. HIV-infected individuals should receive injectable polio vaccine (IPV) instead of oral polio vaccine (OPV) if polio vaccine is indicated, MMR (even though live vaccines are generally not given to other immunocompromised persons), Td, pneumococcal, influenza, HIB, and hepatitis B vaccinations. Household members of HIV-positive individuals and other immunocompromised patients should not receive OPV (Zimmerman and Clover, 1995). Typhoid vaccine may be considered in household contacts of *Salmonella typhi* carriers.

There are rare cases in which BCG is used to prevent the spread of TB (Centers for Disease Control, 1988). Generally this would occur if a child was exposed to an infected household member who cannot or will not adhere to treatment, or a child who cannot receive long-term primary preventive therapy. Any use of this vaccine should be done in consultation with local TB control experts.

# Infectious Diseases

*Robin K. Avery*

Detection and treatment of infectious diseases, and appropriate patient education, are a crucial part of the screening of newly arrived immigrants (Wilson, 1991; Wolfe, 1992). This is important for the health of the individual and the family, as well as the health of the general public. Although some screening will often have taken place prior to arrival in the United States, screening methods and infectious disease treatments are highly variable from one region to another and deserve a thorough review upon arrival.

This section focuses on the medical history and physical examination in relation to infectious diseases and discusses specific diseases and topics in more detail. Situations where the infectious disease screen is particularly important include pregnancy or contemplation of pregnancy, blood donation, and administration of immunosuppressive medications. Mary Wilson's *A World Guide to Infections* (1991) is a comprehensive and invaluable reference that should be immensely helpful to any clinician treating immigrants.

## History and Physical Examination

The medical history (preferably conducted in the patient's primary language) should ascertain the country of origin, travel history, and intermediate holding camps or other stops because they may have different epidemiology from the original region. The patient should be questioned about her menstrual history, family history, medications, transfusions, and past infections, with particular reference to tuberculosis, hepatitis, and parasitic diseases.

Issues of HIV exposure and testing are highly culturally sensitive. For some groups of patients, questions regarding HIV may best be deferred, preferably until after a therapeutic relationship has been established.

If possible, the clinician should be aware of indigenous treatment practices and the role of traditional healers in the patient's culture of origin. Injections, bloodletting, or other invasive procedures with the use of nonsterilized instruments may contribute to the spread of HIV, hepatitis B, and other blood-borne pathogens. It is important to be aware of procedures that may have been performed prior to arrival, such as female genital mutilation with its attendant risks of pelvic, urinary, and obstetric complications. In addition, a thorough understanding of the patient's beliefs about healing will facilitate the interaction of the individual with the American health care system and lead to greater understanding on the part of both the clinician and the new immigrant.

Table 7.3 summarizes the most common infectious diseases encountered in particular geographic regions. Important elements of the medical history and review of systems are listed in Table 7.4. The history may indicate an urgent need for further evaluation and treatment; common causes of acute febrile illness in immigrants are listed in Table 7.5. The physical exam should be thorough, although it need not be lengthy. Key elements of it are listed in Table 7.6.

## Tuberculosis

TB is highly contagious, particularly when an individual with active cavitary disease is coughing. The HIV epidemic is closely tied to tuberculosis in many parts of the world, and there is growing evidence that TB may accelerate HIV progression, in addition to HIV's predisposing to development of active tuberculosis (Goletti and others, 1996). Immigrants account for a significant fraction of the cases of TB in the United States. In 1989, the overall U.S. TB rate was 9.5 per 100,000 population, but 124 per 100,000 for foreign-born persons arriving in the United States (Centers for Disease Control, 1990a). Foreign-born individuals accounted for 60 percent of the total increase in the number of U.S. TB cases from 1986 to 1992 (Cantwell, Snider, Cauthen, and Onorato, 1994). Chest

## Table 7.3. Geographic Distribution of Major Infectious Diseases.

**Multiple Geographic Regions**

HIV

Tuberculosis

Malaria

Diarrheal disease (bacterial, parasitic, viral pathogens, such as *Salmonella, Shigella, Escherichia coli* strains, *Campylobacter,* giardiasis, amebiasis, rotavirus, others)

Intestinal parasites (for example, *Ascaris,* hookworm, *Strongyloides*)

*Helicobacter pylori*

Typhoid fever *(Salmonella typhi)*

Hansen's disease (leprosy)

Syphilis (in some areas; also yaws, bejel, pinta)

Other sexually transmitted diseases (gonorrhea, chlamydia, chancroid, herpes)

Respiratory pathogens (bacterial, viral)

Toxoplasmosis

Trichinosis

Tetanus

Trachoma

Typhus and other rickettsial diseases

Meningococcal meningitis (outbreaks and sporadic cases)

Rheumatic fever

Hepatitis A, B, C, D, E

Measles, mumps, rubella, influenza, polio

Rabies

**Central and South America**

Amebiasis

Brucellosis

Chagas' disease

Cysticercosis

Dengue fever

Echinococcosis

Histoplasmosis

HTLV-I

Leishmaniasis (including cutaneous, mucocutaneous, visceral)

Leptospirosis

Onchocerciasis

Paracoccidioidomycosis

Schistosomiasis

Viral hemorrhagic fevers, yellow fever

**Africa**

Anthrax

Brucellosis

Cholera (in certain areas and refugee situations)

Cysticercosis

Dengue fever

Dracunculiasis

Echinococcosis

Filariasis

Histoplasmosis (especially *duboisii*)

HTLV-I

Leishmaniasis (cutaneous and visceral)

Loiasis

*(continued)*

**Table 7.3.** (*continued*)

Mycetoma

Onchocerciasis

Q fever

Relapsing fever (*Borrelia*)

Schistosomiasis

Trypanosomiasis, African

Viral hemorrhagic fevers and other viral illness (for example, Rift Valley fever, West Nile fever, yellow fever, Lassa, Ebola)

**Asia: Far East, Southeast**

Anisakiasis

Brucellosis

Capillariasis

Cholera

Clonorchiasis and opisthorchiasis

Cysticercosis

Dengue fever

Echinococcosis

Filariasis

HTLV-I

Japanese encephalitis

Leptospirosis

Melioidosis

Paragonimiasis

*Penicillium marneffei*

Schistosomiasis (*S. japonicum*)

**Asia: India and Neighboring Countries**

Anthrax

Brucellosis

Cholera

Cysticercosis

Dengue fever

Diphtheria

Echinococcosis

Filariasis

Leishmaniasis (cutaneous and visceral)

Mycetoma

Plague

Q fever

Relapsing fever (*Borrelia*)

**Middle East**

Anthrax

Brucellosis

Crimean-Congo hemorrhagic fever and other viral illness

Echinococcosis

Leishmaniasis (especially cutaneous)

Q fever

Relapsing fever

Schistosomiasis

**Eastern Europe**

Anisakiasis

Echinococcosis

Encephalitis (Central European tick-borne)

Hemorrhagic fever with renal syndrome

Lyme disease

Q fever

Rhinoscleroma

*Note:* This is simplified due to space considerations. For a comprehensive listing and discussion of infectious diseases by geographic region, see Wilson, 1991. Diseases mentioned in the table may be present in only some areas of a region.

**Table 7.4.  Medical History and Review of Systems
for Infectious Diseases in Immigrants.**

Country of origin, travel history, intermediate holding camps or other
  stops

Obstetric history, history of female genital mutilation

Previous infections or other medical conditions

Medications, treatments by traditional healers, injections, transfusions

Traumatic injuries (wartime or domestic violence)

Fevers, chills, sweats, weight loss

Problems with eyes or ears, vision or hearing

Cough, sputum, hemoptysis, shortness of breath, chest pain

Nausea, vomiting, diarrhea, abdominal or pelvic pain, increase in
  abdominal girth

Dysuria, hematuria, vaginal discharge, menstrual problems, genital
  ulcers

Breast masses or lesions

Edema, joint problems

Focal weakness, gait difficulty, seizures, headache

Skin lesions, rashes, enlarged lymph nodes, nodules, jaundice

*Note:* This is a very abbreviated summary of a highly complex subject. Clinicians
are strongly encouraged to consult Wilson, 1991, for a comprehensive discussion of these issues.

**Table 7.5.  Some Causes of Acute Febrile Illness in Immigrants.**

Malaria

Typhoid fever

Dengue fever or dengue hemorrhagic fever

Typhus

Tuberculosis

Brucellosis

Leptospirosis

Relapsing fever (borreliosis)

Influenza

Bacterial pneumonia, urinary tract infection

*Note:* See Wilson, 1991, and Gove and Slutkin, 1984, for further details.

**Table 7.6. Physical Examination of the Immigrant.**

---

**General appearance:** nutritional status, wasting (HIV, TB, visceral leishmaniasis, other chronic illness)

**Eye exam:** trachoma, onchocerciasis, loiasis, bacterial conjunctivitis, vitamin A deficiency

**Head and neck exam:** otitis media or externa, perforated tympanic membrane, oral thrush, dental infections (if from endemic regions, mucocutaneous leishmaniasis, rhinoscleroma, rhinosporidiosis, or "leonine facies" of Hansen's disease)

**Adenopathy:** HIV, HTLV-I, Epstein-Barr virus, tuberculosis, Hansen's disease, melioidosis, chancroid, lymphogranuloma venereum, tularemia, plague, many others

**Chest exam, with observation of cough and sputum production:** asthma, bronchitis, pneumonia, pleural effusion, tuberculosis, paragonimiasis, melioidosis, malignancy

**Cardiac exam:** congenital heart disease, rheumatic heart disease, endocarditis, dilated cardiomyopathy

**Abdominal exam:** tenderness, masses, hepatosplenomegaly (schistosomiasis, visceral leishmaniasis, tropical splenomegaly), ascites (advanced liver disease, tuberculous or bacterial peritonitis, malignancy), focal tenderness (bacterial abscess, amoebic liver abscess, appendicitis)

**Gynecologic exam:** genital ulcers (syphilis, chancroid, herpes), cervicitis (gonorrhea, chlamydia), pelvic inflammatory disease, sequelae of female genital mutilation, endometritis (if recent delivery or abortion)

**Extremities:** lymphedema (filariasis), loss of distal digits (Hansen's disease), generalized edema (cardiac or liver disease or postmalarial nephrotic syndrome), Madura foot, dracunculiasis, deformities due to uncorrected congenital abnormalities or trauma

**Neurologic exam:** chronic dementing disease (HIV, African trypanosomiasis, others), focal findings (cerebral cysticercosis, tuberculoma, toxoplasmosis, paragonimiasis, hydatid disease), spastic paraparesis (HTLV-I), asymmetric leg weakness (prior polio)

**Skin exam:** anesthetic lesions (Hansen's disease), ulcers (leishmaniasis), lesions or rashes (lice, scabies, yaws, pinta, cutaneous larva migrans, dracunculiasis, loiasis, onchocerciasis, chromomycosis, mycetoma, myiasis, *Penicillium marneffei);* tache noire with or without rash (acute rickettsial infection)

---

X ray and sputum smears performed prior to arrival should be viewed as preliminary information.

Although individuals with active TB are supposed to complete a course of effective therapy before arrival in the United States, screening after arrival may turn up more patients with active TB. In addition, the incidence of positive PPD skin tests is high in immigrants from certain areas, and those with inactive or latent disease but positive skin tests are candidates for prophylaxis. A study of ninety-nine Vietnamese immigrants revealed that 70 percent were tuberculin positive, and 39 percent required antituberculous medication (mostly prophylaxis) (Nelson, Bui, and Samet, 1997). The initial screen may not be enough; a study of Tibetan immigrants in Minnesota revealed that this high-risk population (98 percent PPD positive) had an 8.4 percent incidence of active TB; about half of the cases were picked up on initial screening, and the other half were diagnosed ten to twenty-seven months after arrival (Truong and others, 1997). However, a review of the current screening system by the CDC suggests that the system identifies most persons who have active TB at that time (Binkin and others, 1996).

Current recommendations for screening include examination of a chest radiograph (brought by the patient or newly obtained) and PPD skin testing; sputum smears and cultures should be obtained from patients with symptoms, compatible history, or radiographic findings. The threshold for repeating the chest X ray after arrival should be low if suspicion of active disease exists. Many of those with suspected active or inactive disease will be referred to the local TB clinic for treatment and follow-up. Individual tuberculosis clinics already will be highly aware of the risk of multiple-drug-resistant TB in many parts of the world, as well as the need to treat active disease with an aggressive multidrug regimen until sensitivities are available. History of previous administration of antituberculous medications is important and has bearing on the incidence of multiple-drug-resistant TB. The choice of a new regimen for that individual should include at least two drugs that she has not received before. The American Thoracic Society/Centers for Disease Control consensus statement (1994) provides detailed recommendations about therapy.

Directly observed therapy (DOT), in which patients take medication in the presence of a third-party observer (such as a health care professional or government agent), has been shown to increase the rate of completion of TB therapy greatly (Weis and others, 1994). This may be particularly important where linguistic and cultural barriers to care occur. Well-designed TB programs also can be a vehicle for health education in general. A model example is a culturally sensitive DOT program in a displaced population in Ethiopia that successfully treated eight hundred patients with a short-course, four-drug regimen with a high rate of completion of therapy. The program increased community morale as well through education, outreach, and use of community health workers (Hodes and Azbite, 1993). A program in Vietnam for prospective migrants bound for the United States screened 39,581 persons, of whom 322 were smear positive, and achieved an 82 percent cure rate, also with a short-course, four-drug, directly observed regimen (Keane and others, 1995). However, many immigrants arriving in the United States will not have had the benefit of such effective screening and treatment prior to arrival.

Tuberculosis presents serious problems for some immigrants because of the stigma attached to it in their home countries. Patients may fear the sequelae of positive testing. This is especially so among those from countries where patients with tuberculosis are still isolated from their families, even long after the initial period of maximum transmissibility.

## Hepatitis and Liver Diseases

Hepatitis A, B, C, D, and E occur with high frequency in certain areas of the world. The impact in terms of chronic disease is most profound for hepatitis B, with the risk for development of chronic liver disease in the HBsAg carrier, the risk for transmission from an infected mother to her neonate, and the risk for hepatocellular carcinoma in long-term carriers. Chronic liver disease due to hepatitis C also is a problem of significant magnitude.

In a group of recent Vietnamese immigrants, 14 percent were HBsAg carriers (Nelson, Bui, and Samet, 1997). A study of Ethiopian immigrants to Israel revealed that serologic evidence for hepatitis B virus (HBV) infection occurred in 35 percent of one-to four-year-olds, and reached 98 percent in individuals over age forty, with 19 percent of children from one to eight years of age positive for HBsAg (Ben-Porath and others, 1986).

Hepatitis B screening protocols have varied from one center to another. One strategy is that of the SFGH Refugee Clinic Newcomers' Program. In this program, all children aged eleven years or under are immunized against hepatitis B, and an HBsAg test is obtained on all individuals twelve years and older from countries with intermediate or high prevalence for HBV carriage (see Exhibit 7.2). Individuals aged twelve to eighteen who are HBsAg negative are vaccinated. Some centers also obtain an HBsAb test and do not vaccinate those who already are surface antibody positive. Those who are HBsAg positive have liver function tests to detect chronic hepatitis, and alpha fetoprotein (a marker for the development of hepatocellular carcinoma) is obtained; household contacts are vaccinated and counseled.

It also is important to counsel the HBsAg-positive person and her family and sexual partners regarding prevention of transmission, and nonimmune family members and close contacts should be vaccinated. Cultural factors contributing to transmission should be considered (Chemtov and Rosen, 1993). In addition to describing transmission by blood and blood products, intravenous drug use, and sexual relations, counseling should include cautioning the individual about such practices as tattooing and ear piercing with shared instruments and sharing needles for legal medications such as insulin and vitamins (Loue and Oppenheim, 1994). Given the development of newer therapies for chronic hepatitis B, such as lamivudine, the purpose of screening increasingly may include identification of individuals who are candidates for treatment.

Hepatitis A and E are primarily enterically transmitted and acute rather than chronic in presentation; many immigrants will already have hepatitis A antibody and thus immunity. Hepatitis D (delta) occurs only in patients with concomitant hepatitis B, with a frequency ranging from less than 1 percent to 40 percent of patients chronically infected with HBV (Wilson, 1991). For certain high-risk persons, from the Amazon basin, for example, it may be important to consider HDV in HBsAg-positive individuals (Wilson, 1991). Hepatitis C is a worldwide cause of chronic liver disease and a major cause of posttransfusion hepatitis. Although therapy with interferon may modify the course of the disease, most screening programs do not routinely include HCV.

Other causes of hepatobiliary problems in immigrants include chronic schistosomiasis (especially *S. mansoni*) with portal hypertension; opisthorchiasis in Southeast Asian immigrants with late biliary complications and possible cholangiocarcinoma echinococcosis (the liver is the most common site for hydatid cysts, and these cysts may rupture into the biliary tree or peritoneum); amoebic liver abscess; occasional migration of *Ascaris* into the biliary tree; and ingestion of toxins.

## Malaria and Parasitic Infections

### Malaria

Malaria is extremely common in transit camps and refugee camps; of 279 Somali refugees in one study, 15 percent had malaria parasites detected on blood smears (Slutsker and others, 1995). In many areas of the world, the most serious form, falciparum malaria, is resistant to chloroquine and may be resistant to other antimalarials as well. Treatment should be based on current CDC guidelines and delineation of areas where resistance occurs (Centers for Disease Control).

*Plasmodium vivax* and *P. ovale* malaria can persist asymptomatically in the liver (the exoerythrocytic cycle) and may cause recurrent febrile episodes long after arrival in the United States. Patients with histories of these types of malaria may be candidates for treatment with primaquine, which eradicates this liver cycle. A glucose-6-phosphate dehydrogenase (G6PD) screen should be performed first, because individuals with a deficiency of this enzyme can have a severe hemolytic reaction to primaquine. G6PD deficiencies are more common in blacks who originate from central Africa and in people of eastern Mediterranean origin, especially Sephardic Jews. Clinicians should be alert for malaria with the onset of any febrile illness, but thick and thin blood smears are not generally considered necessary screening for the asymptomatic patient. Malaria may be transmitted by blood transfusion, and donors who have traveled from endemic areas are usually excluded for a period of time.

## Other Parasites

The stool ova and parasite (O&P) exam is an important part of screening; three sets of stool samples significantly increase yield. Intestinal parasites are exceedingly common among immigrants; in one group in Thailand, 79.3 percent of males and 94.7 percent of female workers had parasitic infections, with hookworm and *Opisthorchis* being the major ones (Pongpaew and others, 1993). The most common in general include *Ascaris* (which is reported to infect more than one-quarter of the world's population), hookworm, *Enterobius* (pinworm), and *Trichuris* (whipworm). Hookworm is important to eradicate because it can cause significant anemia. Tapeworms, particularly *Taenia solium* (the agent of cysticercosis), are important parasites to detect and eradicate. *Entamoeba histolytica*, the agent of amoebic dysentery and amoebic liver abscess, should be treated, but there also are numerous nonpathogenic amoebae that may appear in stool and require no treatment.

Some parasitic infections, such as strongyloidiasis, may persist for long periods of time asymptomatically. It is particularly important to screen immigrants who are going to be treated with immunosuppressive medications (for example, steroids for asthma), given the risk of disseminated strongyloidiasis in such a situation (Longworth and Weller, 1986). Schistosomiasis may also be present over time; evidence of *Schistosoma mansoni* eggs and specific Immunoglobulin E was found in 12 percent and 37 percent, respectively, of Israelis who had migrated from Yemen thirty-eight years previously (Hornstein and others, 1990). If persistent schistosomiasis is detected, it is important to treat with praziquantel and recheck stools to prevent late sequelae of portal hypertension. *Schistosoma haematobium* may produce long-term alterations of the bladder and ureters and may predispose to urinary tract infections, obstruction, and late bladder carcinoma. If it is suspected, *S. haematobium* eggs should be sought in urine samples. Past filariasis may produce lymphedema or elephantiasis of the extremities, with a predisposition to recurrent cellulitis.

An area of active research is the chronic activation of the immune system as a result of multiple parasitic infections. It has been hypothesized that this activation, especially an exaggerated T-helper cell subset-2 (TH-2) response, may have an impact on the course of HIV infection and concomitant immunopathology.

## Gastrointestinal and Diarrheal Diseases

Diarrheal disease is a significant cause of morbidity and mortality in many parts of the world and may be present in epidemic form in refugee and holding camps. Bacterial agents include various strains of *E. coli, Salmonella, Shigella* (which may be multiply resistant), *Vibrio cholerae* (cholera), *Campylobacter,* and others. Rotavirus and other viral causes of diarrhea occur worldwide. Parasitic causes such as amoebiasis, giardiasis, capillariasis, and strongyloidiasis are important to detect and treat. Space does not allow here for detailed discussion of the different symptom complexes that suggest one cause or another, but the stool O&P screen usually is performed for each immigrant. Sensitivity may be increased by obtaining three stool samples when infection is suspected. Persons who are symptomatic may also require rehydration, specific antibiotic therapy, bacterial stool cultures, or other evaluation.

Though not a diarrheal disease, *Salmonella typhi* (typhoid fever) is an important worldwide cause of febrile illness, and the chronic carrier state may persist. A stool culture for *Salmonella* and other enteric bacterial pathogens should be performed on prospective food handlers.

## HIV-1 and HIV-2

With the advent of highly effective combination antiretroviral therapy, there is more reason to screen for HIV in asymptomatic individuals than ever before. With trends in clinical practice emphasizing early reduction in viral load to prevent later destruction of the immune system, there is now a compelling reason to test (Carpenter and others, 1997), if the immigrant has not already been tested as a condition of entry into the United States.

In addition, testing affords the opportunity for early administration of prophylaxis, such as for *Pneumocystis carinii* pneumonia (PCP) in patients with CD4 counts of under 200 or other high risk. Finally, testing a woman who is pregnant or of reproductive age allows for the initiation of therapy, which can drastically reduce the risk of transmission of HIV to the unborn child (Connor and others, 1994).

Ideally, HIV counseling should be given to every individual as part of basic health education. However, there are many cultural and psychosocial barriers to HIV testing and education in immigrants, among them fear of legal and immigration ramifications; fear of violence, abandonment, or reprisals; cultural and social stigmas (Adrien and others, 1996; Almstrom, 1993; Chemtov and Rosen, 1992; Chittick, 1996; Chohan, 1996; Hodes, 1997; Londero and Damond, 1996; Loue and Oppenheim, 1994; Nakyonyi, 1993; Sheran and others, 1994; Soskolne and Shtarkshall, 1994; Spizzichino and others, 1996); and in some cultures the custom of telling the family the diagnosis rather than the patient (Hodes, 1997). These issues must be approached with great sensitivity and understanding, preferably with primary language and peer educators. If time permits, it may be advisable to defer discussion of HIV testing and transmission to a subsequent session once a clinician-patient relationship has been established.

Pre- and posttest counseling are essential. Consideration must be given to the availability of effective medication, the availability of ongoing primary care, and social service support. At an appropriate time, counseling on safer sex precautions, drug and needle transmission, and other educational issues should be addressed. Creative programs to increase accessibility and acceptance of such education are being developed.

West African and Cape Verdean patients may have been exposed to HIV-2; this may not show up on a standard HIV-1 assay and should be specifically requested from the laboratory. Another retrovirus of importance in the Caribbean, Far East, and other areas is HTLV-I, which can cause human T-cell lymphoma/leukemia or tropical spastic paraparesis. This is not routinely included in screening but may be appropriate in symptomatic patients from endemic areas.

## Sexually Transmitted Diseases

Serologic tests for syphilis are recommended, since latent infection is common and appropriate therapy can prevent neurologic and cardiovascular complications, as well as sexual transmission and congenital syphilis (Centers for Disease Control, 1998b). It is important to detect concurrent HIV infection, because syphilis in the HIV-infected patient may present with early neurologic complications or unexpected relapse. Clinicians also should keep in mind that a positive serology may be due to other treponemal diseases such as yaws, pinta, and bejel (Wilson, 1991).

Gonorrhea and chlamydia are important causes of pelvic inflammatory disease and consequent infertility, tubal pathology, and other complications. A pelvic exam should identify symptomatic individuals, but chlamydial infection, in particular, may be asymptomatic. Considerable research has gone into defining the cost-effectiveness of screening and empiric therapy for chlamydial infection in asymptomatic populations, and screening is recommended in sexually active adolescents and young women ages twenty to twenty-four (Centers for Disease Control, 1998b).

Chancroid and lymphogranuloma venereum are common in certain parts of the world and should be evident on physical exam. Diseases causing genital ulcers, such as chancroid, are important cofactors in HIV transmission and should be vigorously treated. Genital herpes may be symptomatic or asymptomatic, and treatment and counseling should follow the standard practice of sexually transmitted disease clinics (Centers for Disease Control, 1998b).

## Special Considerations: Pregnancy, Immunosuppression, Transfusion, and Rheumatic Fever

With the pregnant or potentially pregnant woman, particular attention should be paid to the possible presence of HIV, HBV, and syphilis, since the risk of transmission to the fetus can be greatly reduced with appropriate therapy. Certain infections such as malaria can be extremely severe in the pregnant patient, and febrile illness is of great concern. Chronic infections such as Hansen's disease may worsen during pregnancy.

When immunosuppressive medications such as corticosteroids are to be administered, it is important to rule out tuberculosis and strongyloidiasis, given the risk that these infections will become disseminated or overwhelming in the setting of immunosuppression (Longworth and Weller, 1986). Three stool O&P exams may not be adequate to detect *Strongyloides*. In the high-risk patient, consideration should be given to a serologic test or an empiric course of thiabendazole to eradicate this parasite prior to steroids.

Blood donation for transfusion will likely not be permitted for immigrants from endemic areas in the short term, but the potentially transmissible agents to consider include HIV, HTLV-1, HBV, hepatitis C virus, cytomegalovirus, Chagas' disease, and malaria (Wilson, 1991; Sandler and Fang, 1991). Testing for the first four of these is routinely performed; in addition, Wilson recommends serologic testing for Chagas' disease in any prospective blood donor who has lived in endemic areas of Central or South America (Wilson, 1991). Also, heightened awareness of the possible presence of those diseases is important for patients who have received transfusions prior to entry

Finally, in developing countries, the cardiac sequelae of rheumatic fever may appear at an early age (Hodes, 1988). Young adults and adolescents with valvular abnormalities are at ongoing risk for endocarditis, and should have a thorough dental evaluation and extractions as indicated. Those at risk for endocarditis should be educated about the importance of antibiotic prophylaxis for dental, gastrointestinal, and genitourinary procedures.

## Cross-Cultural Considerations

Cross-cultural considerations have bearing on infectious disease screening in that acute or chronic problems may be undetected or misdiagnosed if the clinician is unaware of certain cultural practices. For example, the medicinal use of capsules of dried rattlesnake flesh for a variety of ailments in Mexico and Central America can cause infection with *Salmonella arizona* (Wilson, 1991). Another example is cutting of the uvula for sore throat, tooth extraction for infants with diarrhea, and many other unexpected health practices in Ethiopian immigrants (Hodes, 1997).

Uvulectomy by traditional healers occurs in many other areas in Africa as well (Katz, 1989). The wording of questions is important. One physician asked a patient about eating undercooked meat; the patient said no, but did not connect this with the *raw* meat that she regularly ate and that likely caused her toxoplasmosis (S. Schmitt, personal communication).

Explanations of the screening process, as well as diagnoses and proposed treatments, should be presented in a culturally sensitive manner. Acceptance of therapy will depend on the manner in which it is explained, offered, and followed. Wherever possible, DOT can greatly increase adherence and prevent confusion and medication errors. In addition, the availability of short-course or simplified therapies for common endemic diseases is important for the clinician to know. A very effective example is single-dose azithromycin treatment for trachoma, which replaces the previous six-week course of topical or oral tetracycline (Bailey, Arullen-dran, Whittle, and Mabey, 1993); similarly, single-dose azithro-mycin is effective for treatment of chlamydial infection and chancroid (Centers for Disease Control, 1998b).

## Conclusion

Diagnosis and prevention of infectious diseases is important not only to the care of the individual patient, but to the health of the family, the patient's future children, and the community as a whole. Because the screening process and discussion of the individual infections can be a confusing and frightening experience, the screening should be conducted in a welcoming and sensitive manner, and should be seen as an opportunity for conveying important messages about health education and prevention. If it is possible for the screening process to lead directly into a primary care relationship, this is ideal, but even if not, the manner in which it is conducted will set the tone for the interaction of the new immigrant with the health care system.

# Nutritional Assessment and Dietary Intervention

*Marion M. Lee and*
*Shirley Huang*

A thorough assessment and understanding of immigrant women's dietary intake permits more complete delivery of health care. In all cultures, food is more than a nutrient. It may signify prosperity, good health and strength, or love; it may be a distraction, the centerpiece of family gatherings, or serve as a stress release (Sanjur, 1995). Foods that are consumed and preferred are based on their physical and cultural availability (Garcia and Warren, 1992). Therefore, an understanding of the needs, preferences, and beliefs of certain immigrant groups with regard to food will allow health care providers to target dietary intervention plans to improve the health of immigrant women.

## Acculturation, Disease, and Nutrition

A relationship exists among diet, nutrition, health, and disease (U.S. Surgeon General, 1988; Willet, 1990). Disease patterns in immigrants to the United States, whose food consumption remains consistent with their traditional culture, more closely resemble those of the home country. More acculturated immigrant Japanese were more likely to suffer similar kinds of illness to Americans (Kagan and others, 1974). A typical Asian diet consists primarily of rice, vegetables, and noodles; the major ingredients of the American diet are animal protein, fats, and sugar. This shift in diet results in an increase of body weight, coronary heart disease, stroke, and certain types of cancer.

In the United States, dietary intake and nutritional factors have been associated with six of the ten leading causes of death: hypertension, coronary heart disease, cancer, cardiovascular disease, chronic liver disease, and adult onset diabetes (U.S. Surgeon General, 1988). Diets high in saturated fat and cholesterol contribute to atherosclerotic disease. High fat consumption also has been associated with an increased incidence of breast, colon, and prostate cancers (World Cancer Research Fund, 1997).

Using general characteristics to define immigrant populations can be dangerous because of the numerous differences that exist. Diseases and customs that apply to one immigrant group may not hold true for another group within this general category. An increased rate of mortality from heart disease is seen in Japanese Americans, and hypertension is particularly prevalent among Filipinos (Guillermo, 1992). Hypercholesterolemia is a prevalent problem among Japanese Americans, Filipino Americans, and Native Hawaiians (Guillermo, 1992; U.S. Department of Health and Human Services, 1990). Differences exist in Hispanic populations. Within Hispanic subcultural groups, culture and ethnicity play a particularly important role in patterning food behavior (Sanjur, 1995; Fieldhouse, 1986). Therefore, health care providers need to integrate knowledge of differing dietary beliefs and practices in order to implement appropriate therapy.

The problem of obesity in the Hispanic population is multifactorial, reflecting genetic, environmental, cultural, and socioeconomic factors. Romero-Gwynn (1992), who studied obese Mexican Americans living in California, found that these immigrants have become acculturated and given up much of their traditional diet in exchange for one higher in fats and sugars. The changes include an increased consumption of flour tortillas, which are higher in fat than traditional corn tortillas; decreased use of lard, but increased consumption of margarine, butter, vegetable oil, mayonnaise, salad dressing, and sour cream; increased consumption of sliced white bread; increased consumption of sugar-rich drinks and condiments; increased consumption of ready-to-eat breakfast cereals; and decreased consumption of chilies and many traditional dishes with vegetables. The resulting diet is lower in fiber, beta-carotene, and specific nutrients provided by vegetables.

Dietary intervention and behavior intervention programs can be useful adjuncts to teaching. A weight loss manual with information on nutrition, exercise, food lists, and recipes; bilingual videotapes; food records; and cooking demonstrations may assist in addressing obesity and associated health-related problems in immigrants (Garcia and Warren, 1992; Romero-Gwynn, 1992).

Kunstadter (1997) analyzed the epidemiological consequences of migration and rapid cultural change among Hmong refugees in Fresno, California. Compared to nonrefugee Hmong in Thailand, an increase was seen in the rates of upper respiratory infections, gastrointestinal complaints, hypertension, stroke, diabetes, depression, neoplasms, and allergies in the immigrant group. Dietary changes among the Hmong immigrants reflected an increase in fat and salt. A possible explanation for these changes may be that in Thailand, the cost of meats was greater than the cost of vegetables, while in California, the prices were more comparable. The increase in meat intake among the immigrant Hmong may contribute to the increased rates of hypertension, diabetes, and cancer that are reported in the study.

A study comparing dietary habits, physical activity, and body mass index among Chinese in North America and China (Lee and others, 1994; M. M. Lee, 1994) showed that differences in the nutrient intake of Chinese living on the two continents suggest possible explanations for observed differences in chronic disease rates between the two populations. North American Chinese eat more meat and dairy products and consume about 35 percent of total calories from fat. Chinese immigrants to North America often go through a gradual and continuous progress of assimilating a Western lifestyle, although not entirely abandoning their native habits.

## Dietary Assessment

A clinical nutritional status assessment involves a combination of methods. An initial clinical exam consisting of a medical history, evaluation of dietary intake, and physical exam is followed by and augmented with anthropometric measurements and laboratory tests (Pressman and Adams, 1990; Terry, 1993).

Initially, a comprehensive interview including health, social, and family history should be obtained to better understand lifestyle, psychological, and eating patterns that may influence the nutritional status of the patient. Social conditions involving food should be emphasized and analyzed. The questions to be asked in eliciting the history are listed in Exhibit 7.3. These questions can be used to identify high-risk patients who may require further evaluation by the primary care physician or referral to a dietitian or nutritionist for further assessment.

A comprehensive analysis includes a physical exam in addition to a clinical history. The examiner should pay particular attention to the skin, eyes, lips, mouth, gums, tongue, hair, and nails, since these areas of the body often will display signs of malnutrition (Terry, 1993; Austin, 1978). In addition, the patient's height, weight, blood pressure, glands, subcutaneous tissue, musculo-skeletal system, gastrointestinal system, nervous system, and car-diovascular system must all be examined carefully to assess for physical abnormalities that may be related to poor or inadequate nutritional intake. Many signs may be mild or nonspecific, and they may be attributable to nonnutritional factors.

Further evaluation of the patient's dietary intake can be ob-tained by a variety of techniques, including food frequency ques-tionnaires, twenty-four-hour diet recalls, and a three-, five-, or seven-day food diary (Willet, 1990). Several screening tools focus-ing on a particular nutrient, such as fat, fiber, or calcium, have been developed for the general population as a quick means of gathering and evaluating eating patterns (Block and others, 1995).

Twenty-four-hour diet recalls provide quick and rough esti-mates of nutrient intakes (Willet, 1990). Patients are asked to re-call all foods, beverages, and additives consumed at meals and snacks in a specific twenty-four-hour time period. Information about preparation methods and eating habits should be obtained. Problems with this method include errors in recall, poor estima-tions of serving size, and poor generalizability from a specific day to overall dietary habits. The patient may keep a three-, five-, or seven-day food diary to provide a prospective recording of all foods, beverages, and additives consumed within a specific time

## Exhibit 7.3. Questions for a Dietary History.

1. How often does the patient eat?
2. Is food available regularly?
3. Who buys the food?
4. Who prepares the food?
5. What cooking and storage facilities are available?
6. Is food eaten mainly at home or away from home?
7. Is food eaten alone or with others?
8. Does the patient use any special diet?
9. Does the patient take any dietary supplements? If so, which ones?
10. Does the patient drink alcohol? If so, how much and how often?
11. Does the patient take medications or use any drugs (prescription and nonprescription)?
13. Does the patient have any allergies?
14. What foods are eaten daily?
15. What are the patient's favorite foods?
16. Does the patient have excess cravings for sweets, bread and butter, salt, coffee, fried foods, junk foods?
17. Are there particular foods that make the patient feel better or worse?
18. Does the patient snack between meals or at bedtime? If so, how often?
19. Does the patient ever binge?

period. Although this method provides more accurate quantitative information, the same problems, (omissions, poor serving size estimations, and so forth) may arise. Prior to employing these methods, it is important to determine whether the patient can read and write and is able to keep records accurately.

Information about dietary intake can be analyzed using food consumption tables, food groups, or computer analysis. Food consumption tables provided by the U.S. Department of Agriculture (USDA 1976–1987; Adams, 1975) and manufacturers' nutrition labels offer nutrient values for various foods and beverages. After the nutritional composition of each recorded food item is obtained, the nutrient composition of the overall diet can be calculated by a computer program (Block and others, 1995). This can be compared with the recommended dietary allowance (RDA), the standard for evaluation of dietary intake (National Research Council, 1989).

Food intake also may be evaluated through the use of food groups and determining how many servings were consumed from each basic group. *The Food Guide Pyramid* (U.S. Department of Agriculture, 1992) is available in many languages and cultural adaptations, including Spanish, Chinese, and Arabic. Evaluation using the food groups provides a general guideline of nutrient adequacy of the overall diet and serves as a basis for patient education. However, it does not determine whether the patient's food intake is deficient in any particular nutrient.

Anthropometric and body measurements are sensitive to dietary intake and may be useful in the assessment of nutritional status (Pressman and Adams, 1990; Frisancho, 1990). Height and weight, triceps skin fold (TSF), and midarm muscle circumference (MAMC) are the most commonly used measurements. Weight measurements allow for the calculation of relative weight ([current actual weight/desirable weight] x 100). Relative weight greater than 120 percent is defined as obesity. Body mass index above 27 (25 for Chinese) is considered overweight, and anything in excess of 30 is defined as obesity. TSF and MAMC measurements serve as estimates of fat stores and skeletal protein. Perhaps more important, waist and hip measurements should be taken. For women, a waist-to-hip ratio greater than 0.8 indicates abdominal obesity, a risk factor for coronary heart disease, stroke, type 2 diabetes, and some cancers (including breast).

Laboratory tests such as serum albumin, serum transferrin, and total lymphocyte counts may be used to determine nutritional status (Pressman and Adams, 1990; Shils and Young, 1998); however, confounding factors such as the number of hours since the patient last consumed food may make these tests unreliable.

All patients should be counseled if they have obesity, hypertension, diabetes, or high cholesterol. Specific diets are used for common chronic diseases—for example:

*Obesity:* Weight loss

*Hypertension:* Low sodium diet and weight loss

*Diabetes:* Low calories and weight loss

*High cholesterol:* Low fat and low cholesterol

The primary care provider must be able to assess the patient's motivation before specific diets and behavioral changes are implemented. Only motivated patients should be started on formal dietary therapy. When dietary therapy is begun, follow-up visits should be scheduled regularly. Serial measurements of body weight and regular clinical assessments should be performed. Meetings with dietitians and peer support groups should be suggested to improve adherence. Direct feedback should be given to the patient with support and reinforcements. Patients who fail to show any improvement in three months should be tried on a more quantitative approach with the assistance of a dietitian.

The primary care provider may help the patient establish an environment that offers a range of healthy foods and reinforces good nutrition. Patient empowerment must be stressed. Small and sustained changes in weight must be accepted and should elicit satisfaction. Change comes gradually, something both patients and providers must keep in mind.

## Conclusion

*Healthy People 2000* (U.S. Department of Health and Human Services, 1990) stresses the importance of understanding the needs of different immigrant populations in order to target health programs and dietary interventions. The report emphasizes the challenge that lies in developing an understanding and refining knowledge of different cultural and ethnic groups in order for health policies to be translated into effective community prevention programs and clinical preventive services.

The key components of successful dietary intervention involve the development of awareness and sensitivity in working with patients. Cultural differences in behaviors, feelings, and preferences must be respected, and socioeconomic and environmental issues relevant to particular ethnic groups must be understood. Rosenstock's health belief model (Rosenstock, Strecher, and Becker, 1988) stresses the importance of individual perceptions and of demographic, personal, situational, and social factors that affect an individual's ability to follow a therapy (Garcia and Warren, 1992; Sanjur, 1982). The primary care provider or dietitian must explain the diet rationale, using language that the client can easily grasp, and explain the need to modify harmful behaviors in a way that will increase the likelihood of action. To increase recent women immigrants' adherence to dietary intervention, the provider must:

- Understand the woman's past.
- Address her fears and anxieties and increase her perception of control over the outcome of events.
- Encourage the patient to maintain a traditional diet. Knowledge about price differences is important in understanding the reasoning behind the dietary choices of immigrant populations and may assist the provider in addressing dietary issues and implementing dietary intervention plans to improve the health of immigrants.
- Set up support networks by involving family members, relatives, neighbors, and friends. Involving family members, the primary social support, greatly increases adherence.
- Be a partner with the woman, thoroughly describing benefits and risks, and offering trade-offs and compromises.

If the provider follows these guidelines and offers a concrete, tangible approach rather than abstract suggestions, immigrants' adherence to dietary intervention will be increased.

# Chapter Eight

# Prenatal and Reproductive Health Care

*Francesca M. A. Taylor*
*with Ruby Ko*
*and Marilyn Pan*

Human migration may change the setting of a woman's life, but it does not notably alter her advance through the life phases typically established by her gender. The concerns and needs of immigrant women related to pregnancy and reproduction will be fundamentally similar to those of all other women seeking healthful family formation. Health-seeking behavior for perinatal and reproductive needs also will be colored by immigrant women's coping skills for accessing and utilizing care.

The benefits to be reaped from an integrated approach to care are plentiful, ranging from cost savings on expensive intensive care hospitalizations to better maternal, child, and family health status. The risks that accompany provision of fragmented care or denial of access to care are great.

## Contraception

Immigrants to the United States have brought with them various birth control practices, some traditional and folk oriented, and some modern. Modern contraceptive methods have been introduced and implemented in many countries, and cultural preferences or habits have developed in each country depending on the availability, cost, and acceptability of the methods introduced. Immigrant women frequently know about and request modern methods of birth control in U.S. health care settings, and differences in requests often mirror the beliefs and habits of each group.

In Chinese American communities, oral contraception generally is avoided because of a perception that "hormones are not good for you." Husbands or other male partners use condoms in acknowledgment of this belief. If a Chinese woman wants to use a method that is coitus independent, she may prefer an intrauterine device (IUD) or implanted sustained-release-hormone device even though the latter contains a hormone. Because of China's restriction on family size and widespread publicity about birth control, Chinese immigrants usually are quite aware of contraceptive methods.

Latina immigrants usually are familiar with hormonal contraception and favor the Depo-Provera injection *(la inyeccion),* which is given monthly in their home countries. The Latino preference for injectable medication rather than pills fits with this method. In my experience, Latinas typically avoid the diaphragm, and the education and demonstration session needed to teach its insertion may be surprisingly lengthy. Time is required to teach women how to touch their genitalia and to accustom themselves to feel the anatomical landmarks necessary for correct insertion and removal of the diaphragm. Sometimes there is much distress and embarrassment about touching and inserting fingers into the vagina *"Eso es feo!"* ("It's dirty") is a typical protest.

Birth spacing and family formation are pursued differently by different immigrant groups. On average Latina women are younger than non-Latina women at the age of first pregnancy and have more children (Juarbe, 1995). Therefore, reversible contraception is preferred initially. Following the birth(s) of the desired number of children, Latinas typically opt for long-term reversible contraception, such as IUDs or sustained-release devices, or for tubal ligation. When Latinas opt for abortion, it is usually because of an unplanned pregnancy. In contrast, Caucasians and Asians more typically postpone starting their families and so more frequently obtain abortion when nulliparous. Male sterilization is accepted and used in many Asian and Caucasian groups, but sterilization, when chosen by a Latino couple, usually is designated for the woman.

## Support for Choice in Contraception

In Chinese culture the decision to use contraception usually is made in egalitarian fashion, and most pregnancies are spaced. For Latinas, decisions about contraception and abortion are felt to belong primarily to the woman (Amaro, 1988). Nonetheless, Latina patients do report husbands' and partners' using condoms, and when they refuse other forms of contraception, typically report, *"El me cuida"* ("He takes care of me").

## Barriers to Contraceptive Use

Many immigrant women desire clear and accurate information about contraception and family planning, and they seek professional assistance and knowledge from clinicians as well as informally obtaining it from friends and family. Family planning programs that offer multilevel educational materials coupled with personal counseling interviews have been shown to aid women in choosing a method that suits their individual needs. When these programs include specially modified outreach and education to teenage and minor women, contraceptive effectiveness increases. When programs include language-specific and culturally sensitive counseling for family planning, effectiveness also increases. One study found that freestanding or nonprofit clinics were perceived by patients to offer language-specific services more than private physician practices, and those services are a significant aid to improving utilization of services (Silverman, Torres, and Forrest, 1987).

Culture affects contraceptive use and effectiveness. For example, use effectiveness of condoms has been relatively poor among Hispanic men (Jones and Forrest, 1989). Among unmarried women, contraceptive failure is greater for all non-Caucasian groups compared to Caucasians. However, marital status creates a significant difference for Hispanics, with contraceptive failure rates uniformly lower than for other minority groups (Jones and

Forrest, 1989). Religion has been found to have a less significant effect than might be anticipated. Although Roman Catholicism remains the predominant faith of Hispanic and Latino peoples, with well-publicized proscriptions against almost all forms of contraception, Latinos have not allowed church dictates to prevent them from using contraception, including permanent sterilization (Amaro, 1988).

## Therapeutic Abortion

Although abortion remains illegal or heavily regulated in many countries from which immigrants originate, it is practiced in most countries throughout the world, and many immigrant women understand that the procedure is available in the United States. Although views and values regarding elective abortion differ from one culture or religion to another, women of all cultural groups and religious affiliations seek and obtain abortions.

Abortion rates are unknown for specific immigrant groups; however, a higher rate of abortion is found among all minority women in the United States (Koonin, Smith, Ramick, and Strauss, 1998). Minority women have proportionately more unintended pregnancies, which lead to both more abortions and more unplanned births. The higher rate of unplanned pregnancies is due partly to greater proportions of women who do not use birth control and partly to higher contraceptive failure rates in these groups.

Access to abortion is restricted by a lack of public funding for the procedure and restrictions (which differ from state to state) such as parental or spousal notification or consent laws and mandatory waiting periods. Information about abortion is more available in freestanding nonprofit clinics than from private offices, and the procedure itself is most often performed in outpatient surgical centers or clinics by physicians who do abortions as a separate practice from their other medical work.

For centuries, women have obtained abortions through networks and word-of-mouth referral to midwives and other traditional practitioners. In many ways, the outpatient clinics and systems that provide abortions fit well with women's historical demand for the service in a private, confidential, separate environment. Most women who have abortions do not obtain them from their regular primary care providers. Immigrant women often have had abortions illegally and clandestinely in their countries of origin, or have known family members and friends whose lives have been affected by illegal abortion. Although legal abortion is not unduly difficult to obtain in urban areas, its absence from mainstream health care continues to make it vulnerable to ongoing political efforts to recriminalize it. Immigrant women, especially those who are undocumented, suffer most when access to a specific health care service becomes more regulated or sharply restricted. Abortion would be no different from other forms of reproductive health care in that sense.

## Prenatal Care

Prenatal care may be less available or accessible in the countries of origin from which current U.S. immigrants come. Births at home, attended by midwives or family members, are more the norm in most cultures. Length of stay or time since arrival in the United States appears to affect the time of entry into prenatal care: recent arrivals and undocumented women tend to initiate prenatal care after the first trimester (Chavez, Cornelius, and Jones, 1985), while immigrant women who have been living in the United States for longer periods begin prenatal care earlier. As with other traits, initiation of prenatal care varies among immigrant groups. Mexican American and Central and South American women are more likely to begin care after the first trimester than Cuban American women, and Chinese and Japanese women are more likely to seek early care than Native Hawaiian or Filipino women (Ventura, Martin, Curtin, and Mathews, 1997).

Regardless of their length of stay in the United States, most urban immigrant women integrate into institutional prenatal and delivery care rather than opt for home birth. However, various family members may be present in the delivery room, and birthing units in hospitals that accommodate family members during labor are favored by immigrant women.

Modern childbirth preparation and prenatal classes that integrate spouses or other partners, as well as other family members, are frequented by immigrant women, who increasingly seek access to information about the process of birth and earlier prenatal care. In some cultures, male partners seem to experience some embarrassment in attending classes on childbirth. Chinese women who take advantage of prenatal education classes often attend with female support persons, as husbands may be reluctant to attend.

## Folk Traditions About Pregnancy

Pregnant Chinese women believe it is taboo to attend funerals because they will expose the baby to the realm of the dead and may cause untoward effects for the child later. Moving into a new house or hammering are thought to cause birthmarks and thus are avoided.

Many people of Hispanic origin place food and nutrition practices in a framework known as the hot-cold theory of illness and disease (Murillo-Rohde, 1980). When there is adequate or healthy balance of temperature and humidity in the body, the body is warm and somewhat wet. Where an imbalance is perceived to occur, the body may be excessively hot, or dry and cold, or something else. Foods are thought to play a role in rebalancing the body because they can be typified as hot or cold. When an illness is thought of as a hot illness (such as fever, ulcer, or inflammation), the treatment should be cold food or medicine, and vice versa. During pregnancy, Latina women typically avoid hot foods and medications, believing this will prevent the baby from having skin rashes or eruptions (hot problems). Cool preparations are preferred.

The hot-cold theory is used in Chinese culture as well. For the Chinese, childbirth is considered a cold condition and must be treated with hot food. Cabbage is a food to be avoided during pregnancy as it may cause flatulence. An undesired outcome of this flatus may be false contractions.

Another folk belief of Latino culture involves *antojos* (cravings), in which it is thought that a pregnant woman should obey cravings she may have for specific foods. If she does not follow these urges, the baby may be born with characteristics of the particular food; for example, the infant may have strawberry spots if the mother craves strawberries but does not or cannot consume them during her pregnancy (Burk, Wieser, and Keegan, 1995).

Adherence to food cravings during pregnancy also is valued among API groups, for similar reasons. During the postpartum period, on the other hand, Latina women avoid cold foods because it is believed that cold substances will keep the uterus from expelling the blood (lochia) and evacuating all its contents following birth. Similarly, cold foods are avoided during menses so as not to impede complete emptying of menstrual blood from the uterus.

## Nutrition Education

Nutrition education is optimal when it is tailored to meet the specific dietary characteristics and risk profiles of the targeted cultural group. For pregnant Latina women, the risk of cholelithiasis is increased compared with non-Hispanic women, and gestational diabetes is two to three times more prevalent than in non-Hispanics (Council on Scientific Affairs, 1991; Ginzburg, 1991). Nutrition education designed to support prevention of these illnesses functions best when it informs patients about foods and nutrient amounts that are culturally familiar and also meet criteria for weight maintenance and special metabolic requirements. When this guidance and advice is first taught to individuals from the cultural group and then presented by them in a class format that integrates communal and collaborative techniques, the acquisition and retention of information is greater and the advised eating behavioral changes are more readily adopted.

## Infectious Disease Prevention

Prenatal screening with purified protein derivative (PPD) testing is valuable, particularly to identify younger patients who will be candidates for prophylactic isoniazid after delivery. Partners of migrant workers may be at higher risk for tuberculosis (Poss and Rengel, 1997). Screening for sexually transmitted diseases, including chlamydia, gonorrhea, and human immunodeficiency virus (HIV), is a typical part of prenatal screening.

HIV and acquired immunodeficiency (AIDS) syndrome disproportionately affect minority and immigrant women. Hispanics account for 14 percent of all reported AIDS cases, 21 percent of AIDS cases among women, and 22 percent of pediatric cases

(Council on Scientific Affairs, 1991). The ability to accomplish significant antiretroviral preventive treatment during pregnancy makes it even more compelling to provide sensitive and consistent counseling about voluntary prenatal HIV testing.

## Preterm Labor and Pregnancy Complications

Infant mortality is the most widely used indicator of population health (Becerra, Hogue, Atrash, and Perez, 1991). Low birth weight is an additional measure of pregnancy outcome. When these indicators are used, Latinas consistently have infant mortality and birth weights that are comparable to Caucasians and decidedly better than for African Americans, despite the fact that they often have less health insurance coverage and poorer access to care (James, 1993). Some researchers have hypothesized that the spiritual or religious grounding of Latino communities and families may play a role in this striking phenomenon (Magana and Clark, 1995). Other research suggests that better nutritional intake and lower prevalence of smoking and alcohol use are the explanatory factors (Guendelman and Abrams, 1994).

## Prenatal Diagnosis of Birth Defects

Most cultures, primitive and modern, understand that birth defects occur. Risk for certain defects, for example, neural tube defects, has been shown to vary across ethnic groupings and by immigration status (Shaw, Velie, and Wasserman, 1997). When a defect occurs, the parents frequently search for a reason or explanation, which may be an important part of the process of grieving over whatever loss the defect engenders for the child or family.

Pregnant immigrant women accept alpha-fetoprotein and triple marker screens as an initial step in the diagnosis of fetal anomalies such as neural tube defects or Down's syndrome during pregnancy. However, a positive result can be devastating for the woman and her family and partner.

Subsequent steps in prenatal diagnosis become challenging as the woman copes with the shock of a potential problem in her fetus. Although most immigrant women accept ultrasound in furthering the diagnostic process, many refuse amniocentesis, preferring to believe that the screening tests have been erroneous or that there will be no gain from a study that they perceive as invasive and dangerous (Gaviria, Stern, and Schensul, 1982).

### Traditional Customs

Many cultures have folk traditions for preventing birth defects. In Latino cultures, women use a safety pin affixed to the front panel of their underwear (sometimes two safety pins are used and fastened in the shape of a cross) to protect the fetus from a cleft lip or palate, which they believe could be caused by a lunar eclipse (Villaruel and Ortiz de Montellano, 1992). This concept originated with the Aztecs, who thought that an eclipse resulted from a "bite" being taken out of the moon; if a pregnant woman saw the phenomenon, her baby would have a bite taken out of its mouth. It also has been observed that Latina women refrain from cutting their hair during pregnancy due to the belief that "cutting the hair cuts the vision" of the developing baby.

### Pregnancy Termination

Although it never is easy to end a pregnancy, planned or wanted, that has become unsustainable or unwanted because of a fetal defect, the decision can take on symbolic dimensions for immigrant women, especially those who have lost other children or family members. The hope and sense of renewal that pregnancy and an anticipated baby represent for an immigrant family become fragile as the promise of success in the new country and the desire for an improved future seem shaken by events that are not surmountable, even with modern medical technology and practice.

## Prenatal Care Adherence

Perceptions of prenatal care may vary among new immigrants. Women who come from remote or economically depressed regions in their country of origin may view prenatal care as important but somewhat of a luxury. Often there is a perception that it is worthwhile, but early entry into care may be a low priority. The problem is that the more valuable screening tests and procedures cannot be done for patients who wait until the fourth or fifth month to begin care.

Lower use of preventive services may be due in part to cultural perception of time orientation, which varies considerably among different immigrant groups. Present-time orientation signifies a more loosely structured and less rigid concept of time that is found more commonly among newer immigrants, and represents an area where medical culture often conflicts with the culture of recent immigrants. It can affect interactions with the health care system through tardiness for appointments, missed appointments, failure to seek preventive health services, or low adherence to medications and treatment plans. Pregnant women with present-day orientation may delay or sometimes even discontinue prenatal care because they feel well and do not perceive services to be useful (Burk, Wieser, and Keegan, 1995).

For the U.S. health care system, with its future-time orientation, emphasizing compulsive usage of all measured time intervals, facilities and providers who are caring for immigrants must allot additional time for educating their patients about the importance of timely preventive care, early treatment, and adherence to care instructions. Community health workers, who can act as cultural brokers to translate information between health care providers and patients, are very useful in prenatal and postpartum care. Sometimes patients resist accepting care within the Western system due to ambivalence or fear of mistreatment, or simply because the system represents an uncomfortable place to receive what are usually intimate or personal services.

Historically, when state funding for prenatal care for all women in need, regardless of citizenship status, increased, maternity services became more available and accessible, with a resultant increase in utilization and predicted diminution of perinatal complications. However, government funding for maternity care for low-income women has not entirely ensured access to services. Undocumented immigrant women fear and lack knowledge about how to enroll for Medicaid and as a result may enter care later than is optimal. Some women obtain insurance initially but subsequently lose it, usually because of a failing of the complex and bureaucratic state insurance system. This leads to missed appointments and gaps in care, with only a portion of screening services completed prior to delivery.

In one study, noncitizen immigrant women accessed prenatal care for five to six months of their pregnancy; those who were citizens and covered by the same government-funded insurance were able to obtain seven months of prenatal care (Norton, Kenney, and Ellwood, 1996). With recent changes in noncitizen eligibility for government-funded programs, this gap in access is likely to widen (see Chapter Four).

Occasionally patients become so disenchanted with the process of applying for medical assistance, or so fearful of deportation, that they take the position of "wanting to pay for it by myself." Although some are able to cover prenatal visits and tests on a cash-pay basis, few can rally the funds to pay for expensive testing or for hospital delivery (especially operative delivery, if that is required).

## Substance Use During Pregnancy

Patterns of substance abuse vary with age, cultural or ethnic background, socioeconomic status, and country of birth. In Latino culture, a discrepancy has been noted between U.S.-born women and immigrant women, with illicit drug use affecting perinatal outcomes for a high-risk group of U.S.-born Latinas aged twenty-five to thirty-four years who received no prenatal care and experienced a consequent increased complication rate (Vega and others, 1997). In contrast, alcohol use during pregnancy was demonstrated to be equivalent among both U.S.-born and immigrant Latinas. In another study, African American women in Los Angeles County had higher rates of alcohol, tobacco, and substance use than either Mexican American or Mexican immigrant women. No significant differences were noted between Mexican American and Mexican immigrant women (Zambrana, 1991).

## The Experience of Birth

Immigrants often have used home birthing in their country of origin, and many view hospital care as an improvement. Still, the desire for a homelike environment is strong, and the presence of spouse and often family is critical (Khazoyan and Anderson, 1994). Encouragement and the expression of faith that "everything will turn out normal" are important supports that Latinas and many other women want to receive during parturition. There also is a desire to hear reassurances of love and affection from the spouse or partner. Programs that utilize *comadres* (indigenous community workers who support women during the perinatal period) and institutions that provide midwifery services have been well accepted in the Latino community.

Labor support persons also are valued in Chinese culture. Usually the mother's mother or mother-in-law is the labor coach; the spouse or male partner is present for the delivery but arrives relatively late. This custom may be due to values of stoicism or not allowing the experience of pain to be evident to others, even one's spouse. Chinese husbands seem to need encouragement to touch their wives or express comforting communication to the woman when others (health providers) are present. Chinese women are reluctant to walk during labor, preferring to stay in bed. Herbal remedies and acupressure on the back, sacral area, and small toe are preferred remedies for pain.

## The Fourth Trimester: Postpartum

In Latino culture, the first forty days postpartum is referred to as *la cuarentena* (the quarantine); it is a time set aside to permit the mother to recuperate from pregnancy and delivery and to adapt to the new infant and new family relationships. Certain dietary and activity restrictions are typically observed during this time (Gaviria, Stern, and Schensul, 1982).

Chinese women perceive that the hot-cold balance of the body needs rebalancing after parturition. "Hot food" is preferred because it is believed to help replenish blood loss. Ginger is a favored ingredient, thought to be good at "getting rid of the cold." During their postpartum stay, many Chinese patients insist on eating foods brought from home to the hospital. They do not consume fruits or vegetables during the first month postpartum. Some special foods are eaten and shared with loved ones. The Taiwanese eat sesame chicken, while the Cantonese use vinegar, peanuts, pigs' knuckles, and eggs. Vinegar in a broth with pigs' knuckles is believed to help transfer calcium from the knuckle bones and so assist the woman in meeting a perceived heightened calcium requirement. Dong Quai (better known in Western culture as angelica root) and chicken wine also are taken to increase body heat and reduce anemia.

## Folk Beliefs

Many traditions about children and child rearing are passed through generations of mothers. Among Latinos there is reference made to *caida de mollera* (fallen fontanel), which is believed to be caused by holding or picking up a baby improperly, moving or carrying it roughly, bouncing it while playing, or separating it from its milk bottle or the mother's breast too quickly (Burk, Wieser, and Keegan, 1995).

Binding of the umbilicus after birth is a frequently observed custom among Latinos (Zepeda, 1982). Many of the special binders (*fajeros*) are elaborately decorated with fine embroidery and other ornamental items and are given as gifts for the new baby. The purpose of the binder is to prevent bulging or herniation around the navel and also to "keep the intestines from falling out." Many mothers feel that binding is better than the usually recommended airdrying of the umbilical stump after birth, and some place oils on and around the stump. Infections or other skin irritations are seldom observed in babies who have had the binding, but on occasion an omphalitis can develop. Respect for the practice can be balanced with friendly advice to keep the binding relatively loose and to use *fajeros* made of cotton and other light materials.

## Lactation

Latina immigrants strongly believe in the importance of natural breast milk as a source of nutrition for the baby. However, there also is an entrenched perception that formula contains advantageous factors and that the baby "has to get used to the bottle eventually." Consequently the trend among new as well as longerterm immigrants is to give both breast and bottle. This practice continues to reinforce traditional positive values toward *la leche de madre* (mother's milk), but it interferes with lactation physiology and in some cases may contribute to early cessation of milk production.

Rates of breast-feeding among immigrant Vietnamese women in Western countries are low compared to those in Vietnam. One study suggested that the switch to bottle feeding is part of the process of adaptation and acculturation in the new country (Rossiter, 1992). This corroborated earlier findings that immigration status was the main factor influencing the change to bottle feeding in this group because of perceptions of the practice in the new country and an expressed motivation for freedom and convenience (Henderson and Brown, 1987).

Preferred eating practices during lactation also have been encountered among other API groups. For example, Filipina women are known to consume soups in large quantity while breast-feeding and to take in extra fluids to maintain balance in the body.

## Infertility

The crisis of infertility for immigrant couples takes on diagnostic difficulty and challenges treatment plans. Most public insurance plans do not cover infertility services, and immigrant women, if they can access these services at all, usually are treated at teaching hospitals where an interest exists in acquiring patients for physician training or for research. Although the care rendered frequently is optimal, access may be piecemeal (Ginzburg, 1991).

## Adoption Practices

Adoption is a critical means of family formation; for immigrant women this may be an important option that is not as well recognized as it might be.

Informal adoption, which may include adoption by blood-related kin, as well as informal adoption of children who have been orphaned during an extended migration, also occurs more frequently than in the United States. Haitian women adopted children of mothers who died in boat crossings between Haiti and the United States. In Latin American countries, kinship networks tend to be very large and to include *hijos de crianza* (informally adopted children) as kin.

Children from all ethnic and racial backgrounds need adoptive parents. Greater numbers of adoptable children in the United

States come from minority backgrounds. Although there has been significant outreach and participation among African Americans for adoption of babies within that community, there has been a relative paucity of work on the role of health care and social work professionals in developing similar, programmed promotion of adoption among Latino Americans and other groups. Many Latino infants and children find caring adoptive homes with parents who are not of Latino background. Although this has been helpful for many children and adoptive parents, it also would be helpful to publicize and support more adoptions within Latino cultural communities programmatically.

Children who are brought to the United States as international adoptees also represent a new immigrant group. Varied social and cultural factors interplay in these adoptions, but many healthful families are formed by this process. Children arriving from developing countries typically need attentive follow-up for infectious diseases such as hepatitis and tuberculosis, as well as behavioral development. Some groups may need more cautious surveillance for fetal alcohol syndrome or malnutrition.

## Conclusion

Many challenges in immigrant health care that seem new or unprecedented have been faced and surmounted in the past. The United States is, and will remain, a nation of immigrants. As we form policies and programs for the future, we must be informed with a perspicacity that comes from knowing the past. Health care providers can be potent advocates for their patients in the face of attempts to destroy access to prenatal care and other crucial health services, including choice among reproductive options and contraception.

# Chapter Nine

# Chronic Diseases

# Cardiovascular Disease

*Susan L. Ivey and*
*Gerrie Gardner*

Cardiovascular diseases (CVD) are the leading cause of death across all racial categories used in death certificate reporting in the United States. Coronary heart disease (CHD) and cerebrovascular disease kill nearly as many Americans as all other diseases combined. In 1996, nearly half a million people, roughly half of them women, died from CHD (Peters and others, 1997). CHD deaths are common in all ethnic groups. There are many theories about the reasons underlying the high prevalence of CHD in the United States compared with other countries. Westernization, urbanization, smoking, dietary fat intake, physical inactivity, and stress may all play a role.

CHD mortality rates usually have been examined by gender and certain racial and ethnic categories, but not by immigrant status, obscuring variation within categories. This limits our ability to understand factors related to acculturation and recency of immigration. In addition, it sometimes is difficult to determine which differences among countries relate to actual prevalence differences and which are reflections of large numbers of deaths that are coded as "unknown cause."

Although prevalence data on specific immigrant groups are sparse, we can infer from other data that CHD often becomes more common after migration to the United States (Polednak, 1989; Kagan and others, 1974). Little is known about CHD in specific subpopulations of immigrant women. Perhaps more than any other disease, understanding CHD and its related risk factors requires the inclusion of acculturation variables in national surveys. Determination of which ethnic groups are at current or future risk is important for providers and policymakers alike (Wild and others, 1995).

## Predisposition or Environment?

Coronary heart disease and other diseases that increase the risk of CHD (diabetes, dyslipidemias, and hypertension) have known genetic bases. However, rates of cardiac disease among certain ethnic groups increase following migration to countries where CHD rates are high (such as the United States), indicating a substantial influence of environmental factors such as tobacco use and dietary fat intake (Polednak, 1989). Multiple studies have shown that hypertension, truncal obesity, sedentary lifestyle, smoking, and hypercholesterolemia are significant markers for risk of CHD. Certain of those risk factors may be more common in specific ethnic groups.

In the past, mortality related to cardiovascular deaths has been underreported due to poor record keeping or incorrect diagnoses on death certificates, especially for Hispanic populations in the southwestern states (Mitchell and others, 1992). Reliable mortality statistics and survey and morbidity data (such as self-reported functional status) generally are available for Caucasian populations, and there is a growing body of information on CHD in African Americans. However, surveys of CHD in Latinos and Asian Americans have been conducted only recently, sample sizes usually are small, and they often are limited to one or a few states.

Prevalence is not static. Within one to two generations, cardiovascular disease patterns can change dramatically, as demonstrated by the Ni-Hon-San study of Japanese men postmigration and studies of African Americans (Kagan, 1974; Polednak, 1989; Gillum and Liu, 1984; Hames and Greenlund, 1996). Whether these changes are related to dietary change or changes in other risk factors is unclear. Overall, mortality rates from CHD are improving. Despite a continuing decrease in the age-adjusted death rate from heart disease between 1994 and 1995, Anderson, Kochanek, and Murphy (1997) concluded that cardiovascular diseases were the primary cause of death for women across all racial groupings in the United States.

Differences in actual values displayed in Tables 9.1 through 9.4 relate to varying methodologies among studies. (The numbers cannot be compared across tables due to differing methods of analysis in different studies.) For instance, some studies have looked at deaths from CHD alone, while others include deaths for other cardiovascular diseases, such as stroke or rheumatic heart disease. In addition, data may be age adjusted to standard U.S. populations from 1940, 1980, or 1990, which makes the reported rate incomparable to mortality rates that use other age-adjustment techniques.

Given this caveat, in a CDC report that used 1990 data on ischemic heart disease (Centers for Disease Control, 1994a), age-adjusted death rates per 100,000 U.S. population varied from 73.7

**Table 9.1. Age-Adjusted Mortality Rates for Ischemic Heart Disease and Stroke for Women, by Race.**

| Female | White | African American | Native American/ Alaskan | API |
|---|---|---|---|---|
| Ischemic heart disease | 130.2 | 148.3 | 74.5 | 73.7 |
| Stroke | 45.8 | 68.7 | 31.4 | 43.7 |

Note: Rate per 100,000 persons adjusted to the 1980 standard U.S. population.
Source: Centers for Disease Control, 1994a, Table C-2.

**Table 9.2. Age-Adjusted Mortality Rates for Ischemic Heart Disease and Stroke for Women, by Hispanic/Non-Hispanic Origin.**

| Female | Hispanic | Non-Hispanic |
|---|---|---|
| Ischemic heart disease | 147.1 | 131.8 |
| Stroke | 45.4 | 47.9 |

Note: Rate per 100,000 persons adjusted to the 1980 standard U.S. population.
Source: Centers for Disease Control, 1994a, Table C-4.

**Table 9.3. Age-Adjusted Mortality Rates for Cardiovascular Disease for Women, by Race, 1995.**

| Female | All Races | White | African American | Hispanic | API |
|---|---|---|---|---|---|
| Cardiovascular disease | 100.4 | 94.9 | 156.3 | 68.1 | 57.3 |

*Note:* Rate per 100,000 population adjusted to the 1940 standard U.S. population.
*Source:* National Center for Health Statistics, 1996–1997.

for Asian American women to 148.3 for African American women (see Tables 9.1 and 9.2). In that analysis, Hispanic women had slightly higher rates after age adjusting to a 1980 standard U.S. population than did white women (Centers for Disease Control, 1994a). In 1995, rates per 100,000 U.S. population varied from 156.3 deaths per 100,000 for African American females to 57.3 for API women adjusted to the 1940 standard population (see Table 9.3) (National Center for Health Statistics, 1997). For Hispanic women (which includes various racial groupings) the rate was 68.1, lower than that for white females. A study of racial patterns of CHD mortality, which used National Health Interview Survey (NHIS) data and linked them to the National Death Index, showed that black women had higher rates of death from CHD than did white women, and Hispanic women had lower CHD mortality (Liao and others, 1997).

These findings highlight the controversy on actual prevalence of CHD in Hispanic women who, until recently, were thought to have lower mortality rates from CHD compared to black and white women (Aronow, 1992). Genetics and family history have been hypothesized to contribute to the lower rate of CHD in this ethnic group. However, other sources have reported CHD mortality rates for Hispanic women that are slightly greater than those for non-Hispanic women (of all races) (Centers for Disease Control, 1994a).

State-level data offer similar paradoxes. Despite adverse cardiovascular risk factor profiles, such as higher levels of obesity and diabetes, Mexican American women in Texas appeared to have

**Table 9.4. Age-Adjusted Mortality Rates of Women, by API Subgroups as Compared to Other Races, 1992.**

| Female | White | African American | API | Chinese | Japanese | Hawaiian | Fili-pino | Asian Indian | Korean | Samoan | Viet-namese |
|---|---|---|---|---|---|---|---|---|---|---|---|
| Ischemic heart disease | 226.0 | 144.8 | 57.3 | 72.1 | 84.7 | 115.4 | 48.3 | 33.0 | 42.8 | [a] | 31.7 |
| Cardiovascular disease | 322.7 | 238.9 | 86.9 | 107 | 136.6 | 193.1 | 80.4 | 44.1 | 62.1 | 102.3 | 44.9 |
| Cerebrovascular | 47.5 | 44.6 | 30.4 | 36 | 61.2 | 44.4 | 27.2 | [a] | 16.5 | [a] | 20.1 |

[a] = inadequate number of deaths in this category for analysis

*Note:* Deaths per 100,000 specific population, adjusted to 1990 U.S. census data.

*Source:* Based on a sample from seven states reported to the National Center for Health Statistics in 1992.

similar age-adjusted rates of myocardial infarction (MI) to whites and CHD mortality roughly equal to rates of white women (Goff and others, 1993a). Among patients admitted for MI, however, Mexican American women had higher short- and longer-term mortality rates than non-Hispanic white women (Goff and others, 1993b).

The API population has lower mortality from CHD in all age groups compared to whites, African Americans, Hispanics, and Native Americans in the United States (Centers for Disease Control, 1994a). In a detailed study of mortality among APIs from the seven states with the largest populations of this group, the overall mortality rate from all CVD was 106.2 per 100,000 in 1992 (Hoyert and Kung, 1997) (see Table 9.4). This study showed marked variation among API subgroups, but the finding must be interpreted with the caveat that it was adduced from the death certificate data of only seven states. Data were age adjusted to the 1990 census. Despite limitations, the study results constitute a good example of variation in CVD rates within a single "race" category—in this case, API. Further studies of ethnic and immigrant populations with careful age adjustment are needed. Similar variation among other racial and ethnic groupings, as well as by generation of immigration, is plausible.

Use of the overarching term *African American* obscures immigrant groups within this racial category. Recent immigrants from Africa and the Caribbean, as well as from Latin America, may have African heritage. African Diaspora groups are more likely to metabolize sodium less efficiently, theoretically providing an advantage to individuals from hot climates. As a group, these persons have higher rates of hypertension. U.S. Filipinos also have high rates of hypertension, approaching those of African Americans, but a lower incidence of death from cerebrovascular disease and CVD (Polednak, 1989). There is a persistent difference in all-cause CVD mortality between African Americans and whites (Pappas and others, 1993); mortality rates from CVD in African Americans that appeared to improve in the 1970s seemed to have leveled off in the 1980s.

Differences in mortality rates may be explained in part by immigration characteristics that moderate lifestyle and risk factor changes. For example, Japanese immigrants to the United States have decreased risk of cerebrovascular accidents, but increased risk of CHD compared to their native Japanese counterparts. The Ni-Hon-San study demonstrated an increase in the incidence of coronary artery disease in male Japanese familial immigrants who migrated to Hawaii and then to California (Polednak, 1989; Kagan and others, 1974). South Asians have a higher risk of insulin resistance and centripetal obesity, and appear to have increased risks for CHD (Enas and others, 1996). Korean immigrants in New York City had an increased risk for cerebrovascular disease and stroke, but showed very low rates of death secondary to ischemic heart disease (Stellman, 1996).

## Risk Factors

Assessment of CHD risk factors should include questions about tobacco use, dietary intake, family history, physical activity, lipid disorders, and diabetes. Menstrual history and history of premature surgical menopause by hysterectomy or bilateral oophorectomy should be ascertained. Tobacco use, obesity, and estrogen status are discussed below; hypertension and diabetes appear later in the chapter.

## Tobacco

Tobacco use and environmental tobacco smoke contribute significantly to rates of CHD. Although less acculturated women typically smoke less than acculturated women, their partners may be heavier smokers (Perez-Stable, VanOss Marin, and Marin, 1993). As women acculturate, they are more likely to smoke. (The opposite trend exists for men.) Thus, recent immigrant women may be at risk of adopting smoking. Concern has been expressed that there is underreporting, reflecting social desirability among certain cultures that women not smoke (Perez-Stable, VanOss Marin, and Marin, 1993). Studies that used biologic markers (such as serum cotinine) also showed that Mexican American smokers may be underreporting the number of cigarettes smoked per day (Perez-Stable, VanOss Marin, and Marin, 1993).

Data from the NHIS show a pattern of higher rates of current smoking among Puerto Rican women than either Cuban American or Mexican American women (Centers for Disease Control, 1994b). Another study on Puerto Rican women in Boston and Hartford, Connecticut, showed higher levels of smoking for this subgroup compared to national smoking rates (Smith and McGraw, 1993).

The NHIS reported that API women tend to have a low prevalence of smoking: 7.8 percent for the years 1987–1991 combined (Centers for Disease Control, 1994c). It appears that rates are higher for U.S.-born Asian American women than for Asian-born women (Chen, 1993). When surveys are conducted in native Asian languages, they reveal higher cigarette smoking rates than for surveys conducted in English (Centers for Disease Control, 1992a); the reason for this is unclear. There also is variation in smoking rates among API groupings. For example, in a recent study by the National Asian Women's Health Organization (1998), Vietnamese women reported lower smoking rates (2 percent) than Korean women (4 percent).

Eastern European immigrants also may have high-risk profiles. Russian and Ukrainian immigrants have been shown to have lifestyle habits such as smoking, high dietary fat intake, and low levels of physical activity that are associated with increased risk of CHD (Duncan and Simmons, 1996). Similarly, Roma (gypsy) women may be more likely to smoke, have hypertension and high cholesterol, and be physically inactive (Polednak, 1989).

## Obesity and Insulin Resistance

Overall, the U.S. population has higher rates of obesity than in the past. Based on physical examinations of a civilian sample of Mexican American women, levels of obesity increased from 41.4 percent in 1982–1984 to 51.8 percent in 1988–1994 (National Center for Health Statistics, 1997). Diabetes mellitus also has a high prevalence in the Mexican American population. Diabetic Mexican American women are three times more likely to have MIs than nondiabetic Mexican American women. Therefore, the theoretical cardioprotective effect of Mexican American heritage and family support may be partially mitigated by the increasing prevalence of diabetes in this population (Kovar, 1992).

Native Hawaiian, Tongan, and Samoan women also have higher rates of obesity. However, CHD rates among Native Hawaiians appear to be lower than the rate of Caucasian women, although they are higher than overall API rates (Hoyert and Kung, 1997). Asian Indians appear to have higher rates of non-insulin-dependent diabetes mellitus, high-risk lipid profiles, and insulin resistance. However, they have much lower rates of smoking and obesity, which appears to afford them some level of protection from CHD (Enas and others, 1996). In the Behavioral Risk Factor Surveillance Survey, physical inactivity has been noted to be higher among certain Asian groups (Centers for Disease Control, 1992b). This risk factor is one of the least studied among immigrant groups, possibly due to language barriers that prevent participation in surveys.

## Primary and Secondary Prevention

Unless women perceive CHD to be a threat to them, they are unlikely to undertake preventive interventions when they are young or to respond appropriately to symptoms of CHD when they get older. Education about CHD is vitally important for immigrant women. By supporting healthy habits such as not smoking, or eating less fat and providing culturally competent information on the need for periodic cholesterol screening, diabetes screening, and early intervention, we have a unique opportunity for primary prevention of CHD in many immigrant groups.

Demonstration projects have developed programs for CHD prevention in specific ethnic groups, such as Latinas and African American women, with attention to incorporating cultural sensitivity and culturally tailored media messages to improve participation and adoption of components such as low fat diets, higher levels of physical activity, tobacco resistance, or smoking cessation (Centers for Disease Control, 1998c; National Institutes of Health, 1997; Perez-Stable, VanOss Marin, and Marin, 1993). Evaluation of these programs is in progress.

## Effects of Estrogen and Hormone Replacement

CHD risk increases over the postmenopausal years. In some, if not most, cultures, menopause is viewed as a normal life occurrence, and no medical treatment (such as hormone replacement) is considered. This is a common view in both Asia and Eastern Europe

(Davis and others, 1994). Women who have had premature surgical menopause (oophorectomy) also are at higher risk for early CHD. Estrogen appears to have a protective effect on lipids, and it optimizes vasomotor stability and endothelial function.

Certain groups of women tend to ingest higher levels of phytoestrogens (naturally occurring "plant hormones" that are similar to estrogen), which are commonly found in foods containing soy protein (Reinli and Block, 1996). Asian women who eat tofu and other soy products report lower rates of flushing perimenopausally. Whether such a diet is protective against cardiac disease is under investigation (Clarkson and others, 1998; Wagner and others, 1997).

The benefits of hormone replacement therapy (HRT) must be balanced against increased risk of uterine cancer and possible effects on the growth of other estrogen-sensitive tumors such as breast cancer. The clinician must individualize recommendations for HRT for each patient based on her risks and benefits.

## Assessment of Symptoms

Women with CHD may have unusual symptoms with angina or MI. Some women have typical left-sided chest pain with radiation to neck, jaw, shoulders, or arms. Others may have dyspnea as their anginal equivalent. Other descriptions include nausea alone, reflux symptoms, chest heaviness (which may not be attributed to angina), and even feelings of unrest or doom. Symptoms may be associated with exertion or emotional stress. Diabetics, hypertensives, and the elderly, who are most at risk for MI, have more silent ischemia (Valensi and others, 1997).

Cultural factors determine when and how patients report both symptomatology and pain. (Cultural differences in interpretation of somatic sensations are discussed in Chapter Two.) Diagnosing CHD in immigrant women can be problematic when patients describe their symptoms in their native languages. Further, terms referring to the heart may have culturally embedded meanings that do not correspond to cardiac symptomatology, as in the case with which this book begins. Descriptions of symptoms should be reviewed with the translator and accompanying friends or family members to elucidate the cultural meaning of symptom description.

## Myocardial Infarction

Women experience less favorable outcomes from MI than men, and African Americans have worse outcomes than white women. Some recent data suggest that Mexican Americans have worse outcomes than non-Hispanic whites, at least in Texas. Although mortality from MI has decreased dramatically since the Framingham study reported this discrepancy, post-MI mortality gaps between men and women (men fare better) and between different ethnic groups (Caucasians fare better than African Americans or Hispanics) continue, even after adjusting for age, although socioeconomic status often explains much of the difference.

Some of the difference in post-MI mortality has been hypothesized to relate to treatment differences. Appropriate referral of women and minorities for thrombolysis and interventional cardiac procedures (angioplasty, coronary artery bypass surgery) has been documented to be lower than for Caucasian men (American Medical Women's Association, 1996; Goldberg and others, 1992). This bias against appropriate referral and treatment appears to have multiple factors, including racism and sexism.

Asian women have lower average body weights. Despite the recognition that weight-adjusted dosage schedules of thrombolytic agents were likely to decrease bleeding complications in women, the National Registry of Myocardial Infarctions, in 1996, documented that fewer than 10 percent of patients receive weight-adjusted dosages.

Coronary revascularization procedures (Goldberg and others, 1992), completion of cardiac rehabilitation programs after MI (Cannistra and Balady, 1995), and outcomes for coronary artery bypass surgery are lower for African Americans (Gray and others, 1996). Outcomes post-MI were shown to be worse for Mexican Americans compared to non-Hispanic whites from Texas (Goff and others, 1993b).

Underutilization of medical and surgical therapies affects not only women's mortality but their morbidity, functional status, and quality of life, including sexual functioning, mood, and outlook.

Since these variables also are culturally imbued, information on all aspects of these therapies should be made available to immigrant women to ensure informed decisions on the use of medical and surgical interventions for CHD, within their own cultural frameworks. The provider should maintain awareness that these decisions can be complicated by the potential lack of insurance coverage for recommended treatment.

## Future Directions

Lifetime risk for CHD in women is 31 percent, far higher than the risks for hip fracture and breast cancer. It appears that health care providers have done an inadequate job of educating women about their biggest health risk. Despite the fact that CVD is the leading cause of death for women of all races, until recently most of the information about prevention, recognition, management, and prognosis of CHD was based on studies of Caucasian men. New research must focus on the determination of differences in prevalence, risk factors, and treatment among populations of women, including immigrant women.

Prevalence patterns for specific diseases tend to change as new immigrants acculturate to Western environments. Therefore, research from other countries is not sufficient to tell us about the health of new immigrants in the United States. Future research should seek to assess changes in prevalence and determine the efficacy of culture-specific programs, thereby improving the ability to prevent, diagnose, and treat CHD in immigrant women when they are younger, have less advanced cardiac disease, and are less likely to have comorbid conditions.

Cultural stereotypes can keep optimal care from being delivered to groups of women early enough to prevent mortality and morbidity from CHD. Differentials in socioeconomic status are key markers for health status differences. Targeting health care alone will not be sufficient without similar attention to improving the socioeconomic status of immigrant and refugee women and ensuring access to health care for all.

Prevention research needs to identify primary and secondary prevention methods that will allow women of many different ethnic and cultural backgrounds to receive information that incorporates traditional dietary practices whenever possible, respects cultural preferences, and is language accessible. Providers must support immigrant women to make healthy choices in diet, physical activity, and tobacco resistance in order to combat the negative components of acculturation.

# Hypertension

*Dina Lieberman,*
*Mary L. Del Monte,*
*and Eugenia L. Siegler*

Management of hypertension is difficult under the best of circumstances. Hypertension causes no symptoms until target organs are severely damaged, and patients often are reluctant to adhere to medication regimens and lifestyle modifications when they feel well. These problems are compounded in immigrant populations, when language barriers, family and social stresses, and cultural practices may exacerbate hypertension or interfere with treatment. The terms *hypertension* and *high blood pressure* may not translate well into other languages or may be interpreted to mean tension or stress—something to be coped with rather than actively treated. For these reasons, effective treatment of hypertension in immigrant populations presents special challenges to clinicians.

## Incidence and Consequences

The Sixth Report of the Joint National Committee on Prevention, Detection, Evaluation, and Treatment of High Blood Pressure (JNC VI) defines hypertension as fulfilling any one of three criteria: (1) systolic blood pressure of 140 mmHg or above, (2) diastolic blood pressure of 90 mmHg or above, or (3) a patient's taking medication for hypertension (National High Blood Pressure Education Program, 1997). JNC VI divides hypertension into three stages, based on the degree of elevation of blood pressure. The decision to treat a patient pharmacologically is based on both the blood pressure stage and the presence of end organ damage or additional cardiovascular risk factors.

As many as 43 million Americans may be hypertensive (Burt and others, 1995). The prevalence and incidence of hypertension increase with age. Through middle age, hypertension is more common in men than in women. Because the rate of increase in blood pressure with age is higher for women than for men, by the seventies, hypertension is more common in women than in men (He and Whelton, 1997). Prevalence also varies with ethnic group. Among women, for example, the age-adjusted prevalence of hypertension in the Third National Health and Nutrition Examination Survey (NHANES III, Phase I, 1988–1991) was 31 percent for African Americans, 21 percent for whites, and 21.6 percent for Mexican Americans (Burt and others, 1995).

The health consequences of hypertension are protean. High blood pressure can lead to coronary artery disease, left ventricular hypertrophy, congestive heart failure, cerebrovascular disease such as stroke or transient ischemic attack, nephropathy, peripheral arterial disease, and retinopathy (National High Blood Pressure Education Program, 1997). Concomitant factors such as diabetes mellitus, hyperlipidemia, and smoking add to the risk of cardiovascular disease. The prevalence of these comorbidities varies widely, depending on socioeconomic status and country of origin, further complicating population-based policy decisions about whether and how aggressively to treat hypertension in ethnic groups.

Fortunately, hypertension is a modifiable risk factor for disease; treatment improves mortality and morbidity. Prevention or treatment of hypertension reduces the incidence of cardiovascular disease and stroke (He and Whelton, 1997). Treatment of hypertension with angiotensin-converting enzyme inhibitors slows the progression of renal failure and congestive heart failure (Giatras, Lau, and Levey, 1997). Nondihydropyridine calcium antagonists may also prevent or slow deterioration of renal function in diabetics (Bakris and White, 1997).

# Role of Ethnicity in Hypertension Control and Impact

Although treatment of hypertension is efficacious, blood pressure control remains suboptimal. The percentage of Americans who were aware of their hypertension increased from 51 percent in the mid-1970s to 73 percent in the late 1980s, and the percentage whose blood pressure was adequately controlled increased from 10 to 55 percent. This improvement may have peaked, despite increased efforts by the National High Blood Pressure Education Program to increase provider and public awareness of hypertension and its consequences; in Phase 2 of the NHANES III survey (1991–1994), these percentages dropped slightly to 68.4 percent and 27.4 percent, respectively (National High Blood Pressure Education Program, 1997).

There are gender and racial disparities in awareness and control as well. African American women have the greatest degree of awareness and control—nearly 80 percent and 30 percent, respectively; Hispanic men have the lowest percentages—approximately 45 percent and 10 percent, respectively (Burt and others, 1995). Among Spanish-speaking populations, there is further disparity between levels of control. In the Hispanic Health and Nutrition Examination Survey (HHANES), fewer than 10 percent of Hispanic men, regardless of country of origin, had their blood pressure under control. Among the women, degree of control was quite variable: 34 percent for Mexican Americans, 14 percent for Cuban Americans, and 28 percent for Puerto Ricans (Crespo, Loria, and Burt, 1996). Less is known about hypertension in Asian and Pacific Islander Americans. Although the overall prevalence of hypertension in Asian Americans appears to be lower than other groups, there are ethnic differences within this population; one study documented higher rates of hypertension in Californians of Filipino origin than in those from Japan or China (Klatsky and Armstrong, 1991).

Degree of acculturation, socioeconomic status (SES), and education may also influence the prevalence of hypertension, its control, and its impact. For example, higher education and SES were associated with lower blood pressure in Mexican American women living in San Antonio (Hazuda, 1996). In a follow-up of the Multiple Risk Factor Intervention Trial, degree of blood pressure control and income also were found to account for a large proportion of the excess risk of end-stage renal disease in hypertensive African American men (Klag and others, 1997). In addition, SES has been found to account for much of the difference in functional consequences (although not the prevalence) of hypertension and other chronic diseases when Hispanic and African American populations were compared to whites (Kington and Smith, 1997). Not surprisingly, there is a consensus that improvements in hypertension awareness and treatment adherence in populations of lower socioeconomic status will necessitate more focused and intensive educational programs (National High Blood Pressure Education Program, 1997).

## Implications for Patient Care

Hypertension cannot be evaluated alone; both severity of blood pressure and the presence of comorbidities and other risk factors such as age together determine the nature of treatment. From the public health perspective, a population may show relatively low levels of hypertension, but if other comorbidities have a higher prevalence, aggressive blood pressure control may still be warranted. For example, although prevalence of hypertension in Hispanics as a group is approximately the same as that of whites, there is a much higher prevalence of type 2 diabetes mellitus and obesity (National High Blood Pressure Education Program, 1997). When dealing with the individual patient, such comorbidities may make achieving optimal health difficult. The presence of diabetes, in particular, warrants aggressive therapy of hypertension, yet the patient may not understand why medications are necessary when the blood pressure is only modestly elevated. In addition, the presence of these comorbidities may reflect a lifetime of inactivity and poor dietary habits. Such habits are hard to break, yet lifestyle modification plays an essential role in treatment, and the patient's inability to make significant changes can become a source of friction with the provider.

Regardless of ethnic group or gender, lifestyle modification is essential to effective control of hypertension and treatment of many other cardiovascular risk factors. JNC VI recommends the following: (1) weight loss for overweight patients, (2) limited alcohol intake, (3) increased physical activity, (4) reduced sodium intake and adequate intake of dietary potassium, calcium and magnesium, (5) smoking cessation, and (6) reduced intake of saturated fats and cholesterol (National High Blood Pressure Education Program, 1997).

Patients may use herbal remedies for hypertension, or they may ingest other herbs or supplements that can elevate blood pressure. It is unrealistic for clinicians to know the content and effects of all of these remedies, but they should take a thorough history to determine what patients are using. Resources are available for clinicians to determine the hemodynamic impact of herbs and other alternative remedies (Eisenberg, 1997).

Studies have documented ethnic differences in response to antihypertensive therapy (Hui and Pasic, 1997; National High Blood Pressure Education Program, 1997), and clinicians often choose medications based on these data. However, the presence of target organ damage and concomitant risk factors are far more important in determining the choice of agent (Jamerson and DeQuattro, 1996). The JNC VI guidelines are sensitive to the needs of different ethnic groups, and they remain the most thorough and research-based recommendations available (National High Blood Pressure Education Program, 1997).

Several years ago, the National Heart, Lung and Blood Institute held a two-day workshop entitled, "Epidemiology of Hypertension in Hispanic Americans, Native Americans, and Asian/Pacific Islander Americans." In their summary of the workshop, Havas and Sherwin (1996) urged that data collection be repeated, systematic, and standardized. In addition, they called for nationwide efforts to improve hypertension awareness and control.

# Diabetes Mellitus

*Elizabeth J. Kramer and William B. Bateman*

Diabetes is widely prevalent among a number of ethnic groups, and, although scant, there is some evidence that incidence increases among immigrants as they acculturate to an American lifestyle. Among new immigrant populations, the disease is particularly prevalent among Hispanics. Puerto Rican and Mexican American adults have rates of diabetes that are approximately twice those of non-Hispanic whites. Further, the age-adjusted prevalence of overweight among Hispanic women is 37 percent for Puerto Ricans, 39 percent for Mexican Americans, and 34 percent for Cuban Americans, compared with 24 percent for non-Hispanic whites (National Coalition of Hispanic Health and Human Services Organizations, 1995).

The high prevalence of diabetes among Hispanics is of sufficiently great concern that the U.S. Department of Health and Human Services established the following objectives for that population group in Healthy People 2000:

1. To reduce diabetes among Puerto Ricans to a prevalence of no more than 49 per 1,000 from a baseline of 55 per 1,000 aged twenty through seventy-four in 1982–1984
2. To reduce diabetes among Mexican Americans to a prevalence of no more than 49 per 1,000 from a baseline of 54 per 1,000 aged twenty through seventy-four in 1982–1984
3. To reduce diabetes among Cuban Americans to a prevalence of no more than 32 per 1,000 from a baseline of 36 per 1,000 aged twenty through seventy-four in 1982–1984

Progress has been less than optimal. The prevalence of diabetes among Mexican Americans increased from 54 per 1,000 in 1986 to 66 cases per 1,000 in 1994 (U.S. Department of Health and Human Services, 1997). The prevalence of overweight among Hispanic women ages twenty and older increased from 27 percent in 1985 to 33 percent in 1993. The target for the year 2000 is 25 percent (U.S. Department of Health and Human Services, 1997). For Mexican Americans, diabetes-related age-adjusted mortality remained just about constant, dropping to 55.6 from a baseline of 55.7.

In the Hispanic Health and Nutrition Examination Survey, Mexican American people with type 2 diabetes were found to have a high degree of truncal adiposity. They also have an increased risk of diabetic retinopathy, particularly the severe forms. Among Puerto Ricans, the rate of diabetes rose from 42.0 to 57.8. Part of this increase is a reflection of better reporting of Hispanic origin on death certificates in New York City, where the majority of mainland Puerto Ricans live (U.S. Department of Health and Human Services, 1996). The year 2000 goal for individuals with diabetes to attend classes in management of their condition is 75 percent. In 1994, 26 percent of diabetics received such education (U.S. Department of Health and Human Services, 1996).

Healthy People 2000 identified an objective for reducing the prevalence of diabetes among blacks, which includes many African, South American, and Caribbean islander immigrants, to a rate of 32 per 1,000 from a baseline prevalence of 36 per 1,000 blacks of all ages in 1987. Although the percentage of blacks who attended diabetes educational programs increased from 34 percent in 1991 to 50 percent in 1994, mortality from diabetes increased from 67 per 100,000 in 1986 to 73 in 1994 (U.S. Department of Health and Human Services, 1996). Over the past three decades, diabetes and other chronic disorders have emerged as the major causes of adult morbidity and mortality in the Caribbean Islands (Mahabir and Gulliford, 1997).

Healthy People 2000 does not provide diabetes objectives for Asian immigrants, who numbered nearly 7 million from more than twenty population groups in the 1990 census, and whose numbers are growing. However, a survey of second-generation Japanese Americans in Seattle who were between the ages of forty-five and seventy-four found that 20 percent of men and 16 percent of women were diabetic, compared to 12 percent and 14 percent, respectively, for Caucasians of similar age and 5 percent and 4 percent, respectively, for residents of Tokyo. A comparison of physical characteristics of Japanese women in the United States and in Japan shows that U.S.-born women were heavier and taller than native Japanese women. Weight gain is a powerful risk factor for diseases such as type 2 diabetes, coronary heart disease, and hypertension, and it appears to be associated with urbanization and Westernization for this as well as other ethnic groups. Asians constitute an ethnic group that seems to be especially at risk. This may be due to the presence of the "thrifty" genotype, which leads to the concentration of weight gain in visceral fat deposits in susceptible populations and is postulated to be related to populations who have survived for generations with inadequate food supplies. That, in turn, is associated with insulin resistance, hyperinsulinemia, and dyslipidemia, all risk factors for type 2 diabetes and cardiovascular disease (Fujomoto and others, 1995).

## Use of Traditional Medicines in Immigrant Populations

In cultures other than our own, treatment of diabetes usually consists of a mixture of traditional treatment and Western medicine. This section discusses the use of traditional medicine among Chinese, Latinas, and Caribbean blacks.

### Chinese

In a comparative study of Chinese Canadian and European Canadian women in Canada, more than 80 percent of the Chinese Canadian women, all of whom were using Western biomedical treatments, believed that herbs such as ginseng are useful in the management of diabetes and had used or were using them. However, none of the women used traditional remedies to replace Western biomedical treatments. Of significant interest, 86 percent of the women discontinued or said they would discontinue taking the traditional remedies if their physicians directed them to do so.

The quality of the relationship a woman reported having with her health care provider, support from family and friends, and biomedical knowledge were the key variables in daily management of the disease. Knowledge depended on the patient's ability to access resources, which was dependent on language skills; 83 percent of the Chinese Canadian women spoke only Cantonese, whereas all of the European Canadians were fluent in English. The majority (73 percent) of the Chinese Canadian women reported that they did not find instructions for such things as regulating diet, administering medication, and monitoring blood sugar clear (Anderson and others, 1995).

The Chinese use many herbs and decoctions. Frequently neither providers nor patients know what they actually contain, especially those that come from China.

## Latinas

Some Latinas attempt to control diabetes with folk remedies such as a shake consisting of radishes and cactus, and a tea made from coconut root (Gordon, 1994). Aloe and garlic are other popular remedies. These vegetable-based remedies are not thought to be harmful. As a result of high retention of ethnic identity, Mexican Americans may exhibit traditional health beliefs and practices, and they are likely to engage the services of folk healers (Zaldivar and Smolowitz, 1994).

## Caribbean Blacks

In a study of 204 men and 418 women in Trinidad and Tobago, 264 (42 percent) reported using bush medicine (herbal remedies from medicinal plants) to treat their diabetes; of those, 41 percent (107) used them at least weekly. Use was more frequent among African Trinidadians and persons of mixed ethnicity than among Indo-Trinidadians. This practice reflected an informal pattern of self-care that rarely involved practitioners of folk medicine and prevailed despite a relatively advanced health care system that includes universal access to free prescription pharmaceuticals. The choice of remedies was influenced by patients' ethnic group and educational attainment.

The study in Trinidad and Tobago documented that the plants used to treat diabetes, at least in Caribbean Islanders, may have significant hypoglycemic effects. Preparations from medicinal plants also may have toxic side effects, and patients who use bush medicines may modify their use of and responses to formal treatments. Mahabir and Gulliford (1997) suggest that use of bush medicines is influenced by the patient's type of symptoms and the type of formal treatment he or she is receiving.

## A Pilot Study Relating to Diabetes in Chinese Immigrants

The Chinese language contains two words for diabetes: the traditional medical name is *xiao-ke*, which means, "wasting and thirsting," and the modern term, *tang-neo bing*, which means "sugar urine illness." Discussion of diabetes by its traditional name appears in all the earliest texts, including the *Nei Jing*, a classical Chinese medical text. Traditionally it is divided into three types—upper, middle, and lower—each of which corresponds to a disproportionate emphasis on the three main symptoms: thirst, hunger, and excessive urination. Deficient yin usually is associated with all three types. However, a traditional diagnosis of "wasting and thirsting" may include illnesses other than the modern entity of diabetes. The opposite also is true: someone with *tang-neo bing* would not necessarily have *xiao-ke*. Traditional Chinese medicine does not acknowledge the existence of the pancreas (Kaptchuk, 1983).

We work in a clinic where approximately 25 percent of the patients are first- and second-generation Chinese immigrants, and approximately 5 to 10 percent of them are illiterate. Although we do not have good numerator data, diabetes appears to be as prevalent in our Chinese patients as it is in the rest of our multiethnic patient population, of whom 55 percent are Latino. There is a dearth of culturally competent, language-specific educational materials for this group.

As a first step to developing a comprehensive educational program for Chinese immigrants, we conducted a small pilot study, which consisted of interviews with a convenience sample of thirty patients with the diagnosis of type 2 diabetes who attend our general medical clinic, thirty additional patients who do not have diabetes, and a focus group of Chinese American health care providers with whom we work. An interpreter was used for the interviews. The purpose of the study was to develop greater insight into the knowledge, attitudes, beliefs, and health care practices of this population with regard to their diabetes.

Patients and members of the nondiabetic comparison group were asked a series of questions relating to the definition of diabetes, its etiology, symptoms, side effects, treatment, and dietary modification. In addition, this group was asked whether they knew anyone who had diabetes. Health care professionals were asked what in their experience requires special attention when teaching Chinese Americans about diabetes.

Nearly one-third of the patients, and an equal proportion of comparison group members, did not know what diabetes is or what causes it, much less how it should be treated. Although some mentioned that sugar and starch should be restricted, the lay groups surveyed knew little about the disease and its management. What they seemed to know most about were the complications.

The professional group corroborated these responses, listing diet, exercise, blood glucose monitoring, and complications as major problem areas that need to be addressed. They further informed us that available materials and the dietitian are not helpful because of language problems. Colleagues expressed serious concern over their patients' health care practices, particularly the use of herbs, which may be purchased in pharmacies or herbal shops in Chinatown, brought back from China by relatives or friends, and sometimes obtained through the mail. Concern focused on two issues: not knowing what the herbal remedies contained and the fact that some patients with symptoms of non-insulin-dependent diabetes mellitus try herbal remedies before they seek Western medical care.

## Conclusion and Recommendations

There is a strong need for culturally competent, culture-specific educational materials about diabetes for patients. Videotapes and audiotapes probably will be more helpful than printed materials, although posters might be another way to approach the content. In addition, health care providers must work closely with patients, adapting therapeutic regimens to the beliefs and practices of the patients with whom they work. For example, nutritionists and dietitians should adapt the traditional Chinese diet to one that is suitable for diabetics, rather than expecting Chinese patients to accept a Western diet. Providers can counsel patients to eat more vegetables and less rice and to cut back on other potentially harmful foods. Since women usually prepare the meals for their families, they also can be taught that a healthy diabetic diet is a healthy diet for the entire family.

Patients must be strongly cautioned about the use of herbal preparations and decoctions, particularly if they are taking prescription medication for their diabetes or other conditions. Insulin-dependent diabetics and those who are taking oral hypoglycemic agents should be strongly advised not to stop their allopathic medication and to report the use of any unprescribed medications to their health care providers.

Educational materials for Latinos should be customized to incorporate the mores of the particular culture from which patients originate, and these materials should be evaluated, comparing them to the commonly used translations of materials designed for fully acculturated Americans. Visual materials may be extremely helpful, along with targeted media messages that use celebrity spokespersons or otherwise provide *personalismo* (Perez-Stable, VanOss Marin, and Marin, 1993). Health care costs are two to three times greater for people with diabetes than the average for the total population. The American Diabetes Association estimates that the total cost of diabetes in the United States is $92 billion. These astounding costs, combined with the high prevalence of the disease in rapidly growing immigrant groups, points to the need for public health primary prevention education campaigns about diabetes and its risk factors. These, too, must be culture and language specific.

# Breast and Cervical Cancer

*Barbara A. Wismer*

Periodic screening of women for early detection of breast and cervical cancer is recommended by the U.S. Preventive Services Task Force (1996). Early detection can reduce breast cancer mortality by up to 30 percent and cervical cancer mortality 20 to 60 percent. Mammography, with or without clinical breast examination (CBE), is recommended for women aged fifty to sixty-nine, every one to two years. Data about whether women between the ages of forty and forty-nine who are of average risk should be screened are conflicting (Harris and Leininger, 1995). Although there is insufficient evidence, there are other grounds for screening high-risk women under age fifty and healthy women aged seventy and older. More specific recommendations for immigrant women have not been made, although being born in Northern Europe or North America is a strong risk factor for breast cancer (Kelsey, 1993).

Papanicolaou (Pap) testing is recommended at least every three years for all women who have a cervix and have been sexually active (U.S. Preventive Services Task Force, 1996). Although the evidence is insufficient, there are other grounds for discontinuing testing after age sixty-five in those women who have had regular testing that has always been normal.

Healthy People 2000 health promotion and disease prevention objectives for the nation are for at least 80 percent of women aged forty and older to have a mammogram and CBE; 60 percent of women aged fifty and older to have them in the past one to two years; 95 percent of women aged eighteen and older with an intact cervix to have a Pap test; and 85 percent to have one in the past one to three years (U.S. Department of Health and Human Services, 1990). Latina women are one of the special target populations for these tests.

## Incidence and Mortality Rates

Little is known about the incidence and mortality rates of breast and cervical cancer among immigrant women in the United States. Some national data are available on Latina and API women, the racial and ethnic minorities that comprise a large proportion of the population of immigrant women and are largely composed of immigrant women. In general, breast and cervical cancer are important causes of death for these groups of women, although mortality rates are lower than those of white women (Truman, Wing, and Keenan, 1994; Keenan, Murray, and Truman, 1994).

In California, where a large proportion of the Latina and API populations reside, breast cancer was the most common cancer for both of these groups, even though average age-adjusted invasive breast cancer incidence and mortality rates from 1989 to 1993 were significantly lower for Hispanic and "Asian/Other" women compared with white women (Perkins, Morris, and Wright, 1996). Cervical cancer incidence and mortality were significantly higher for "Hispanic" and "Asian/Other" women. (See Table 9.5.)

**Table 9.5.  Average Annual Age-Adjusted Breast and Cervical Cancer Rates per 100,000 Women, California, 1989–1993.**

|  | Invasive Breast Cancer | | Cervical Cancer | |
|  | Incidence | Mortality | Incidence | Mortality |
| --- | --- | --- | --- | --- |
| Asians/others | 61 | 13 | 11.8 | 3.3 |
| Blacks | 96 | 32 | 11.8 | 5.0 |
| Hispanics | 68 | 18 | 17.3 | 4.2 |
| Whites | 117 | 27 | 7.3 | 2.1 |

Note: Age adjusted to 1970 U.S. standard population.

Source: Perkins, Morris, and Wright, 1996.

Within API subgroups, there is evidence to suggest that breast cancer incidence varies by recency of immigration, with higher rates in successive generations of women (Kelsey and Horn-Ross, 1993). Rates also vary significantly among API subgroups (Perkins, Morris, Wright, and Young, 1995). From 1988 to 1992, breast cancer incidence rates were higher for Japanese and Filipino and lower for Chinese, Southeast Asian, and Korean American women, compared with all "Asian/Other" women. Cervical cancer incidence rates were higher for Southeast Asian and lower for Chinese and Japanese American women.

## Screening Estimates

Information about breast and cervical cancer screening behaviors of immigrant women generally is not available. National surveys suggest that variation in screening practices by race and ethnicity has decreased over time (Martin, Calle, Wingo, and Heath, 1996). In California, the 1993 and 1994 Behavioral Risk Factor Surveys (BRFS) revealed that "Hispanic" and "Asian/Other" women were less likely than white women to have mammography (Davis, 1996). (See Table 9.6.) In Hawaii, the 1993 survey revealed that Filipino and Hawaiian women were significantly less likely than white or

### Table 9.6. Women Age Fifty and Older Reporting Mammogram, California, 1993–1994 (N = 1,188).

|  | Mammogram Ever (%) | Mammogram Within Past Two Years (%) |
|---|---|---|
| Asians/other | 68.3 | 56.6 |
| Blacks | 89.9 | 80.1 |
| Hispanics | 76.2 | 65.8 |
| Whites | 87.4 | 76.3 |

*Note:* Weighted to the age distribution of the 1990 Census California population.

*Source:* Davis, 1996.

Japanese women to have mammography, and Filipino women were significantly less likely than white women to have Pap testing (Hawaii, 1996). (See Table 9.7.) In Florida, according to the unpublished 1996 BRFS, Hispanic women were less likely than white women to be tested. (See Table 9.8.)

These large surveys often do not sample adequate numbers of women from racial and ethnic minorities to allow for meaningful analysis. Also, because they are conducted in English, only occasionally in Spanish, and not at all in other languages, these surveys tend to exclude recent immigrants, who are less likely to speak English. Immigrant or racial and ethnic minority populations are challenging to study. This is in part because representative population-based sampling is difficult since there are relatively small numbers of immigrants in the general population, and surveys must be bi- or multilingual.

Studies of populations that include large proportions of immigrants, and that are population based and include bilingual surveys, reveal low rates of screening compared with predominantly white populations and, within these populations, lower rates of screening among first-generation immigrants. Several

### Table 9.7. Women Reporting Mammogram or Pap Test, Behavioral Risk Factor Survey, Hawaii, 1993.

|  | Mammogram Ever (%) (n = 1,223) | Pap Smear Ever (%)[a] (n = 1,017) |
|---|---|---|
| Filipinos | 44 | 77 |
| Hawaiians | 46 | 95 |
| Japanese | 63 | 93 |
| Others | 51 | 93 |
| Whites | 57 | 98 |

Data for Pap smear weighted to the gender, age, and race distribution of 1990 Census Hawaii population.

[a] Women without a hysterectomy only.

**Table 9.8. Women Reporting
Mammogram or Pap Test, Behavioral
Risk Factor Survey, Florida, 1996.**

|  | Mammogram Plus Clinical Breast Examination Ever (%)[a] (n = 1,223) | Pap Smear Ever (%)[b] (n = 1,513) |
|---|---|---|
| Blacks | 76.1 | 89.9 |
| Hispanics | 75.7 | 84.9 |
| Others | 78.1 | 86.6 |
| Whites | 81.2 | 96.5 |

*Note:* Weighted data. Data unpublished.

[a] Women age forty and older only.

[b] Women without a hysterectomy only.

surveys have been conducted in California. One that was completed in 1994 revealed that Latina, Chinese, and Vietnamese American women, most of whom were born outside the United States, were significantly less likely than a comparison group of white women to ever or recently have mammography, CBE, or Pap testing (Hiatt and others, 1996). In another 1994 survey, Korean American women, most of whom were born in Korea, had lower rates of testing than women of all races and ethnicities (Kang and others, 1997). A 1993 survey of Latina women revealed that first-generation immigrants, most of whom were born in Mexico, were significantly less likely to ever have had a Pap test than U.S.-born Latinas or white women (Hubbell, Chavez, Mishra, and Valdez, 1996a). On the East Coast, a study in the early 1980s of black women in Brooklyn, most of whom were born in the Caribbean, revealed that those born outside the United States were less likely to ever have a Pap test (Fruchter and others, 1985). The generalizability of this study may be limited because the sample consisted of women who were participating in a screening program.

# Screening Behaviors of Immigrant Women

Immigrant women have unique cultural, linguistic, and financial factors, which may vary by country of origin, that may contribute to lower use of testing (Gany and Thiel-deBocanegra, 1996). They also may have different levels of knowledge and types of attitudes about cancer and screening. For example, they may rely on traditional medicine, or they may not have preventive health orientations. Many do not speak English well, if at all. Immigrants often work long hours, have low incomes, and lack health insurance. The relative importance of these and other factors is not known and seems to vary among racial and ethnic groups.

Several studies of Latinas, most of whom were born in Mexico, have investigated correlates of breast and cervical cancer screening. One study in Texas found that women with less knowledge about breast and cervical cancer and screening were less likely to be tested (Suarez, Roche, Nichols, and Simpson, 1997). Women who were born in Mexico or did not speak English well in general had less knowledge. However, most measures of acculturation were not associated with breast and cervical cancer screening behaviors after controlling for sociodemographic and access factors, with one exception: those with Mexican family attitudes (extended family and male authority) were more likely to have had mammography (Suarez, 1994).

A study in California found differences in knowledge and attitudes about cervical cancer in Latina immigrants compared with U.S.-born Latinas and white women (Hubbell, Chavez, Mishra, and Valdez, 1996a). Immigrants were more likely to think of certain accepted factors (such as early onset of sexual intercourse) and unaccepted factors (such as abortion) as risks. They were less likely to know that other accepted factors (such as family history) were risks. They also had different attitudes. Compared with white women, knowledge and attitudes were more often associated with lack of Pap testing for Latinas, even after controlling for sociodemographic, access, acculturation, and other knowledge and attitude characteristics. Paradoxically, Latinas who correctly knew that cervical cancer was associated with various aspects of sexual behavior were less likely to be screened. Therefore, the authors suggested that since sexual activity may be a private and sensitive topic, attempts to improve screening behavior should not emphasize that cervical cancer is a sexually transmitted disease. These Latinas also were less knowledgeable and had less favorable attitudes about breast cancer (for example, preferring not to know if they had breast cancer, being afraid to tell their husbands if they had breast cancer, and needing a mammogram only for a lump) than white women (Hubbell, Chavez, Mishra, and Valdez, 1996b). Among Latinas, acculturation was an independent correlate of these types of knowledge and attitudes.

A study of Vietnamese American women, many of whom were first-generation immigrants, suggested that sociodemographic and acculturation factors were more important correlates of breast and cervical cancer screening than attitudes and beliefs or access (McPhee and others, 1997). Women age forty and older who had less education or had immigrated more recently were less likely to have had mammography in the past two years. Women who were younger or older, never married, had less education, immigrated more recently, had no regular doctor, or had a Vietnamese doctor were less likely ever to have had a Pap test. The authors hypothesized that Vietnamese doctors may have less training in preventive medicine (most are trained in Vietnam), have less time for screening tests (many see patients on a drop-in basis), or be more sensitive to women's personal modesty. Cancer fear, fatalism, and Eastern orientation were not associated with receipt of either test. The most frequently cited reasons for not having the tests were not needing the test if healthy, worry about cost, the test not being recommended by a doctor, and not having time.

A study of Korean American women in California, also predominantly foreign born, suggested that sociodemographic and access factors, more than knowledge and attitudes or acculturation, predicted screening (Wismer and others, 1998a, 1998b). Women age fifty and older who were either unmarried or not employed, had not had a recent routine checkup, or had cost as a barrier to health care were less likely to have recent mammography. Women who were either unmarried or not employed, older, had not had a recent routine checkup, had private or no health insurance, or had a transportation barrier were less likely to have a recent Pap test.

Neither cancer knowledge and attitudes nor proportion of life spent in the United States were related to testing.

Another study of a convenience sample of older Korean American women in California, all born in Korea, revealed that women were more likely to ever have a mammogram if their doctor recommended the test, they were comfortable asking for a mammogram, more friends or relatives had had one, or did not have a transportation difficulty (Maxwell, Bastani, and Warda, 1998). In general, knowledge, attitudes, and barriers did not vary with acculturation, except that traditional women were less likely to have a doctor recommend the test and more likely to have a transportation barrier.

A similar study of a convenience sample of older Filipino American women in California, all born in the Philippines, also showed that women were more likely ever to have a mammogram if their doctor recommended the test, they were comfortable asking for a mammogram, or they did not have a transportation difficulty (Maxwell, Bastani, and Warda, 1998). Filipino American women also were less likely to have the test if they believed that it was necessary only in the presence of symptoms. Traditional women were more likely to have this belief and less likely to be embarrassed about getting a mammogram. There were no other differences in knowledge, attitudes, or barriers with level of acculturation. The generalizability of these last two studies may be limited because results were based on convenience samples.

More research needs to be done to identify predictors of and barriers to screening, which may vary by immigrant group. Available data suggest that sociodemographic characteristics, level of acculturation, knowledge and attitudes, and access to health care may affect breast and cervical cancer screening behaviors of immigrant women. Programs to improve screening should address pertinent determinants of screening and be tailored to the unique cultural characteristics of the target population (Hiatt and others, 1996).

# Osteoporosis

*Eugenia L. Siegler and*
*Elizabeth J. Kramer*

Osteoporosis is a "disease characterized by low bone mass and microarchitectural deterioration of bone tissue, leading to enhanced bone fragility and a consequent increase in fracture risk" (Consensus Development Conference, 1991). How one defines osteoporosis clinically is somewhat more controversial. Before accurate means of measuring bone density were readily available, many defined osteoporosis by its end result, the development of nonviolent fractures. More recently, there is consensus that low bone mineral density itself establishes the diagnosis of osteoporosis (Ross, 1996).

The World Health Organization has defined three categories of bone loss, based on comparisons to bone mineral density of healthy adults thirty to forty years of age (Kanis and others, 1994). These cutoffs, shown in Table 9.9, were derived from studies of postmenopausal white women and may not be relevant to other ethnic groups (Raisz, 1997).

The prevalence of osteoporosis increases with age. Women are at higher risk for osteoporosis than men. Approximately one-third of women in their sixties are osteoporotic, and 70 percent over age eighty have osteoporosis. (Looker and others, 1995; Ross, 1996). Osteoporosis is a devastating disease because it increases the likelihood of disabling fractures. Although most lay and professional people are aware of the link between osteoporosis and fractures of the hip, the spine is the most common site, and wrist fractures also are common. More than half of all women in the United States can

## Table 9.9.  Bone Loss Categories.

| Category | Bone Mineral Density |
| --- | --- |
| Osteopenia (Low bone mass) | Between 1 and 2.5 standard deviations below the mean |
| Osteoporosis | More than 2.5 standard deviations below the mean |
| Severe osteoporosis (established) | More than 2.5 standard deviations below the mean with a history of nonviolent fracture |

*Note:* Healthy young adult as reference.

*Source:* Kanis and others, 1994.

be expected to fracture an osteoporotic bone in their lifetimes (Ross, 1996).

The incidence of hip fractures is three times greater in women than in men. Hip fractures are the most feared complication of osteoporosis because they result in an increased mortality rate two to five times that of an age- and sex-matched population, especially in the first year after the fracture (Ross, 1996). Half of those who sustain hip fractures lose their ability to walk independently (Marotolli, Berkman, and Cooney, 1992), and nearly 20 percent require long-term care (Chrischilles, Butler, Davis, and Wallace, 1991).

A single hip fracture can result in more than $20,000 in direct medical costs (U.S. Congress, Office of Technology Assessment, 1994). The total cost of osteoporosis and associated fractures in the mid-1990s was estimated to be between $10 and $12 billion (Lindsay, 1995). If the disease is not contained, these costs will continue to rise severalfold over the next few decades; the cost of hip fractures alone may be greater than $240 billion by the year 2040 (Lindsay, 1995).

Ethnicity influences a patient's risk for osteoporosis. Data from the third National Health and Nutrition Examination Survey (NHANES III, 1998–1991) document that white women have a higher prevalence of osteoporosis than do black women, but approximately the same prevalence as Mexican American women (Looker and others, 1995). Asian women also are at increased risk of osteoporosis, although there are controversies about bone mineral density measurement and standardization in this population (Tobias, Cook, Chambers, and Dalzell, 1994). Increased risk of osteoporosis does not correlate perfectly with increased fracture risk, which must also take risk for injury into account. For example, despite the overall decrease in bone density compared to white populations, Japanese have a lower incidence of hip fractures, probably secondary to a lower rate of falls or differences in hip geometry, or both (Ross, 1996).

Ethnicity is not the only determinant of osteoporosis risk. Because bone density peaks in the twenties (Recker and others, 1992), nutrition and exercise during the first few decades play a pivotal role in determining risk for osteoporosis (Heaney, 1987). This may be especially important in immigrant women, who may have endured years of financial hardship or nutritional deprivation when young. Many other risk factors have been described for osteoporosis (Dempster and Lindsay, 1993). The major ones are use of medications, such as corticosteroids, anticonvulsants, or excessive doses of thyroxin; estrogen deprivation from eating disorders, endocrine disorders, or early menopause; cigarette smoking; excessive alcohol use; and limited physical activity (Ross, 1996).

## Screening Considerations

There are several reasons to screen for osteoporosis: (1) lifestyle modifications can reduce the rate of bone loss, (2) pharmacologic therapies are available to improve bone density and reduce the rate of fractures, and (3) in individuals with established osteoporosis, reduction of the rate of falls or interventions designed to reduce injury from falls also may reduce the likelihood of fractures.

All screening begins with the history and physical examination. History should cover exposure to all of the major risk factors, as well as previous history of fracture and family history of osteoporosis. Clinicians should pay special attention to the patient's dietary and physical activity habits throughout life, especially youth and early twenties, to determine if the patient started her thirties with adequate bone density. The history offers an opportunity for education about adequate dietary calcium, vitamin D, and exercise. Physical examination can be useful to assess the patient's overall nutritional status and to search for bone loss as evidenced by dorsal kyphosis or documented loss of height.

The decision to offer bone mineral density testing to all peri- and postmenopausal women is controversial (Raisz, 1997); it is unrealistic to assume that it will be universally applied even in high-risk populations. Nonetheless, it can be an essential educational tool, especially for women at high risk for osteoporosis who lack motivation to treat it because they do not feel ill. Bone mineral density testing also is very useful to assess the effectiveness of treatment regimens; chemical markers of bone resorption may one day become more cost-effective and simpler tools to monitor therapy (Raisz, 1997).

## Prevention and Treatment

The mainstay of osteoporosis prevention and treatment is adequate calcium and vitamin D intake (Raisz, 1997). Counseling patients about adequate calcium intake requires sensitivity to dietary preferences, intolerances, and native cuisines. Lactose intolerance is common in African and Asian populations, and even with the advent of lactose-free milk, patients may have developed a learned aversion to milk products. Even within ethnic groups, calcium sources may differ widely. For example, corn tortillas are an important source of calcium for Mexican American women, but not for Cubans and Puerto Ricans (Looker and others, 1993). In general, women's dietary calcium intake is inadequate, regardless of age or ethnic group (Looker and others, 1993), and the clinician should be prepared to describe the advantages and disadvantages of calcium and vitamin D dietary supplements. The Osteoporosis and Related Bone Diseases National Resource Center has published fact sheets on the Internet for general use, as well as information directed specifically toward African American, Asian, and Hispanic women (Osteoporosis and Related Bone Diseases National Resource Center, 1998). The National Osteoporosis Foundation also has materials available in print and on the Internet (National Osteoporosis Foundation, 1998).

The clinician should counsel patients regarding exercise, emphasizing the need for weight-bearing activities. The importance of weight bearing may come as a surprise to patients, especially those who like to swim. For elderly patients with functional impairments, physical or occupational therapy may be helpful to reduce pain from osteoporotic fractures and the risk of falling.

Many medications are now available to treat and prevent osteoporosis (Raisz, 1997): estrogen, bisphophonates (alendronate is now also approved for prevention as well as treatment of osteoporosis), calcitonin, and selective estrogen receptor modulators, which appear to lack the carcinogenic effects of natural estrogens (Delmas and others, 1997). Fluoride has been used successfully, but is extremely difficult to dose, and not a first-line agent in the United States.

## The Future

In the next century, the potential functional and financial costs of osteoporosis are huge. Already, there are means of identifying and treating this disease. The Women's Health Initiative, a multimillion-dollar project sponsored by the National Heart, Lung and Blood Institute, will be an important source of new information about preventing osteoporosis through diet and hormone replacement therapy in different ethnic groups (Women's Health Initiative, 1997). It has three parts: (1) a randomized clinical trial of sixty-seven thousand postmenopausal women that examines hormone replacement therapy, dietary modification, and calcium/vitamin D supplementation; (2) an observational study that will examine the relationship between lifestyle and risk factors and disease outcomes in one hundred thousand women; and (3) a community prevention study, which will examine the effect of health programs that encourage women to adopt healthy lifestyles. The role of ethnicity will be studied in all three of these projects, and the information should assist practitioners in tailoring care to their patients' individual needs.

# Part Three

# Emotional, Psychosomatic, Behavioral, and Mental Health Problems

# Chapter Ten

# Domestic and
# Sexual Violence

# Domestic Violence

*Shobha Srinivasan*
*and Susan L. Ivey*

The family is a major source of protection and support for most people, particularly in times of crisis (Doherty and Campbell, 1988; Gurin, 1985). Unfortunately for some, however, it may be a source of stress, violence, and abuse (Straus and Gelles, 1988). Individuals are more likely to be abused physically and verbally within the confines of the family than anywhere else in society (Gelles and Cornell, 1990). Estimates are that one out of four women in the United States will experience violence at the hands of her household partner during her lifetime (Schornstein, 1997).

Domestic violence is defined as any violence within the patient-defined family—physical, sexual, verbal, and psychological—that poses a threat to a woman's mental and physical well-being. Most studies of domestic violence focus on wife/spouse/partner abuse. However, in-laws also may play a significant role, as in the case of wife abuse and bride burning in India (Fernandez, 1997). Therefore, the definition of domestic violence needs to include abuse by all family members. In addition, accidental injuries that occur in the course of nonphysical events (such as a quarrel) must be considered in the context of abuse. Injuries resulting from pushing, shoving, or holding, even if there was no intent to injure, may indicate a potentially violent household. For immigrant women, legal or civil rights violations, which may range from withholding a passport to coercive threats, including turning someone in to the Immigration and Naturalization Service, may signal a woman's lack of control in a relationship and can be considered a form of non-physical abuse.

Women's organizations, health care professionals, and international organizations, such as the United Nations, have shifted the debate on domestic violence to a public arena, arguing that violence in the family has psychological, physical, health, and social consequences not only for the woman, but for other family members as well.

In general, there are not enough services that effectively address the full range of problems associated with domestic violence. The situation is worse for immigrant and refugee women because of their unique psychosocial and cultural needs. Available services must become more culturally competent in order to be effective resources for immigrant women. Health care practitioners need to be especially sensitive to both the presentation and the needs of immigrant women who may have been abused.

## Prevalence of Violence

While the status of women may be lower in many other countries, U.S. society is particularly violent (Acierno, Resnick, and Kilpatrick, 1997). Most studies have found that domestic violence cuts across racial and ethnic lines, varies by socioeconomic status of the partner, and is linked with alcohol use (Bachman and Saltzman, 1994; Acierno, Resnick, and Kilpatrick, 1997; Barnett and Fagan, 1993). Unfortunately, reliable prevalence rates of domestic violence in immigrant and refugee women are unavailable. The National Crime and Victimization Survey indicates that women of all races and ethnic groups are about equally vulnerable to attacks by intimate partners (U.S. Department of Justice, 1995). It is estimated that 5 to 10 percent of women who present to emergency departments are recent victims of domestic violence (Abbott and others, 1995).

Anecdotal data make comparisons or generalizations extremely difficult. For example, the significant increase in the number of shelters that serve API women either suggests an increasing prevalence of domestic violence in this population (Abraham, 1995; Kanuha, 1994) or reflects the growing API population (U.S. Bureau of the Census, 1994). Nonetheless, shelter providers and clinicians have argued that the prevalence of domestic violence is likely to be higher in immigrant and refugee communities due to migration-related stressors, the redefinition of familial roles, frustrations in seeking employment, the loss of status associated with downward mobility, and the resulting shame and loss of face.

## Obstacles to Obtaining Care

The U.S. Bureau of Population, Refugees, and Migration (1997) notes that refugee women are vulnerable to violence, such as threats, assault, and rape, at every stage of their flight, and this is compounded by violence within the family. As a result, these women suffer from high rates of posttraumatic stress disorder and depression (Frye and D'Avanzo, 1994; Chung and Kagawa-Singer, 1993). Inability to communicate with service providers, fear of discrimination, and cultural norms that prescribe self-sacrifice and modesty about their bodies (True and Guillermo, 1996; Luluquisen, Groessl, and Puttkammer, 1995), compounded by lack of understanding of Western medicine, ignorance of their medical and legal rights, and fear that seeking government assistance may lead to deportation (Mayeno and Hirota, 1994) impede their ability to obtain help. Help seeking may be intimidating for women in lesbian relationships, because of the censure that exists regarding homosexual practices (Marin, 1997; Kanuha, 1990). In addition, managed care systems may not allow sufficient time for interaction between health care practitioners and patients, making establishment of rapport and elucidation of a history even more difficult. Health care providers and the health care system must be especially culturally sensitive to victims who do seek help (Campbell and Campbell, 1996; True and Guillermo, 1996).

## Culture, Gender Roles, and Meanings of Abuse

It has been argued that asking women about domestic abuse is in itself an intervention (Heise, 1994). Studies have indicated that the identification of domestic violence is higher if women are explicitly asked whether they are being abused (Olson and others, 1996; Quillian, 1996; Poirier, 1997). However, whether this is true for immigrant women is unknown. Most immigrant and refugee women from Asia, Africa, and Latin America are from traditional societies with restrictive gender roles (Chin, 1994; Song-Kim, 1992). Traditional gender role socialization allows men to criticize, chastise, and strike women for whom they have responsibility (Yim, 1978). This is considered acceptable behavior in those cultures. Immigrant and refugee women sometimes live in larger households where resources are shared by extended family members. In these cases, the perpetrator may be an older male sibling, or an adult who serves as guardian and has the power and control or is the main economic provider in the family. Thus, in response to a pointed closed-ended question from an interviewer such as, "Were you beaten by your spouse?" a respondent might answer no since the perpetrator of violence was not her spouse but someone else in the household, whom she feels she cannot betray. Women who are beaten and shouted at may not recognize their experiences as abuse.

Although there are literal translations for the word *abuse* or *assault* in some languages, it may not be used in relation to domestic violence. Women may use other terms to describe their experiences of abuse and battering (Marin, 1997).

## Role of Tradition

In contrast to Western culture, which highly values individualism, immigrant and refugee women often come from traditional cultures, where a woman seldom is given any private, individual space. Immigrants from Africa, Asia, and Latin America often live with their extended families and extended kinship networks, where the family's well-being takes precedence over an individual's rights (Pereira, 1997). Women especially are socialized to be self-sacrificing and to consider the rights of the family as a whole over their own.

The probability that an immigrant or refugee woman will disclose an experience of violence often is minimized when the abuser accompanies her wherever she goes because of religious principles or traditions, not allowing her to move freely in public, treating her as though she is shy and wary, or even providing translation services for her benefit. In such situations, neither the health care provider nor the patient is likely to be able to discuss possibilities of abuse.

In addition, immigrant and refugee women who are socialized in traditional gender roles may not be willing to confide their problems to male health care practitioners or to people outside their own race or ethnic group. It is highly inappropriate to ask the family member who accompanies the woman whether there is abuse in the family; that is tantamount to asking the husband whether he abuses his wife.

## Legal Barriers

Immigrant and refugee women may not want to disclose that they are living with violence at home when their immigrant status is dependent on their marriage (Takagi, 1991; Narayan, 1997). Many immigrants are not aware that the Violence Against Women Act (1994) allows victims of domestic violence, even if undocumented, to seek lawful permanent residence status through self-petitioning or suspension of deportation. A memorandum issued by the Immigration and Naturalization Service (Orloff and Kelly, 1995) allows women to seek political asylum in the United States for problems related to gender persecution (Orloff and Kelly, 1995; Schornstein, 1997), although providing proof of the need for asylum often is a cumbersome and involved process (Schornstein, 1997). Immigrant women may recognize the inconsistencies between recent legal provisions and the general tone of the national discourse on immigration reform and therefore may not reveal their victimization due to fear of deportation. Barriers to accessing resources, which may have increased with welfare and immigration reform, may deny immigrant women an opportunity for identification, protection, and possible asylum.

## Western Model of Services

The Western model of intervention is individually oriented. Immigrants from Asia, Africa, and Latin America have a strong familial and collective sense of self (Hsu, 1985). The individually oriented method of interceding in cases of domestic violence usually is to provide choices that encourage women to leave the abusive situation. However, making that choice implies having viable options for a better life and knowledge of the consequences of those choices. For a woman who is socialized into the traditional ideals of being a good wife and mother, which include the sacrifice of personal freedom and autonomy, leaving her husband and family often is not a viable option (Agger, 1992; Dasgupta and Warrier, 1996). Issues of shame and embarrassment add to the reticence of both patient and provider in broaching the subject of domestic violence. Women also fear retaliation and increased abuse if they attempt to disclose the violence or leave the abusive situation, adding to the difficulty in eliciting a history of abuse.

Marriage brings many immigrant and refugee women a certain social standing and acceptance in their own ethnic or cultural milieu. Divorce and separation are not viewed positively, even if women are attempting to leave abusive situations. Further, many immigrant women do not have extramarital support systems. If a woman chooses to leave with her children, she must learn to negotiate the system to acquire housing, employment, and child care, tasks for which she is often ill prepared, especially in an alien society and culture.

Given the role and importance of the family and social networks for immigrant and refugee women, a more effective model of intervention and prevention needs to encompass the client-defined family. Unfortunately, this may be difficult given the structure of medical insurance and benefits; most insurance coverage targets the individual and does not include a client- or patient-defined family.

Although abused women suffer from mental health problems, such as depression and posttraumatic stress disorder (Houskamp and Foy, 1991; Cascardi and O'Leary, 1992), they may be reluctant to seek assistance due to feelings of shame and guilt (Crites, 1987, 1991). They may approach the health care practitioner only after they have failed in their efforts to elicit the support of other family members or community and religious leaders.

Some have discussed the negative attitude of health care institutions and providers toward victims of domestic violence (Kanuha, 1994). Women who do not leave their abusive situations are viewed as passive by U.S. health care providers. These women believe that breaking up the family is neither economically nor socially beneficial for themselves or their children (Browne, 1993), and their familial and collective sense of belonging precludes them from leaving the abusive situation. Thus, their so-called inaction or passivity is in fact a survival tactic in which the women are trying to do the best for their families, even at the risk of continued abuse.

## Consequences of Mandatory Reporting

Certain states require health practitioners to report suspected cases of domestic violence, and there may be penalties for failure to do so (Hyman, Schillinger, and Lo, 1995). Although mandatory reporting to law enforcement has been common for injuries resulting from or related to firearms or other dangerous weapons, extending it to suspected abuse of adult women may undermine basic principles of patient autonomy in decision making. Although it might seem that mandatory reporting would lead to recognition and criminalization of domestic violence, thereby punishing the abuser, the criminal justice system has little, if any, way to protect women from the repetitive behavior of their abusers without permanent incarceration of perpetrators. Negative repercussions, such as the threat or occurrence of retaliatory violence (Hart, 1993), may further discourage abused women from revealing domestic violence to health care providers (Hyman, Schillinger, and Lo, 1995).

Even after health care professionals report a case to local authorities, the woman may not perceive herself as being abused. Many immigrant and refugee women come from war-torn areas where they have witnessed political, economic, and social strife. They mistrust government and its various arms, so the consequences of the reporting (such as visits from police) and the perceived threat of deportation may result in more tension within the family, and possibly more abuse of the women. If men who are not lawful residents are deported as a result of reporting through this mandate, women must face the added burden of breaking up their families and sharing the custody of the children across international lines (Crites, 1987). In the light of these potential consequences, it is important that the decision to make a report to the police or governmental authorities be made by the woman.

Women must be given sufficient time, resources, support, and information about available legal protections in order to reassure them that disclosure of violence to health personnel will be confidential, will be directed toward the woman's safety, and will facilitate communication with police when they deem that an appropriate step in changing their life situation.

## The Case of Kiranjit Ahluwallia

Many of the issues discussed are poignantly illustrated in the much-publicized case of Kiranjit Ahluwallia, an immigrant Indian woman in England who lived in an abusive situation for ten years (Ahluwallia and Gupta, 1997). Tired of the battering, she allegedly set fire to her abuser, her husband, who subsequently died from the burns. Kiranjit was accused, convicted of manslaughter in the first degree, and remanded to jail. In the hearing and conviction, the prosecution contended that she was culpable since during the ten years of her marriage, she had made no attempts to leave the abusive situation or to get help from social workers. It was further contended that the act of setting her husband on fire was deliberate and intentional, and therefore punishable.

Her case was subsequently reopened and defended by the Southall Black Sisterhood, a women's organization. Her culturally sensitive lawyers and psychologists gathered evidence to show that Kiranjit belonged to a culture that was dominated by the concept of family shame, and family honor, or *izzat*. She also was afraid that she would not be given custody of her children in case of a divorce and thus did not even consider seeking help from social workers, neighbors, or anyone else outside her own family. The defense argued that Kiranjit had developed battered woman's syndrome, in which her consciousness became inured to the consequences of her actions. After considering the cultural context, the judge ruled to acquit Ahluwallia.

This case illustrates the role of tradition in hindering immigrant women from accessing services. It highlights the initial cultural insensitivity of the Western system of care and justice in interceding with cases of domestic violence and shows how a more culturally sensitive understanding finally led to Ahluwallia's acquittal.

## Screening Issues

Health care providers of all types must be trained to screen for domestic violence and to be culturally competent when eliciting a history of abuse from immigrant women. Use of standardized protocols in some hospitals has been shown to increase the accurate identification of physical abuse of women by their husbands, boyfriends, or other intimates (McLeer and Anwar, 1987). Such protocols have been required by the Joint Commission on Accreditation of Healthcare Organizations since 1992.

In screening the immigrant woman, the first task is to establish appropriate translation services that do not depend on family members or friends. This is critical to gain the trust of the patient and to be able to reassure her of the confidential nature of the questioning. Translation can be challenging in settings where few immigrants of a specific language group are seen. It also can be difficult to find private time with a patient who is a victim of battering. It is not uncommon for batterers to insist on remaining with the victim the entire time, to relate the history, and to assume a "protective stance" in the presence of the providers. When the index of suspicion is high, potential victims must be removed from all family company long enough to get unfiltered information. This situation can require a great deal of resourcefulness on the part of the clinician and staff. Training staff ensures that a mechanism for separating suspected victims is in place.

Providers should use routine screening questions that first orient women to the context of violence ("violence is common") and then elicit closed-ended responses (Acierno, Resnick, and Kilpatrick, 1997). These questions should be thought of as another "vital sign." A number of screening protocols for domestic violence have been developed (American College of Emergency Physicians, 1995; American Medical Association, 1992a; Dutton, Mitchell, and Haywood, 1996; Furbee, Sikora, Williams, and Derk, 1998). The protocol used by George Washington University Medical Center is shown in Exhibit 10.1.

# Exhibit 10.1. Screening Protocol for Domestic Violence.

*Introduction*

1. These days many people are exposed to violence in some form.
2. Violence is a health risk and can result in physical and emotional problems.
3. It is our routine procedure to ask adult patients about their exposure to violence.
4. If you are a violence victim, we can better help you if we know it.

*Questions:*

1. In the past 12 months, has anyone threatened you with or actually used a knife or gun to scare or hurt you?

   Last 12 months?     Yes     No

   If "yes" to 12 months, last 1 month?     Yes     No

2. In the past 12 months, has anyone choked, kicked, bitten or punched you?

   Last 12 months?     Yes     No

   If "yes" to 12 months, last 1 month?

3. In the past 12 months, has anyone slapped, pushed, grabbed or shoved you?

   Last 12 months?     Yes     No

   If "yes" to 12 months, last 1 month?     Yes     No

4. In the past 12 months, has anyone forced or coerced you to have sex?

   Last 12 months?     Yes     No

   If "yes" to 12 months, last 1 month?     Yes     No

5. In the past 12 months, have you been afraid that a current or former intimate partner would hurt you physically?

   Last 12 months?     Yes     No

   If "yes" to 12 months, last 1 month?     Yes     No

   If "yes" to any of 1–5, then ask:

6. What is your relationship with the person who has hurt you?

   \_\_\_\_ Current or former intimate partner

   \_\_\_\_ Other family member

   \_\_\_\_ Acquaintance or friend

   \_\_\_\_ Co-worker

   \_\_\_\_ Stranger

   \_\_\_\_ Other (specify)

7. Have the police been notified within the last month about any of these experiences?

*Source:* Dutton, Mitchell, and Haywood, 1996. Used with permission.

In addition to acute injuries that should raise suspicion of domestic violence enough to prompt immediate questioning (see Exhibit 10.2), domestic violence can be a frequent cause of other somatic complaints, including headache and migraine, abdominal pain, chronic pain, and sleep disruptions. Behavioral problems include anxiety and depression, suicidality, posttraumatic stress disorder, and substance and eating disorders (Kilpatrick, Resnick, and Acierno, 1997).

Thus, multiple clues may guide the provider to suspect that a patient is experiencing violence in her home. Specialists from different disciplines may see patients with varying patterns of presentation. Many of the sequelae of domestic violence result in loss of work time and loss of productivity, at great cost to businesses and society (Dunham and Leetch, 1996; McAfee, 1994).

## Conclusion

It is imperative that domestic violence in the immigrant and refugee population be understood and addressed from a culturally relevant, sensitive, and competent perspective. Health care

### Exhibit 10.2.  Medical Clues Raising the Suspicion of Domestic Violence.

Central patterns of injuries

Contusions or injuries on the head, neck, abdomen, or face

Injuries suggestive of combative posture (injuries to palms of hands, extensor aspect or ulnar side of forearm, boxer's fractures)

Type or extent of injury inconsistent with the patient's history of injury

Substantial delay from time of injury to time of care seeking

Injuries occurring during pregnancy

A pattern of repeated visits to the emergency department

Evidence of alcohol or drug use

Arrival in the emergency department for suicide attempt or gesture

Sexual assaults and partner rape

*Source:* Adapted from American College of Emergency Physicians, 1995, and American Medical Association, 1992a.

providers of all types are integral to the provision of care of women and families in domestic violence situations. Team rather than individual care models provide the advantage of case management and improve communication among all service providers. Providers need to understand the role and relationship of the perpetrator and the victim within a cultural context. Written clinical screening protocols should be implemented at all health facilities. Providers must be cognizant of the laws related to domestic violence and their ramifications for women who seek assistance. In addition, health care providers should advocate for victims and participate in training members of the criminal justice system about domestic violence and the repetitive behavior of perpetrators. Culturally competent health care involves understanding the meaning of abuse within the victim's cultural framework, the role of tradition, the legal system, and the specific circumstances of each immigrant woman. The Fourth International Women's Conference (Beijing) concluded that violence is harmful for women and that strict cultural relativism no longer is applicable to domestic violence.

# Sexual Violence, Rape, and War

*Kaila Morris Compton*
*and Deanna Chechile*

The historical use of rape as an instrument of war has a long and ignominious story that stretches across cultures, time, and space from the crusades, to the world wars, to Vietnam, where "rape reared its head as a way to relieve boredom as American GIs searched and destroyed in the highlands of Viet Nam" (Brownmiller, 1975, p. 23).

The uses and functions of rape in war are multiple. Coercive prostitution mollifies the weary or demoralized soldier, as witnessed in the case of Korean "comfort women," the Eritrean prostitutes during Ethiopian occupation, and practices of the United Nations troops during Bosnian "peacekeeping." Systematic rape of the enemy's women constructs a reign of terror, often through public spectacle, and symbolizes the absolute dominion of the conqueror. For example, the Hutu genocidal campaign focused on the "dangerous and arrogant sexuality of Tutsi women," whose rape signified the destruction of the community (Susskind, 1997–1998, p. 8; Ranck, 1998). This tactical function also has been expressed in terms of racial purification, as seen in the Serbian policies of "ethnic cleansing," where the trilogy of the rape-impregnation-motherhood of Croatian women has been directed toward the creation of a "pure" Serbian state with ethnicity traced according to patriarchal lines (Stiglmayer, 1994).

The question that seldom is raised is why rape and other forms of sexual violence against women are the chosen tools of genocidal destruction when torture and murder would achieve the same end. Considering both the function and meaning of rape within the context of war requires recognition of the gendered power relations and the intersectional nature of the violation. A woman might be raped because of her gender and her nationality, ethnicity, or religion. The erasure of rape in war as a gender-specific crime is evinced in its conspicuous absence from the international humanitarian legal regime.

## Rape and the Refugee Experience

The threat of sexual violence is an infrequently discussed yet ubiquitous aspect of the refugee experience as well. Like many soldiers in war, a large number of border guards, police, and others who manage or come into contact with refugees (including other refugees) treat the rape of refugee women as an employment benefit. There are few, if any, reliable sources of protection from or control of this type of sexual violence. Refugee women generally are unaware of or do not trust any exiting authority to which they could report, or they consider the social consequences of revealing their stories to be unbearable. For many women, a discovered rape can lead to a life of exile from family and community, with prostitution as the only means of survival.

A careful reading of refugee narratives reveals routes of flight planned to minimize number of rapes, women as victims of multiple bandit-rapists along the route of flight (Ngor with Warner, 1987, p. 380), and women being forced to have sex to cross a border (Aitchison, 1984, p. 26) or to get food in a refugee camp (Camus-Jacques, 1989, p. 146). The United Nations estimates that at least 39 percent of Vietnamese women who fled by boat were abducted or raped by pirates at sea (Desjarlais and others, 1995, p. 188). In general, statistics are few and unreliable because of international attitudes toward rape, women's shame and fear, and the absence of adequate procedures and protections for reporting.

Regarding Eritrean and Ethiopian refugee women in Djibouti in the early 1980s, Aitchison (1984) reports that women and girls were typically separated from male asylum seekers for "questioning" and frequently raped, sometimes being held for days or weeks and passed from guard to guard. Subsequently, women refugees in Djibouti were reportedly vulnerable to random arrest and rape by police. Sexual abuse also was routine for women who found employment as domestic workers. Aitchison writes of women who became prostitutes because of the experience of being raped repeatedly and its social and psychological consequences.

Somali women who sought refuge in Kenya in 1992 also have been the targets of sexual violence, reportedly perpetrated by bandits in search of food, money, and sex (Africa Watch Women's Rights Project, 1993). In the Horn of Africa, where female genital mutilation is common, rapists often tear or cut infibulation scar tissue of infibulated, unmarried women to facilitate the rape.

## Psychosocial and Physical Health of Rape Survivors

Health care providers must recognize the ubiquity of rape in situations of conflict and displacement and learn effective methods for responding to the needs of survivors and their families. Shame and self-blame are common responses among rape survivors. In addition, depression, posttraumatic stress disorder, and recurring somatic symptoms are common. Among immigrant and refugee women, these reactions may be compounded by sociocultural considerations. Cultural responses to rape vary, and the social consequences can be severe. An understanding of the significance of the rape trauma within the parameters of the woman's cultural system is imperative.

The failures and deficiencies of formal legal systems in developing culturally sensitive and appropriate procedures, forums, and support systems for rape survivors to bring forth their stories of survival and seek justice are well documented. The lesson for providers is twofold. First, silence on the part of an immigrant or refugee patient who has fled a site of violence does not necessarily indicate that she has not experienced rape or other forms of gender violence. Second, the health care provider should attempt to learn about the cultural system of the patient and understand the impact of rape on the individual, her family, and the community. Interviewing techniques, including format and privacy concerns, should be carefully designed. Issues of translation, body language, and somatization acquire heightened significance in this context. Finally, medical and psychological reports and expert testimony serve as pivotal evidence in asylum cases. Health care providers can assist victims of politically related sexual violence in their claims for asylum by acting as expert witnesses or by learning to evaluate and document evidence for this purpose (Laws and Patsalides, 1997).

# Female Genital Mutilation

*Kaila Morris Compton*
*and Deanna Chechile*

The culturally sanctioned excision of parts of the female genitalia, including the clitoris, is a complex source of stress and violence for some immigrant women in the United States. Female genital cutting, usually referred to as female circumcision (FC) or female genital mutilation (FGM), is a practice used to define gender, sexual, and social identity in some twenty-eight African and Middle Eastern countries. FGM is performed most often expressly to control female sexuality and reproduction. Although it results in significant psychological and physical trauma, as well as immediate and long-term morbidity and mortality, it also is embedded in cultural definitions of personhood, morality, and suitability for marriage. Although some women and men from cultures where FGM is practiced are speaking out against it, women themselves are frequently involved in the perpetuation of FGM because of its relationship to socioeconomic survival and membership in a cultural group.

The social and cultural imperatives associated with FGM take on new and sometimes intensified significance for immigrants

Thanks to Susan Ivey, Jean Fourcroy, Meserek Ramsey, Erissica Razak, Suellen Miller, Lynne Wilcox, and Wanda Jones for their comments and suggestions in the preparation of this section.

and refugees. FGM often is upheld as a critical practice for maintaining ethnic identity and moral behavior within a new sociocultural context, such as the United States, where premarital sexual experimentation is normative. Furthermore, the notion of individual rights and autonomy, the foundation of American society, threatens the fabric of social organization in cultures where family and community are the primary decision-making units and men hold absolute control over women's bodies. Finally, women immigrants who have undergone FGM or believe that their daughters' moral, cultural, and socioeconomic survival depend on it confront a society in which FGM is considered an extreme form of child abuse and in which their own bodies incite shock and outrage from health care providers.

New legislative enactments, or the creative application of extant child abuse laws, have been devised to prohibit FGM domestically in at least twelve countries, including the United States, Sweden, the Netherlands, Australia, Switzerland, Belgium, the United Kingdom, and France. These laws do not apply extraterritorially, and if they do, as in Australia, enforcement is quite difficult. With respect to immigration policy, Western countries are confronted with the international dilemma of asylum claims premised on the grounds of FGM.

FGM also is a domestic issue for women and girls with or at risk of FGM, and for the health care providers who serve these immigrant populations. Shame, legal consequences, and the inadequate training and education of health care providers about FGM have a negative impact on health care–seeking behavior. Low utilization rates of health care service not only endanger the health status of immigrant women and girls, but also make detection and prevention difficult since the health care setting is often the only site of detection and a critical site for primary prevention. Provision of sensitive care and counseling requires an understanding of the social and cultural significance of FGM to women, their families, and their communities. Consequently, demographic and epidemiologic surveillance among immigrant communities must be conducted not only to identify high-risk populations, but also to include them in efforts to develop appropriate health care services and strategies for public education and behavioral change.

## Definitional Overview of FGM and Its Effects

The World Health Organization (1996) has categorized FGM into four different forms that vary greatly in degree of severity and attendant consequences:

Type I      Excision of the prepuce with or without excision of part or all of the clitoris

Type II     Excision of the clitoris with partial or total excision of the labia minora

Type III    Excision of part or all of the external genitalia and stitching or narrowing of the vaginal opening (infibulation)

Type IV     Unclassified: includes pricking, piercing, stretching, or incising of the clitoris and/or labia; cauterization by burning the clitoris or surrounding tissue; scraping or cutting of the vaginal orifice or surrounding tissue; introduction of corrosive substances into the vagina to cause bleeding for the purpose of tightening or narrowing it; other procedures that fall under the above definitions.

The term *female circumcision* implies an inaccurate analogy between FGM and male circumcision (itself a controversial practice). As Nahid Toubia (1994, p. 712) points out, "Clitoridectomy is anatomically equivalent to amputation of the penis." More severe forms of FGM are equivalent to removing the penis, its roots, and parts of the scrotal sac. There are significant differences: the penile urethra travels through the penis, while the clitoris and female urethra are separate structures; and the scrotal sac covers the testes, while the ovaries do not lie underneath the labia majora. However, consideration of embryological development, especially with regard to nervous tissue, suggests that the glans penis and clitoris are analogous sites of sexual sensation.

In practice, the degree of tissue removal in FGM is variable. Traditional practitioners of FGM may or may not have any experience or training and use a variety of instruments, such as razors, knives, scissors, broken glass, and sharp rocks. In most cases, the procedure is performed without anesthesia, and the struggling of the infant, child, or young woman makes any kind of accuracy impossible.

FGM is practiced across socioeconomic lines and among different religious and ethnic groups. Although the form and timing of FGM vary according to geography and ethnic membership, the procedure generally is performed on girls between the ages of three and eight. However, FGM may be performed on a newborn, on a bride's wedding night, or during late pregnancy before the birth of a first child. Anecdotal evidence suggests the average age has been declining in some countries of origin and in immigrant communities in Western countries in recent years. Presumptively, girls are easier to control physically during the procedure at a younger age. Furthermore, this approach combats the inverse correlation between educational attainment and FGM.

## Health Consequences of FGM

The health risks associated with FGM are immense, consisting of both immediate and long-term physical and psychological consequences. The form of FGM practiced, the degree of sterility of the conditions, the expertise of the practitioner, the health status of the girl, and the extent to which she resists the procedure correlate with the outcome. The causal nexus between FGM and health consequences has not been clinically documented in any systematic manner, and many women who have undergone the procedure do not link secondary health problems with earlier FGM.

The most exigent short-term complications from all types of FGM are hemorrhage, severe pain, shock, and sometimes death. Following the procedure, girls are at risk for urine retention and sometimes dehydration from the withholding of fluids. Other short-term effects are septicemia, fever, tetanus, gangrene, and genital infection.

Long-term complications include urinary tract infections, urethral and vaginal stenosis, retention of urine and menstrual blood (hematocolpos), fistula, birth complications, dyspareunia, infertility, and other sexual and psychological consequences (Fourcroy, 1983; Toubia, 1994). Infibulation generally creates more long-term health problems because it obstructs the passage of fluids. Moreover, the massive scar tissue and the small opening left after infibulation can result in obstructed and protracted labor, risking the lives of the mother and child in childbirth. Vaginal tearing may occur if deinfibulation is delayed or not performed. Reinfibulation is commonly performed following delivery, reestablishing the small posterior opening.

## Psychological Consequences of FGM

The psychological ramifications of FGM are not documented in any systematic way, although Toubia (1994) has witnessed chronic depression and anxiety among infibulated women in Sudan. However, many women may sublimate psychological effects in acceptance of cultural norms. Still, a sense of betrayal may persist throughout life, particularly since one's own family actively participates in the procedure (Toubia, 1994). This sense of betrayal is a consequence of the fact that a trusted caregiver often physically forces the child to undergo extreme pain and lies to the child to coerce cooperation. It could be argued that not submitting a child to a ritual required for cultural membership and marriageability also could be experienced as a kind of betrayal, but this remains undocumented in the ethnographic and anecdotal sources regarding FGM.

## Historical and Contemporary Justifications for FGM

Although no direct trajectory or single rationale exists for the practice of FGM, it is best understood as a practice resulting from the juncture of religion, culture and tradition, and socioeconomics. FGM predates both Islam and Christianity, and it is practiced among all religious groups, including Christians, Jews, Muslims, animists, and indigenous religious traditions. Despite the fact that no textual basis exists for FGM in either the Koran or the Bible, adherents who practice FGM cite religious belief as a rationale for the practice. Absent any religious mandate for FGM, however, both the Koran and the Bible place a high premium on chastity, virginity, and the suppression of female sexuality, common explanations for FGM.

From the perspective of culture and tradition, FGM effectively operates as a centripetal force that ensures group identity. A woman who forgoes FGM will be ostracized, deemed unsuitable for marriage, and seen as willfully deviating from the community ethos. FGM is associated with health, beauty, femininity, fertility, and moral behavior. In some FGM-practicing cultures, the clitoris is seen as a masculine appendage because it hangs down between the legs. In many of the communities that practice FGM, marriage signals full social integration and constitutes a woman's only viable means for economic security. If FGM has a cultural function in the maintenance of honor, respectability, and power relations, it also has a profoundly economic function for those practitioners whose livelihoods and status depend on it (Lightfoot-Klein, 1989; Walker and Parmar, 1993).

## Prevalence of FGM in the United States

The CDC estimates that in 1990 there were 168,000 girls and women with or at risk for FGM living in the United States (Jones and others, 1997). An estimated 45 percent of the women and 44 percent of the girls live in eleven metropolitan areas, including New York, Los Angeles, the San Francisco Bay Area, Atlanta, and Washington, D.C. The authors point out that the CDC estimate is indirect, derived from a statistical analysis based on two data sources: a public use data set from the 1990 U.S. census based on a 5 percent household sample, and country-specific prevalence estimates compiled by Toubia for the Research, Action, and Information Network for Bodily Integrity of Women (RAINBO). They also identify immigration and acculturation as key challenges to assessing the prevalence of FGM. However, the CDC analysis provides the best estimate based on available data at this time.

## Legislative Response in the United States

The United States has adopted a twofold approach to address FGM: implementing special legislation prohibiting the procedure domestically and reexamining the parameters of asylum laws. The proposed Federal Prohibition of Female Genital Mutilation Act of 1995 was incorporated in the Illegal Immigration Reform and Immigrant Responsibility Act of 1996 (PL 104–208, sec. 644–645, 10 Stat. 3009, 3708–3709), which directs federal authorities to inform new immigrants about the ban against FGM (8 U.S.C.A. sec. 1374) as well as the criminal penalty for such practice. Drawing on the strengths and learning from the weaknesses of the British legislation prohibiting FGM, the U.S. law not only criminalizes the practice of FGM on girls under the age of eighteen, but also mandates a demographic and epidemiologic study to identify high-risk communities, followed by implementation of educational and outreach programs to those target populations. Still, the marginalization of the high-risk immigrant and refugee communities due to poverty, linguistic, and ethnic isolation exacerbates problems of both access and enforcement of the legislation.

Federal law criminalizes circumcision of a female minor: "Whomever knowingly circumcises, excises, or infibulates the whole or any part of the labia majora or labia minora or clitoris of another person who has not attained the age of 18 years shall be fined under this title or imprisoned not more than 5 years, or both." Only two exceptions permit genital surgery on a minor female: if it is (1) "necessary to the health of the person on whom it is performed" or (2) "performed on a person in labor or who has just given birth and is performed for medical purposes connected with that labor." Neither instance of this medical necessity exemption has been tested yet in the courts. Federal criminal law does not recognize any exemption on the basis of religious or cultural belief.

Seven states (California, Delaware, Wisconsin, Minnesota, Tennessee, Rhode Island, and North Dakota) have enacted legislation proscribing the practice of FGM on minors; a few states also prohibit the practice after the age of majority. As distinguished from federal law, which imposes criminal liability only on those individuals who actually perform FGM, some states extend liability to persons who allow or permit FGM to be practiced on a child in their custody.

The passage of recent legislation prohibiting FGM raises compelling medicolegal issues. Indeed, the criminalization of FGM poses difficult questions concerning what acts are specifically covered within the meaning of the legislation and what constitutes "permitting" or "allowing" FGM to occur within the meaning of state statutory prohibitions against it. The law also lacks specificity with regard to how the Department of Health and Human Services

(DHHS) will implement and monitor compliance with the law (Omnibus Consolidated Recisions and Appropriations Act of 1996, Pub. L. No. 104-134, S 519(e)(b)(2), 110 Stat. 1321, 250-251).

Similarly, reporting requirements for health professionals who encounter FGM on a minor or suspect that a child is at high risk for FGM must be developed since the legislation is conspicuously silent on this point (Dorkenoo, 1994). Of course, any reporting mechanism must be connected with a child protection system sensitized to issues confronting immigrant families and the dynamics of FGM (Key, 1997). Finally, a criminal conviction also may adversely affect the resident status of immigrant families since the passage of the Illegal Immigration Reform and Immigrant Responsibility Act of 1996 seeks, through expedited removal proceedings, to prevent the naturalization of any immigrant convicted of an aggravated felony in the United States, including crimes against children (8 U.S. Code sec. 1228).

## Health Policy and Clinical Guidelines

Clinical protocols and public health initiatives must be developed to ensure culturally sensitive quality care and to promote prevention in FGM-practicing immigrant communities in the United States. For providers, ethical issues arise regarding patient confidentiality and the potential endangerment of women, girls, and family unity due to criminalization, stigma, and shame.

The 1996 federal legislation mandates the DHHS to identify potentially FGM-practicing communities and to develop outreach and education in collaboration with community members. The legislation also mandates the DHHS to develop recommendations for medical education on FGM. To date, the DHHS has held ten community meetings in different regions in the United States. In addition, it has surveyed all American medical and osteopathic schools and has organized a task force to develop an appropriate curriculum. However, the education of providers in health care settings, as well as nonphysician providers, has yet to be addressed; training nurses and midwives is critical.

Many national and state medical professional organizations, including the American Medical Women's Association, the American Medical Association, the American Nurses Association, and the American College of Obstetrics and Gynecology, have enacted policies on FGM. The AMA policy (Resolution 513, A-96) condemns FGM as a form of child abuse and suggests that physicians provide culturally sensitive counseling and referral to families who request the procedure. Presumably this approach would support our recommendation for creating a path of referrals for a family with a child who is at risk for FGM. A culturally competent social worker would assume case management, serve as the child protection advocate, and coordinate family and community-based preventive education and individual, family, and group treatment as appropriate to the case.

Culturally competent clinical management of FGM also requires the development of protocols for handling the physical and psychological sequelae of FGM. In addition to the medical knowledge required for routine gynecological examination or assisting labor and delivery of an infibulated woman, familiarity with issues of patient modesty and reluctance to indicate pain is critical for quality care. A small sample of Somali women immigrants in 1985 indicated that provider familiarity with FGM and the availability of women providers were among their greatest health care priorities (Shaw, 1985). The women expressed concern about provider lack of familiarity with the methods and timing for opening an infibulation scar for delivery. Anecdotal evidence from health care providers in the San Francisco Bay Area demonstrates a lack of provider familiarity with FGM, resulting in reactions such as exclamations of horror, panic, and the insensitive display of infibulated women as teaching cases (personal communications with providers from four health care facilities in San Francisco and the East Bay).

Because FGM is now illegal in the United States, providers face ethical dilemmas regarding detection and reporting. The health care setting is critical in the control and prevention of FGM in the United States because it is the primary site of detection. However, providers are reluctant to take steps that will adversely affect care seeking or remove a child from a family, and they tend to resent state intervention in a provider-patient relationship. Harborview Hospital in Seattle attempted to design a less severe substitute procedure for Somali parents who requested FGM for their daughters but abandoned the idea after legal advice and an outpouring of contrary advice and complaints. Nonetheless, health care providers must be educated about and receive training on the new legal mandates prohibiting FGM, and assist in the development of referral networks for at-risk families, similar to their obligations concerning child abuse and domestic violence.

Provision of care to an infibulated adult woman raises the ethical dilemma of whether to reinfibulate after labor and delivery. Some providers perform extended episiotomies or cesarean sections to avoid this issue altogether. Providers who incise the infibulation scar for delivery (the recommended practice) are faced with the dilemma of whether to reinfibulate if the woman so requests. Anecdotal evidence suggests that American providers do reinfibulate, saying that they are "reapproximating the tissue" or simply "putting things back the way they were." Some providers frame the issue in terms of an adult woman's right to choose, while others maintain that "it isn't all that different from adding a few extra stitches," a discretionary practice in American obstetrics that shares the goal of maximizing the husband's sexual pleasure. Further, providers are concerned that refusal to reinfibulate in the hospital in the way prescribed by family and culture will put the woman at risk for having the procedure done under less safe conditions. Whereas mutilation of children can be considered a form of child abuse from an outsider's perspective, reinfibulation of an already mutilated woman with informed consent is not legally considered a form of domestic or other violence against the person.

There appears to be an underground market for medicalized clitoridectomy and infibulation for immigrant families who can afford it. One Somali woman in Los Angeles quoted the going rate as $3,000 (personal communication, 1997). It is unclear whether these practitioners are medical professionals licensed in the United States or traditional practitioners who may have provided such services prior to their immigration to the United States.

Of course, criminalization of FGM does not ensure its eradication. On the contrary, the recent prohibitions may intensify the insularity and marginalization of practicing or at-risk immigrant communities, as evidenced by the divergent anecdotal evidence concerning the incidence of FGM gathered from Western health care providers and members of the immigrant communities, respectively. The inherent problems of detection and enforcement of the prohibition signal the need for developing community-based prevention programs and social service systems from the ground up, in partnership with the affected communities.

## Conclusion

Although the issues of cultural relativism, cultural imperialism, individual rights, and women's rights are tensely intertwined at the core of debates about FGM, the United States (and much of the rest of the Western world) has determined that FGM causes irrevocable and unacceptable physical and psychological damage to women and has mandated its criminal proscription. We need to create ways to work with affected immigrant communities to help them relinquish the practice of FGM while addressing their concerns about the loss of this ritual and avoiding adverse impact on health care–seeking behavior, individual self-esteem, and family unity. This is no easy task, and we are in the early stages of grappling with it. The regional community meetings organized by the DHHS have been a first step in the dialogue. Training of providers and establishment of protocols and referral networks will be key components. Importantly, the affected communities must be involved in the planning and implementation of the services and outreach. Our call is to develop a continuum of care, including culturally sensitive clinical management of FGM, family-centered counseling and referral services, and community-based prevention and outreach in order to facilitate immigrant communities' transition to life without FGM.

# Chapter Eleven

# Depression and Anxiety Disorders

*Lisa C. Tracy and*
*Sandra Mattar*

According to international studies, the Epidemiological Catchment Area (ECA) studies in the United States, and the recent National Comorbidity Study (NCS) (Escobar, 1992; Kessler and others, 1996), depression and anxiety are the most commonly occurring mental disorders among women. Both are more prevalent among women than men, and they often are experienced in association with life stressors (Escobar, 1992; Kessler and others, 1994, Kessler, 1997). Thus, despite the lack of substantive empirical community-based research on immigrant mental health, it is likely and consistent with clinical and empirical knowledge that immigrant women may be at heightened risk for both of these disorders. Recognizing and treating depression and anxiety in immigrant women is complex due to cultural issues and their embeddedness in the multiple stressors these women face.

## Epidemiology of Depression and Anxiety

Congruent with other large-scale epidemiological studies in the United States, the recently conducted NCS found affective and anxiety disorders to be the most common diagnoses in women

Thanks to Anthony T. Ng, who wrote the section on psychotropic medication.

(Kessler and others, 1994). This study used the University of Michigan Composite International Diagnostic Interview schedule, a newer scale based on the Diagnostic Interview Schedule, which was used in the ECA studies (Kessler and others, 1994). In the NCS, 23.9 percent of women had experienced an affective disorder, 8.0 percent had experienced dysthymia, and 21.3 percent had experienced a major depressive episode. More than 30 percent of women had experienced an anxiety disorder in their lifetimes, with the most commonly occurring disorders being social phobia and simple phobia, at 15.5 percent and 15.7 percent, respectively (Kessler and others, 1994). The NCS also found that in the year prior to the study, 14.1 percent of women had experienced an affective disorder, and 22.6 percent had experienced an anxiety disorder.

Reports of the prevalence of mental disorders in ethnic minorities versus non-Hispanic whites are inconsistent (Kessler and others, 1994). The NCS found Hispanics had significantly higher rates of current affective disorders and comorbidity than non-Hispanic whites (Kessler and others, 1994). In contrast, the ECA study found that Mexican Americans had significantly lower rates of major depressive episodes than non-Hispanic whites (Karno and others, 1987). However, the ECA study also found that dysthymia, panic disorder, and phobia were more common in Mexican American women over forty years of age, compared with their younger ethnic counterparts and with non-Hispanic white women who were the same age (Karno and others, 1987). Studies of Asian Americans have found higher rates of depression among women than men, and in some cases reported higher levels of symptomatology than studies of the general population using the Center for Epidemiological Studies–Depression Scale (CES-D) (Ying, 1988). However, research does not indicate higher levels of mental disorders among Asians except in refugees. Studies of refugees, particularly Southeast Asians, reveal high rates of mental health problems, including depression and anxiety, compared to other populations (Vega and Rumbaut, 1991).

The NCS found high levels of comorbidity (Kessler and others, 1994). Depression and anxiety are particularly likely to occur comorbidly with other disorders and with each other (Maxmen and Ward, 1995). Numerous studies have found comorbidity of anxiety, depression, and somatization among refugee populations (Carlson and Rosser-Hogan, 1991; Mghir, Freed, Raskin, and Katon, 1995; Moore and Boehnlein, 1991).

## Risk Factors

HHANES found that higher levels of depression symptoms on the CES-D were associated with being female, lower education and income, and a combination of U.S. birth and an Anglo-oriented acculturation style. With a few exceptions, findings on gender, income, and education are similar to those found in other studies and in other populations (Kessler and others, 1994). However, other studies have found higher acculturation to be associated with better outcomes. For example, in a study of 2,234 Southeast Asian refugees, Ying, Akutsu, Zhang, and Huang (1997) found that a more traditional or separation-style cultural orientation was associated with poorer mental health outcomes. The relationship between acculturation and mental health may vary by migration status and remains an important empirical question.

## Cultural Issues

Defining and measuring mental illness in culturally diverse populations may have limitations in reliability and validity due to linguistic and cultural differences in manifestations of distress and illness (Kleinman, 1988). In many cultures, depression and anxiety are expressed through somatization. Some researchers suggest that many cultures lack the psychological experience or language to express symptoms of distress (Marsella, 1979), and others view psychological versus physical responses as merely different means of expressing distress (Kleinman, 1988). In addition, it is important to note that anxiety symptoms typically are expressed somatically not only in traditional cultures but also in modern Western cultures (Maxmen and Ward, 1995). Corr and Vitaliano (1985) argue that depression is one of many alternative ways of expressing distress. Kirmayer (1996), Kleinman (1988), and others emphasize that sociocultural factors determine the expression of depression and anxiety, both intrapsychically and interpersonally. Amering and Katschnig (1990) argue that anxiety disorders are a universal phenomenon, but the particular contextual correlates and manifestation of anxiety can vary tremendously across cultures.

The understanding of anxiety and depressive disorders across cultures is still debated. However, forms of both types of disorders have been studied in many cultures. In a recent epidemiological study of seventeen hundred Chinese Americans in the Los Angeles area, Zheng and others (1997) found that the most commonly occurring disorder was neurasthenia. Neurasthenia, which occurs in East Asian cultures, has similarities to both anxiety and depressive disorders and manifests in response to shame and conflict surrounding social responsibility and self-presentation (Kirmayer, 1996; Kleinman, 1988). According to Zheng and colleagues (1997), neurasthenia was not comorbid with depression and anxiety. Thus, it would be difficult to argue that neurasthenia or other culture-bound disorders are manifestations of either anxiety or depression as they are defined in the *Diagnostic and Statistical Manual of Mental Disorders* (DSM-IV). Whether anxiety and depressive disorders are clearly distinct phenomena or whether, instead, anxiety, depression, and a host of culture-bound disorders are varieties of manifestations of distress determined by cultural context can be questioned.

Regardless of these debates, somatic complaints among immigrants must be taken seriously and need to be treated as both a physical and a mental manifestation of distress (Good and DelVecchio, 1980). In Kirmayer's words (1996), "Far from being mutually exclusive alternatives, somatic and emotional symptoms coexist and are substantially correlated in the general population" (p. 133). Somatization, neurasthenia, and culture-bound disorders are described in more depth in Chapter Thirteen.

## Psychosocial Context

Premigration, migration, and acculturation stressors are correlated with and hypothesized to be etiological factors in depression and anxiety. The recent trend in immigration and mental health studies is to focus more on the context, that is, on the social and economic stresses that immigrants face, and less on premorbid conditions or predisposing psychological factors (Furnham and Bochner, 1990). The most commonly diagnosed mental disorders among immigrant women occur in such a context and perhaps may best be conceptualized as stress reactions rather than disorders. We do not dismiss the severity and impairment seen in immigrants with serious depression, anxiety, posttraumatic stress disorder (PTSD), and somatization disorders but feel it is important to frame these disorders in the context of the immigrant woman's experience. It also is important to note that emphasizing a stress and coping framework does not negate the significance of biological factors. Stress can bring about biological changes, and biological predisposition contributes to how individual immigrant and refugee women respond to stressors.

## DSM-IV Depressive Disorders

Four types of depressive disorders, or mood disorders, are defined in the DSM-IV (1994): major depressive disorder, dysthymic disorder, depressive disorder not otherwise specified, and bipolar or manic-depressive disorder. Dysthymia and major depression are the focus here. They are distinguished from one another on the basis of intensity, chronicity, and duration of symptoms.

For a diagnosis of major depression to be made, symptoms must be present nearly every day for at least two weeks; in dysthymia the criteria are that symptoms are present more often than not for at least two years. Major depression may include one or more major episodes in which the person's behavior differs markedly from her usual behavior. It also may be a chronic disorder, although the symptoms are more severe than in dysthymia, and the individual may have months of relatively symptom-free functioning. The common symptoms of depression are depressed or irritable mood, fatigue and loss of energy, difficulties with memory and concentration, significant weight or appetite changes, and feelings of low self-esteem, worthlessness, or excessive or inappropriate guilt. In major depression, there may be markedly diminished interest in activities (anhedonia), and frequent thoughts of death and suicide attempts often are present.

### Case Study: Depression

Maria is a forty-two-year-old Mexican mother of two children (ages fourteen and nine). She is married to José, a forty-three-year-old native Mexican who works as a part-time construction worker. Maria was referred to a mental health agency by a county hospital psychiatrist at her discharge following a suicide attempt in which she ingested some pills. Her family had immigrated to the United States two years prior to the admission. At the time of referral, she was unemployed and illiterate, and her immigration status was pending. Maria is a monolingual Spanish speaker.

During her first visit with an agency mental health clinician, she sobbed uncontrollably and complained of feelings of sadness and confusion. The precipitating event for her suicidal attempt was her husband's dismissal from his job three weeks earlier and subsequent excessive drinking. She had been staying in bed during the day feeling weak and tired yet was unable to sleep at night. She claimed she took the pills to get outside attention. She also presented eating disturbances and continued suicidal ideation, but expressed that she would never kill herself because that was against her religious beliefs, and she would not abandon her children.

Upon taking a family and migration history, the clinician learned that Maria had been physically abused by her husband since she married him at the age of fourteen. The family had come to the United States to find a better life. They had lived under extreme poverty in Mexico and were thankful to be living in the United States, especially because of the opportunity for a better education for their children. However, Maria felt very isolated here because she did not speak English, had no family or friends nearby, and was illiterate, and because her husband would not allow her to leave the house for fear of her being exposed to independent women who did not obey their husbands.

Maria was diagnosed with major depression. Treatment consisted of a combined approach including supportive and expressive therapy, psychoeducation, family work, and case management. After spending some time in a women and children's shelter, the family was reunited, and her husband entered treatment for substance abuse and domestic violence. Maria is learning English, has a part-time job, feels hopeful about the future, and is confident she could support herself and her children on her own, if necessary.

## DSM-IV Anxiety Disorders

Several types of syndromes are categorized as anxiety disorders in the DSM-IV: panic attacks, panic disorder, phobias, obsessive-compulsive disorder, generalized anxiety disorder, and PTSD. Because of its particular salience to migrant populations, PTSD is treated separately (see Chapter Twelve).

A panic attack is defined as an experience of "intense fear or discomfort" with four or more of the following symptoms: palpitations, sweating, trembling, difficulty breathing, abdominal or chest pain, dizziness, derealization, fear of losing control or going crazy, fear of dying, paresthesias (numbness or tingling sensations), and chills or hot flashes (American Psychiatric Association, 1994, p. 395). Panic disorder may be diagnosed if the panic attacks recur without warning and the individual experiences at least one month of behavioral change or fear about recurrence of the attacks. Panic disorder may be accompanied by agoraphobia, a fear of being in public places.

Phobia is defined as anxiety provoked in response to a cue, such as an object or situation. Obsessive-compulsive disorder is marked by recurrent intrusive thoughts, images, or impulses that are not "simply excessive worries about real-life problems" (American Psychiatric Association, 1994, p. 422) and that, at some point, the individual realizes are irrational. Generalized anxiety disorder is defined as excessive worry about work or school performance or other life situations that is difficult to control and persists over at least six months, with at least three symptoms of anxiety, such as restlessness, fatigue, concentration problems, irritability, tight muscles and sleep problems, and with impaired social or occupational functioning.

*Case Study: Anxiety*

Ana, a thirty-five-year-old high school–educated asylee from the former Yugoslavia was referred to an agency that specializes in assistance to immigrants and refugees by a county social services worker. In her initial meeting with a mental health clinician, she complained of chest pains, dizziness, insomnia, constant worry, weight loss, heart palpitations, and nervousness, and said she had been experiencing these symptoms since her arrival in the United States seven months earlier. Her speech was somewhat rapid, and she exhibited some paranoid ideation and secretiveness.

Ana was separated from and had lost contact with her only son, aged twelve, who was being cared for in Europe by relatives of her deceased husband, while she pursued a new life for her son and herself in the United States. She was awaiting a change in her immigration status and was not yet eligible to work. Since her arrival in the United States, she had been living with a distant relative, an elderly male, who considered her a burden and provided little emotional or other support. Due to her immigration status, she was ineligible for health and other benefits and had been unable to see a doctor except by a visit to an emergency department. The agency arranged a physical examination for Ana, who was diagnosed with generalized anxiety disorder after other medical disorders were ruled out.

Ana received supportive and cognitive behavioral therapy, psychoeducation, and case management to assist her with contacting her son, finding a new housing arrangement, establishing a social network, and communicating with her immigration attorney. Because her symptoms decreased during the first two months of treatment, medication was not indicated. Since starting treatment, Ana has received her green card, is employed, and is awaiting reunification with her son. She enjoys her life and has a small but growing circle of friends. Her anxiety symptoms remain minimal and are under control.

## Assessment and Treatment of Depression and Anxiety

Diagnosing depression and anxiety in immigrant and refugee women may be complicated due to cultural issues and the presence of comorbid disorders and life stressors. In both case studies, the presentation of symptoms was fairly straightforward, corresponded with DSM-IV diagnostic criteria, and was not confounded by comorbid disorders. Both Maria and Ana experienced significant life stressors that were clearly associated with their depression and anxiety symptoms. Thus, the context of their lives, as well as their psychological and physiological symptoms, became the focus of assessment in treatment.

The traditional assessment process requires some modification for immigrant women. Westermeyer (1993) advises allowing time for the development of trust and rapport and delaying confrontation or psychological interpretation in cross-cultural mental health treatment. The immigrant woman's family context must remain a central focus in assessment and treatment (Tracy, 1997). Westermeyer (1993) also urges that clinicians be aware of cultural variations in the appropriateness of dress and grooming, variation in calendar and time orientation, and knowledge of current events in the United States when conducting a mental status exam. Assessment should cover information on migration history, social systems, concrete needs, cultural values, and significant familial and social networks. In the following sections, issues specific to depression and anxiety disorders are outlined and treatment modalities that are relevant to both are described.

## Depression

Health care providers should be alert to the possible presence of depression and related disorders among immigrants who have repeated somatic complaints such as headache, chronic abdominal pain, or chest pain without resolution. In some cases, depression may be considered a normal consequence of migration and culture shock. However, if symptoms do not remit or serious psychosocial impairment is exhibited, treatment is warranted. Generally a combination of approaches is most effective, and might include medication, supportive therapy, psychoeducation, cognitive behavioral therapy, case management, and family work.

It is particularly important to assess suicidality in the depressed patient. About 15 percent of persons with major depression actually complete suicide; of those, 80 percent have seen a health care provider during the six months prior to the suicide (Maxmen and Ward, 1995). Although cultural values, religious beliefs, and familial commitments among immigrant women may decrease suicide risk, clinicians should still be alert to this possibility.

Maxmen and Ward (1995, p. 233) suggest asking the following questions when there is concern about possible suicidality or depression:

- Do you sometimes have a feeling that life is not worth living, or do you think about death much?
- Do you sometimes think that if you died from an accident or illness tomorrow that it just would not matter? (This is passive suicidal ideation.)
- Have you had thoughts of killing yourself? (This is active suicidal ideation.)

Persons with active suicidal ideation should receive a full risk assessment and be asked additional questions (Maxmen and Ward, 1995, pp. 233–234):

- What has kept you from acting on your suicidal ideation?
- Have you attempted suicide before? If so, by what method?
- Do you have a plan for ending your life?
- Is there a weapon in your home?

Individuals who provide reasons for not acting on suicidal thoughts, such as religious values or family, as in the case of Maria, are considered to be at lower risk. If an individual cannot make a verbal commitment not to harm herself for a designated period, such as one or two weeks, more comprehensive psychiatric assessment and intervention should occur immediately, and hospitalization may be necessary. Maria was able to promise that she would not attempt suicide. Involving the family in providing support is key in suicide prevention (Maxmen and Ward, 1995). Immediate crisis intervention and support are critical when family or other social supports are lacking. Because Maria's husband initially was unwilling to be involved in treatment, the clinician located temporary shelter in a supportive, safe environment for her and her children.

Treatment of depression has several purposes: to educate women about depression and its causes and symptoms, help them feel less isolated, develop better coping skills, learn how to avoid situations that bring on depression, and address losses and other psychosocial problems linked to depression (Maxmen and Ward, 1995).

## Anxiety

The presentation of anxiety disorders among immigrant women is likely to be somatic. Even in the general population, individuals with anxiety disorders are highly likely to present with somatic complaints and to seek treatment for medical conditions rather than seeking mental health services. It therefore is extremely important that primary care providers be familiar with the differential diagnosis of these disorders.

As with any other population, physical causes of somatic complaints among immigrant women must be assessed and ruled out or treated. In assessing immigrant women who report chronic somatic problems, questions about their level of worry, content of the worries, sleep problems, depression, and their perception of the cause of the problems can illuminate the nature of the problem and facilitate appropriate diagnosis. In addition, appropriate early diagnosis of anxiety and depression can prevent inappropriate, extended, and costly medical workups for symptoms that are consistent with somatization.

Medication, psychoeducation, cognitive behavioral approaches, and supportive therapy are suggested methods for treatment of anxiety disorders (Maxmen and Ward, 1995). It is particularly important that somatic and anxiety complaints in immigrant women be explored with respect and compassion; these women may have experienced discrimination and rejection elsewhere, and further insensitive interactions might compound anxiety symptoms. Treatment of anxiety should incorporate referrals for assistance with life skills training and concrete resources, such as English-language classes, immigrant parenting support groups, child care, citizenship education, and job placement. Because immigrant populations often face overwhelming stress, severe anxiety symptoms may not necessarily indicate a need for medication, but rather a need for assistance in resolving some of the stressful situations. In some cases, such as Ana's, resolution of life circumstances, coupled with newly acquired coping skills, will be the most effective treatment for anxiety.

## Treatment Modalities

Various types of interventions are available for the treatment of depression and anxiety in immigrant women. Several approaches may be combined to maximize treatment effectiveness.

### Psychopharmacology

Medication has been shown to be highly efficacious in reversing the underlying chemical imbalance in major depression. Although some patients may not require antidepressant medication, it is generally thought that patients may benefit more from psychotherapeutic approaches when these medications are used in conjunction with other modalities.

Pharmacological treatment of affective disorders began with the use of what are now known as the tricyclic antidepressants (TCA), such as nortriptyline, amitriptyline, imipramine, and desipramine. This class of antidepressants usually requires gradual titration over a period of time to achieve a therapeutic level. Subsequent periodic measurement of plasma drug levels is necessary. Although the tricyclics are effective treatment for depression, they are associated with side effects including sedation, orthostatic hypotension, dry mouth, constipation, and urinary retention, among others. More important, they have serious cardiac side effects related to prolongation of the Q-T interval, which can lead to arrhythmia. Concern about this side effect may limit the use of this class of antidepressant in the elderly and patients with cardiac disease. Cardiotoxicity also is related to the lethality of TCAs in cases of overdose, another concern when using this class of drugs in patients who may be suicidal.

Monoamine oxidase inhibitors (MAOIs) are another class of antidepressants, including phenelzine, tranylcypromine, and procarbazine, that were used more widely in the past. Their cardiac side effects, multiple interactions with other drugs, dietary restrictions, and contraindications to use in patients with preexisting liver disease have limited the use of these medications recently to patients with depression that is refractory to other psychotropic agents.

Tremendous advances in the field of pharmacology have led to the introduction of several new antidepressants. The selective serotonin reuptake inhibitors (SSRIs), such as fluoxetine, sertraline, and paroxetine, have become increasingly popular due to their ease of use, usually once-a-day dosing, and better safety profile compared to the older classes of antidepressants. Although SSRIs have some side effects, such as nausea, diarrhea, insomnia or sedation, and sexual dysfunction, generally they are transient. Education about the medication and support can help patients tolerate the side effects until they resolve.

Recently several atypical antidepressants such as buproprion and nefazadone have been introduced. They also have proved to be effective in the treatment of depression and have low side effect profiles. Attention should be paid to drug-drug interactions, which can influence the therapeutic level of antidepressants and the side effect profile.

Psychiatry's attention to ethnic minorities has increased as interest in cultural diversity and mental health has expanded. In the process, we have learned that there are biological differences in the metabolism of medication among ethnic minorities compared to Caucasians. This often results from differences in the rate of hepatic metabolism of most medications. Therefore, a longer titration period may be necessary, and a lower dose may be sufficient to achieve a therapeutic response in any patient with a lower rate of hepatic metabolism. Further, patients at high risk for previous hepatic dysfunction, such as immigrants from areas where hepatitis B and C are endemic, may warrant screening with liver function studies prior to initiation of therapy.

Other factors that may influence dosage include women's lower body mass index and body fat distribution. Thus, lower doses may be required on the basis of lower body weight and body habitus. Psychotropic medication generally has been avoided in pregnant and lactating women due to concerns about teratogenesis (especially during the first trimester) and transmission of the antidepressant and its metabolites into the mother's milk.

Clinicians need to be sensitive to cultures in which the ability for women to have children is an important concern, discuss these issues even with patients who are not pregnant, and realize that the patient and her family may resist the use of medication for this reason. In women with postpartum depression, the clinician must carefully balance the decision to implement antidepressant therapy with the infant's optimal nutrition and support for breastfeeding.

Finally, it is important for clinicians to be aware of how ethnic minorities view the role of medication in illness. Cultures that view illness as genetic or neurochemical in nature may see a greater role for medication, while others may view medication as being useful only in the acute phase of any illness (Gaw, 1993, p. 416).

### Psychoeducation

Education about the disorder provides a sense of meaning and control over the symptoms, normalizes the experience, provides hope, and sets the stage for the treatment process. Both Maria and Ana received education about their respective mental health problems and were helped to understand how their life stressors were related to their symptoms.

### Cognitive-Behavioral Approaches

Cognitive and behavioral approaches have been shown to be effective for both anxiety and depressive disorders. Use of culturally relevant metaphors to understand and cope with depression also has been successful in the treatment of depressed immigrants (B. Green, personal communication, 1997). Ana's therapist taught her to recognize triggers for somatic stress reactions and to reframe such trigger events cognitively. Through breathing and muscle relaxation techniques, she also was taught to reduce anxiety reactions once they started.

### Supportive, Narrative, and Expressive Therapies

Ego supportive therapy is useful for building on immigrant women's existing strengths (Goldstein, 1995). Narrative therapy provides an opportunity for the immigrant woman to tell and re- shape her own life story. Expressive therapy provides a construc- tive outlet for feelings of anger, frustration, and grief, which might not otherwise have an outlet. Maria explained that sharing her experiences and feelings in therapy was liberating, because she never was allowed to talk about them in Mexico. Maria's depres- sive symptoms dramatically lifted when she gave herself permis- sion to express her angry feelings toward her husband and to confront him in a constructive manner.

### Family Involvement

Involving the family or other significant members of the support network (such as sponsors) is critical because they provide the pri- mary support to immigrant women and also may be contributing to the experience of depression or anxiety. Provision of education about depression, how to provide emotional and practical sup- port, and what behaviors and interactions to avoid is helpful (Maxmen and Ward, 1995). Maria's husband initially was unwill- ing to be involved in Maria's treatment but later agreed to partic- ipate in family sessions and in treatment for domestic violence and substance abuse, all crucial to Maria's recovery.

### Education, Advocacy, Case Management, and Empowerment

Due to multiple stressors, concrete needs, and language and knowledge barriers, it often is essential to provide education and referral resources when working with immigrant and refugee women. Sometimes advocacy on behalf of the patient is required. This ultimately entails case management on the part of the thera- pist. Case management efforts are an important tool for empow- ering immigrant and refugee women and should not be seen as an unnecessary nuisance. In both Maria's and Ana's cases, case management activities were essential elements in the treatment process. These included communication with an immigration attorney; assistance in making overseas contact with Ana's son; and referrals for a variety of other services, such as a shelter, domestic violence and substance abuse treatment, English as a Second Language classes, job leads, housing resources, and health care.

*Grief Resolution*

Grinberg and Grinberg (1989) suggest that refugees and immigrants need a process of mourning. Mourning provides the opportunity to recognize, feel, and express losses that may be at the heart of depressive experiences. Facilitation of traditional grieving rituals can be useful.

## Conclusion

Due to their multiple life stressors, immigrant and refugee women may be at heightened risk for depression and anxiety disorders. Because these disorders manifest in culturally diverse ways, it may be difficult for U.S.-trained professionals to diagnose them in women from non-Western cultures. Regardless of the cultural aspects of symptom presentation, due to the unique circumstances faced by immigrant women, professionals need to modify standard assessment and treatment approaches. With sensitivity, patience, diligence, and respect, professionals can provide effective treatment for anxiety and depressive disorders, enabling immigrant and refugee women to participate fully in their new lives.

# Chapter Twelve

# Posttraumatic Stress Disorder

*Lisa C. Tracy*

Posttraumatic stress disorder (PTSD) has emerged as a particularly significant psychiatric disorder among refugees. In 1984, Kinzie and colleagues first applied the *Diagnostic and Statistical Manual of Mental Disorders* (DSM-III) PTSD diagnosis (American Psychiatric Association, 1980) to Cambodian survivors of concentration camps, initiating interest in cultural dimensions of traumatic stress. Since then, the literature on the study and treatment of PTSD among refugees gradually has increased and become a specialized field of clinical concern. Political refugees are clearly a population among whom PTSD may be prevalent, and there is some evidence that immigrants, particularly immigrant women, are more vulnerable to PTSD when they face stressors in the host country (Webster, McDonald, Lewin, and Carr, 1995).

By definition, PTSD occurs in response to severe stressors; it therefore is important to consider both the risk of experiencing traumatic events as well as the risk of responding to them with PTSD. Both immigrant and refugee women may be at heightened risk of experiencing interpersonal violence and sexual exploitation before and during migration. Once they have resettled, they may be at increased risk due to vulnerability in their status as noncitizens and to gender role conflict in the family. Refugee women from countries where war, severe political oppression, and torture are known to have occurred are particularly at risk for PTSD in response to events that occurred prior to their resettlement. The forms of violence to which some refugees have been exposed often are extreme, and the ways in which PTSD presents in such cases can be extremely severe and difficult to diagnose. PTSD often overlaps with other mental health problems such as depression, other anxiety disorders, somatization, dissociation, and, in some cases, psychotic symptoms. Cultural variation in the expression of distress lends further difficulty to diagnosis and treatment. The following case illustrates this complexity and severity.

Farah, a forty-five-year-old refugee woman with graduate-level professional education, from a war-torn Middle Eastern country, is referred from an emergency department to an agency that specializes in mental health treatment of immigrants and refugees. The referring clinician notes that Farah has been exhibiting severe psychotic symptoms. She appears distracted and at times incoherent and reports that she feels weakness, numbness, and tingling in her arms and legs, and at night she has insomnia, nightmares, and flashbacks of the death of her own child and of another child war victim she assisted during the aftermath of a terrorist attack near the school where she worked. She also hears voices telling her to kill herself. Sensitive, in-depth assessment conducted with Farah and her family in their native language reveals that Farah's husband, brother, and parents had been killed in the war, and a year later, one of her children was hit by random gunfire and died in her arms.

After these familial losses, she had continued her work as academic administrator in a primary school. She was present when fallout from a terrorist attack near the school left a dozen school staff and children critically wounded, and she immediately ran to help. When a child victim close in age to her own recently deceased child died in her arms, she collapsed and was unable to return to work. She and her four surviving children subsequently came to the United States as refugees.

Since her arrival in the United States, Farah has exhibited increasingly severe symptoms such as insomnia, nightmares, lack of awareness of her surroundings (dissociation), somatization, psychotic episodes, and occasional hypervigilant reactions to current stimuli, such as loud noises or scenes of war on television. She is unable to work and depends on her adult children for household management.

Farah was diagnosed with PTSD. The traumatic loss of her own child and the subsequent death of another child in her arms qualified as traumatic stressors. Her symptom profile fits the three major symptom categories of PTSD: reexperiencing by flashbacks and nightmares, avoidance by dissociation and numbing, and hyperarousal as seen in her insomnia and exaggerated response to subsequent stressors.

Other examples of seemingly extreme behavioral manifestations of distress occur among traumatized refugee women. Psychogenic blindness has been documented among Cambodian women survivors of concentration camps (Rozee and Van Boemel, 1990). With an awareness of the intensity of trauma and loss experienced by these women, and sensitivity and humility regarding cultural expressions of distress, such symptom patterns can be recognized as logical reactions and coping efforts in the face of the most horrendous and tragic life events rather than as pathological and bizarre behavior.

## DSM-IV Diagnosis of PTSD

The DSM-IV PTSD diagnosis consists of seven categories of criteria. Criterion A defines exposure to a stressor event in which "the person experienced, witnessed, or was confronted with an event or events that involved actual or threatened death or serious injury, or a threat to the physical integrity of self or others," and the person's response "involved intense fear, helplessness, or horror" (American Psychiatric Association, 1994, pp. 427–428), as demonstrated in Farah's case. Criteria B through D refer to the three major categories of symptoms—intrusive, avoidant, and hyperarousal symptoms—also seen in Farah's case. Intrusive symptoms are those in which an individual reexperiences the traumatic event or events through flashbacks, nightmares, or extreme emotional or physiological distress on exposure to something reminiscent of the original trauma. Avoidance symptoms may include active avoidance of remembering or discussing the trauma, avoidance of things reminiscent of it, inability to remember aspects of it, estrangement from others, diminished interest and range of affect, and "sense of a foreshortened future" (American Psychiatric Association, 1994, p. 428). Hyperarousal symptoms include sleep problems, excessive anger or irritability, problems concentrating, "hypervigilance," and "exaggerated startle response" (American Psychiatric Association, 1994, p. 428). Criterion E requires that the duration of the symptoms be more than one month, and criterion F requires that the symptoms cause "clinically significant distress or impairment in social, occupational or other important areas of functioning" (American Psychiatric Association, 1994, p. 429).

The diagnosis may be categorized as acute, if duration of symptoms is less than three months, or chronic, if symptoms persist more than three months. It should be coded "with delayed onset" if symptoms began at least six months after the stressor event. The major changes in DSM-IV from previous editions include an added discussion of age, cultural, and migration factors; an expanded discussion of differential diagnosis; a revision of the stressor criteria; a refinement of the duration criterion; the addition of a criterion of impaired functioning; and added specifications of acute or chronic subtypes of PTSD. In addition, the DSM authors revised a statement based on the still-controversial hypothesis that previous psychopathology predisposes one to PTSD.

Debate continues over whether posttraumatic stress should be considered pathological given its occurrence in response to terrible events, the validity of the PTSD diagnosis, its applicability across cultures, the distinction of PTSD symptoms from those in other diagnoses, including other anxiety disorders and affective, dissociative, psychotic, and personality disorders (McNally and Saigh, 1993; O'Donohue and Elliot, 1992; Pitman, 1993), and whether there should be several specific diagnostic categories of PTSD, based on type of trauma (Herman, 1993). The cluster of symptoms referred to as PTSD currently are alternatively referred to by many researchers and clinicians as posttraumatic stress syndrome, stress response syndrome, posttraumatic stress reaction, traumatic stress, and posttraumatic stress (Horowitz, 1986; Wilson, Harel, and Kahana, 1988), seemingly in an effort to broaden the emphasis from a specific disorder to a more general phenomenon of a human stress response process.

## Cultural Issues

The validity of the PTSD construct across cultures and situations has been questioned. For example, Eisenbruch (1991) suggests that the concept of cultural bereavement is more appropriate for populations such as Cambodians who have lost homeland, loved ones, and culture on a massive level. However, a recent study supports the validity of the PTSD diagnosis in Vietnamese refugees (Smith-Fawzi and others, 1997), and many researchers and clinicians assert the relevance of PTSD in describing the suffering and symptoms of Southeast Asian and other refugees (for example, Lee and Lu, 1989; Mathiasen and Lutzer, 1992). The cultural bereavement concept is useful. However, in the view of many who work with severely traumatized refugees, although the PTSD concept may still need refinement, it is useful for understanding, assessing, and treating traumatized migrant populations.

## Epidemiology of PTSD

Epidemiological studies of the general population using instruments such as the Diagnostic Interview Schedule (DIS) (Robins, Helzer, Croughan, and Ratcliff, 1981) and the Composite International Diagnostic Interview (CIDI) (Robins, Wing, Wittchen, and Helzer, 1988) have found overall rates of PTSD from 1 to just under 8 percent, with much higher rates among survivors of rape, violent crime, and war combat (Breslau, Davis, Andreski, and Peterson, 1991; Davidson, Hughes, Blazer, and George, 1991; Helzer, Robins, and McEnvoy, 1987; Kessler and others, 1995).

Refugee women who leave war-torn countries in which they may have been exposed to direct combat, rape, sexual assault, and other forms of violence are at great risk for PTSD. Research has revealed high rates of PTSD among refugees fleeing political catastrophe (Carlson and Rosser-Hogan, 1991; Cervantes, Salgado de Snyder, and Padilla, 1989; Dahl, Mutapcic, and Schei, 1998). The most frequently studied refugee populations are Southeast Asians, although other refugee groups, such as Central Americans, Afghans, and Bosnians, also have begun to receive attention in the literature. Carlson and Rosser-Hogan (1991) used the PTSD Symptom Checklist, an instrument based on DSM-III-R criteria and with similar outcomes to the DIS, in a community study of Cambodian refugees, many of them survivors of concentration camps and horrific events during migration. They found PTSD in 86 percent of the sample more than a decade after their arrival in the United States. Ninety percent of the sample met diagnostic criteria in two or more DSM-III-R categories, and 80 percent in three categories. The fact that the majority of this population suffered such a high level of symptomology and that the symptoms had persisted for so long is indicative of the level of trauma Cambodians have experienced.

A study of 258 Central American refugees and Mexican immigrants found that about 50 percent of the Central Americans met PTSD criteria (Cervantes, Salgado de Snyder, and Padilla, 1989). In a study of 209 displaced Bosnian women who attended a psychosocial women's resource center, Dahl, Mutapcic, and Schei (1998) found that 53 percent of the sample experienced posttraumatic stress. These rates of PTSD are much higher than the 1 to 8 percent reported in the general population.

Although many studies of PTSD in refugees have been conducted, less is known about PTSD in immigrants. One recent study compared native and immigrant individuals who experienced a natural disaster in Australia (Webster, McDonald, Lewin, and Carr, 1995). Immigrant women from non-English-speaking countries were at heightened risk for PTSD response (Webster, McDonald, Lewin, and Carr, 1995). In their study of Central American and Mexican migrants, Cervantes, Salgado de Snyder, and Padilla (1989) found that although Mexicans had lower rates of PTSD than their Central American counterparts, their rates of PTSD were still quite high, at 25 percent, well above the PTSD rates in the general population. Thus, it appears that both refugees and immigrants may be at heightened risk for PTSD compared to the general population.

## Traumatic Stress as a Coping Response: Risk and Protective Factors

Applying a stress and coping cognitive processing model (Creamer, Burgess, and Pattison, 1992; Lazarus and Folkman, 1984), the three symptom categories of PTSD—reexperiencing, avoidance, and hyperarousal—can be reframed as ways of coping with the trauma. Reexperiencing may be an attempt to process the event cognitively. Avoidance can be considered a means to reduce distress associated with the event or memories of it, and hyperarousal may be a means to avoid retraumatization (Horowitz, 1986; Tracy, 1997). Janoff-Bulman (1992) argues that trauma is the result of shattered assumptions that the world is just, controllable, and meaningful, and Herman (1992) stresses that interpersonal violence shatters basic trust and connection to others.

Research on PTSD outcomes suggests that the manner in which each individual cognitively processes and understands an event depends on event characteristics, such as level of threat and duration; social support before, during, and after traumatic experiences; the individual's previous history of trauma; developmental experiences and stage; and spiritual strength and practices. It appears that as severity of the event or events increases, other factors become less salient in determining coping and PTSD outcome (McCranie, Hyer, Boudewyns, and Woods, 1992). In a clinical study of 322 Southeast Asian patients, Kinzie and others (1990) found that 93 percent of Mien, 92 percent of Cambodian, 68 percent of Lao, and 54 percent of Vietnamese patients suffered from PTSD. It is thought that the horrendous conditions in Cambodia, and the vast culture shock experienced by hill tribes such as the Mien, contributed to their extremely high rates of PTSD, compared to the lower, though still elevated, rates among the Lao and Vietnamese.

The levels of threat and duration of trauma many refugees experienced often is overwhelming; their experiences may encompass not one circumscribed event, but years of chronic exposure to physical and psychological torture and deaths and brutal murders of loved ones. Under such circumstances, the ability to integrate and apply meaning to events, emotionally and cognitively, and the ability to trust and maintain social bonds are challenged to the point of disintegration. It appears that under some circumstances, such as what occurred in the Cambodian holocaust, PTSD may be a normative response.

# Recognition, Assessment, and Treatment of PTSD

Recognizing PTSD in immigrant and refugee women requires awareness of the context of their lives, knowledge about the variety of manifestations that PTSD can take, and the ability to conduct a culturally appropriate assessment. The discussions of somatization, culture-bound disorders, and neurasthenia in Chapter Thirteen provide further insight into the importance of understanding the possible meanings of physical complaints among diverse refugee and immigrant populations.

Traumatized refugee and immigrant women need to be treated with respect and compassion. Providing too many options may overwhelm a new arrival who is coping with past trauma, PTSD symptoms, and culture shock. Gentle guidance and willingness to take time to listen are needed. Women from many cultures will not discuss events such as rape, lending further difficulty to detection of traumatic roots to symptoms. Physicians and other health professionals need to be aware that forgetfulness, lack of concentration, and nightmares may not be minor complaints or the result of acculturative stress and depression alone, but may be rooted in specific traumatic events and require focused, specialized, culturally appropriate treatment. Kiani (personal communication, 1997) and Shepherd (1992b) emphasize the importance of collecting a complete history, including premigration, migration, and postmigration factors. Shepherd (1992b) suggests using the oral history method, in which the patient is supported in telling her life story, to gather this information.

Undertaking treatment and even simply initiating referrals for appropriate treatment may require patience and diligence. In some areas, there are targeted treatment centers and networks for survivors of torture, most of whom are refugees. However, in many cases, they do not serve refugees and immigrants who may have PTSD but were not subjected to torture. In other areas, culturally appropriate treatment for traumatized refugees can be difficult to locate. There are specialized trauma treatment centers in some urban areas, although such centers do not necessarily have expertise with refugees. Ethnic-specific mental health agencies and agencies that target immigrants and refugees often serve large numbers of traumatized refugees. Their clinical approaches are culturally relevant and may offer a range of language and translation services that are not found in other settings. However, staff may not be specially trained in the treatment of PTSD.

Although there are a number of promising approaches, effective, culturally relevant treatment of refugees and immigrants with PTSD needs further development. The focus of treatment may differ depending on the population or the orientation and capacity of the treatment facility. Essentially there are two stages of treatment. One is gaining control of overwhelming symptoms such as difficulty concentrating, flashbacks, inability to sleep, and exaggerated startle response, all of which can significantly impair basic functioning. The other stage is referred to as *resolution of the trauma*. Resolution generally is accepted as an appropriate goal for work with more circumscribed trauma in Western populations and usually involves remembering and working through traumatic experiences.

The views on resolution as a goal for other populations are varied. It is difficult for women who have experienced pervasive trauma and loss, such as that which occurred in the Cambodian holocaust, to work through multiple experiences of torture, sexual violence, and murder. Verbal orientation and the patient's educational background are considered important factors in determining the approach to treatment, particularly when using narrative or testimonial approaches. Thus, resolution involving remembering, reexperiencing, and verbalizing traumatic events and the feelings they evoke may or may not be an appropriate goal. Another approach, which may be more appropriate for women from traditional cultures, facilitates resolution through such traditional means as shamanic healing or religious practice. Both the goal and type of treatment should take into account the cultural background, individual factors, support system, nature of the trauma experience, and, very important, the capacity of the clinician and service facility to provide consistent, long-term care and support. A combination of approaches such as those described next may be the most useful.

## Psychoeducation

It is important to provide education about the causes and manifestations of PTSD to the patient and her family. It should be explained with sensitivity early in treatment that others have experienced the same problem. In the light of language and cultural barriers, the clinician needs to ensure that the patient and family understand what is being discussed. Such education can normalize the experience, decrease stigma and shame, and provide at least some sense of control and hope.

## Cognitive-Behavioral Approaches

A number of cognitive-behavioral methods, such as breathing, relaxation, and concentration exercises, can help to control PTSD symptoms. These techniques are useful for gaining control over symptoms and should be taught in early stages of treatment.

## Psychopharmacology

Medication can be used to control symptoms of PTSD, but it must be prescribed with awareness that Asian, Middle Eastern, and other non-Western populations may require smaller doses and may experience more side effects than European Americans. Close follow-up, with attention to the possibility of chronic liver problems and decreased metabolism, and to weight-adjusted dosages, can improve medication treatment with culturally diverse populations. Farah is a good candidate for medication to control her symptoms.

## Family Involvement

Because the family is such a central point of identity, support, and conflict for many immigrant and refugee women, provision of services and psychoeducation to family members, and inclusion of family in the treatment process, is important. For example, it would be critical to provide education to Farah's adult children, as well as the patient, about the symptoms of PTSD and its treatment. The family members also could be included in developing the treatment plan, particularly around issues of medication adherence, creating safety, and what to do in an emergency. The adult children may themselves need emotional support as they cope with their own losses and the stress of their mother's disorder.

## Testimony and Oral History Methods

Agger and Jensen (1990) use the testimony method in which survivors of political torture are encouraged to tell their stories in a therapeutic environment, and the story is then used as testimony with the purpose of bringing the truth out and preventing further atrocities against others. This method has been useful primarily with those who have a verbal orientation and a relatively high level of education. Herbst (1992) has used an empowerment-focused oral history method in combination with relaxation and other holistic approaches in work with Cambodian women. In Farah's case, the oral history method may be appropriate due to her high verbal ability. The clinician would slowly encourage the client to tell her own story, carefully monitoring psychotic symptoms and dissociation. The primary focus in initial sessions nevertheless should be controlling symptoms using other approaches.

## Incorporation of Indigenous Healing Practices

Eisenbruch (1991) described a case study of successful shamanic intervention with a Cambodian refugee woman. He argued that among Cambodian and other survivors of concentration camps and war, not only have assumptions of safety, justice, and stability been shattered, but refugees find themselves in a world where their assumptions may no longer be of any practical relevance. The shamanic intervention was a culturally relevant means of restoring shattered assumptions of a just, controllable, and meaningful world and provided nonstigmatizing social support. Shepherd (personal communication, 1997) facilitated a traumatized Cambodian woman's resolution of the murder of her child by locating a Buddhist temple and accompanying her to the temple. Simply providing respectful support of traditional spiritual practices also may be helpful. Work with Farah and her family might include facilitation of culturally appropriate mourning rituals.

## Body Work

Somatic approaches are increasingly used to treat severe PTSD. Faust (personal communication, 1997) has used acupuncture with traumatized refugee women, and many trauma treatment centers incorporate the use of acupuncture, massage, and other forms of body work in holistic treatment plans.

## Structured Support Groups for Traumatized Refugees

The structured support group model, developed by Judith Shepherd in her work with severely traumatized Cambodian women and Vietnamese men at San Francisco General Hospital, can be used in hospital outpatient or inpatient settings and can be adapted culturally. This model is described in detail in Chapter Fifteen.

## Conclusion

PTSD is a significant mental health issue for many refugee and immigrant women. Health care providers need to be aware of the complexity of presentation of PTSD symptoms in this population and provide appropriate screening, emotional support, and referrals. While knowledge about effective treatment for PTSD continues to accumulate, a number of promising approaches can be used to relieve at least some of the suffering associated with PTSD.

# Chapter Thirteen

# Somatization, Neurasthenia, and Culture-Bound Syndromes

# Somatization Disorders

*Cora R. Hoover*

*Somatization* is the name often given to the ubiquitous human tendency to experience and express distress in the form of bodily symptoms. The *Diagnostic and Statistical Manual of Mental Disorders* (DSM-IV) (American Psychiatric Association, 1994) describes several somatoform disorders, including the multisymptom somatization disorder. However, most instances of somatization come to the attention of primary care physicians and do not meet the DSM-IV criteria. Sometimes higher rates of somatization have been found in groups with lower socioeconomic status and in non-Western cultures. For the most part, cultural variations in the patterns of somatization remain unstudied. Somatization is a marker for psychiatric morbidity, especially anxiety and depression, as well as for traumatic life experiences. The subtleties of these links between the body and the mind often are culture specific and may present a particular challenge to practitioners who are working cross-culturally. Most anxious and depressed patients of all cultures present in primary care visits with somatic rather than emotional complaints. Given this tendency, the burden rests on practitioners to inquire about psychosocial problems. Somatizing patients use a disproportionate share of medical services and tend to underuse mental health services. Several treatment approaches to somatization have been proposed, including detection of underlying mental health disorders in primary care, cognitive-behavioral work, and narrative therapy. Further exploration of treatment approaches within the primary care context is needed.

## DSM-IV Somatization Disorder

The DSM-IV describes several somatoform disorders, but such a diagnostic framework does little to suggest etiologic explanations or therapeutic approaches for somatization. The DSM-IV somatoform disorders are somatization disorder, undifferentiated somatoform disorder, pain disorder, and hypochondriasis. The conditions involve "the presence of physical symptoms that suggest a general medical condition . . . and are not fully explained by a general medical condition, by the direct effects of a substance, or by another mental disorder" (American Psychiatric Association, 1994).

Among the somatoform disorders, somatization disorder (SD) has received the most attention, despite its rarity in comparison with other forms of somatization. It is a serious, chronic condition involving "recurring, multiple, clinically significant somatic complaints" (American Psychiatric Association, 1994). Revised and simplified diagnostic criteria for SD in the DSM-IV include all of the following: four pain symptoms, two gastrointestinal symptoms, one sexual symptom, and one pseudoneurological symptom such as a conversion or dissociative symptom (American Psychiatric Association, 1994). Patients with SD tend to seek and receive medical services and may suffer significant morbidity due to invasive testing, unnecessary surgeries, and addiction to pain medication and tranquilizers. Full-blown SD is uncommon, with a prevalence of 0.2 to 2.0 percent among women and 0.2 percent among men (American Psychiatric Association, 1994). The alternative diagnosis of undifferentiated somatoform disorder is applied when a person suffers chronic, unexplained physical symptoms that do not meet the full criteria for SD.

The cutoff for diagnosis of SD in terms of number of symptoms has been criticized as arbitrary. One study of high users of primary care found no significant clinical or behavioral differences between patients suffering four to twelve unexplained symptoms as opposed to those with full-blown SD (Katon and others, 1991). Given this continuum of behavior and symptomatology, Escobar and others (1989) have proposed an abridged construct of SD (the Somatic Symptom Index, or SSI) that technically would fall under the rubric of DSM-IV undifferentiated somatoform disorder. The SSI lists six somatic symptoms for women and four for men. This construct was proposed based on the observation that in a community sample, individuals with less than full-blown SD had "risk factors, service use patterns, and disabilities" (Escobar and others, 1989) similar to those with the full-blown disorder. Escobar and others found a prevalence of 9 percent to 20 percent for the SSI construct in samples surveyed as part of the population-based ECA (Epidemiologic Catchment Area) study done during the 1980s. The prevalence of somatization, as measured by the SSI, was one hundred times that of full-blown SD in the same group. The researchers then pooled data from the Los Angeles ECA site and from a similar study done on the island of Puerto Rico. They found that the odds ratios for having SSI were 1.2 for U.S.-born Mexican Americans, 1.1 for Mexico-born Mexican Americans, and 2.3 for Puerto Ricans, compared with non-Hispanic whites. Among all groups except Puerto Ricans, a positive SSI was more common among women than among men.

## Prevalence of Somatization

Although reports of somatic symptoms are high in all cultures, members of U.S. minority groups and members of non-Western cultures have been said to report more somatic symptoms than members of the majority U.S. culture (Kleinman, 1986; Kirmayer, 1996). Similarly, as part of the recent ECA study, respondents with lower socioeconomic status (SES) were found to report more somatic symptoms than their high-SES counterparts (Simon and VonKorff, 1991). At times, these characterizations may lead to the stereotyping of individual patients as somatizers, at the expense of full medical investigation of a particular complaint. The nuances of the relationship between somatic symptomatology and psychological distress among members of various ethnic groups need to be explored further; at this point, specific patterns of somatization in particular cultures may deserve more attention than comparisons of somatization rates among groups.

Discrepancies in somatic symptom reporting may be due in part to the well-known correlation of SES with physical and mental health (Angel and Guarnaccia, 1989). Immigrants, and especially refugees, also may be at high risk for somatization given their recent experiences of trauma and major life changes (Lin, Carter, and Kleinman, 1985). Castillo, Waitzkin, and Escobar (1994) describe somatization among refugees as "sociogenic" (p. 173) in the sense that stressful experiences lead directly to psychological distress, mental disorders, and unexplained somatic symptoms. Lin, Carter, and Kleinman (1985) found that Asian refugees seeking care at a Seattle health clinic used more health services than nonrefugee immigrants and were significantly more likely than nonrefugee immigrants to present with vague somatic complaints.

## Co-Occurrence of Physical and Psychological Distress

Somatization traditionally has been viewed as a way of defending against difficult emotional experience (Lipowski, 1988, p. 1359), "a process of converting, transferring, or diverting emotional distress into somatic symptoms" (Kirmayer, 1996, p.132). However, recent studies have shown that when they are asked directly, many people who are experiencing a high level of somatic symptomatology also complain of coexisting psychological distress (Escobar and others, 1989; Katon and others, 1991). Researchers have found significant correlations between the number of somatic symptoms and the incidence of psychiatric morbidity, especially anxiety and depression. Somatization also has been found to be associated with the experience of childhood sexual abuse (Morrison, 1989) and posttraumatic stress disorder (Castillo, Waitzkin, and Escobar, 1994).

Data from the ECA study show that individuals who experience one or two unexplained somatic symptoms are four times as likely to be depressed as those who experience no symptoms, and those who experience five or more symptoms are seventeen times more likely to be depressed (Simon and VonKorff, 1991). Similarly, respondents who experience one or two somatic symptoms are eleven times more likely to suffer from panic disorder than those who experience no symptoms, and those who experience five or more symptoms are over two hundred times more likely to suffer from panic disorder. The authors of this study observed that the "expression of overt psychological distress increased steadily with increasing numbers of functional somatic symptoms, and only a small minority of respondents with high levels of somatization did not report overt anxiety or depressive symptoms" (Simon and VonKorff, 1991). This association between physical and emotional distress contradicts the schema in which physical distress substitutes for or defends against psychological distress. Instead it suggests that a process of heightened, simultaneous experience of both forms of distress might be operative for many somatizing individuals. Physical and emotional distress may be seen as occurring in parallel or as intertwined.

The relationship of somatization, distress, and mental disorders may be culturally specific. For example, a recent study of Hispanic women by Deborah Duran of the National Coalition of Hispanic Health and Human Services Organizations showed that the pathways between somatization and psychological distress varied with acculturation (Tucker, 1997). In Hispanic women with low acculturation, distressors such as poverty, domestic violence, and sexual assault led directly to somatization, and less often to depression. For more acculturated Hispanic women, distress was more closely associated with depression, which led to somatic complaints. With respect to ethnic Chinese, May argued in a 1994 article that for this group, the body is synonymous with the self. The lack of a mind-body dichotomy in Chinese culture accounts for traditional Chinese medicine's explaining some physical illnesses in terms of strong emotions and some illnesses in terms of external factors (Tung, 1994).

## Somatization in the Context of Culture

A culturally oriented schema for somatization has been proposed and investigated by other authors (Hulme, 1996; Koss, 1990; Kleinman, 1986; Kirmayer, 1985), many of whom share an anthropological perspective. This schema may prove useful to primary care providers who are caring for somatizing patients. Somatization is understood as a function of coping—an idiom of distress that functions within a particular cultural context to express discontent that may not be expressed easily through other channels. A prominent example of research using this model of somatization is Kleinman's (1986) work on neurasthenia and depression in China. Kleinman found that neurasthenic patients used their disease and illness role as a mechanism to cope with painful and disempowering social circumstances such as forced geographical separation from family or dehumanizing work conditions.

The body is used metaphorically in this last form of somatization (Kleinman, 1986; Lipowski, 1988), although such a metaphorical role should not imply that the symptoms are any less real for the individuals who are experiencing them. Kirmayer (1985) notes that bodily metaphors are a sophisticated and subtle means of communication. Unfortunately, the heightened significance of the somatic symptoms may not be appreciated by members of cultures other than the patient's. For example, Southeast Asian refugees suffering from depression may complain of "weak heart," "weak kidney," and "weak nervous system" (Muecke, 1983); Western practitioners may be confused and baffled by these complaints.

## Somatic Presentation of Mental Disorders

Depression in contemporary Western culture may be anomalous in that it often prominently features "guilt, self-depreciation, and depressed affect" (Katon, Kleinman, and Rosen, 1982), as opposed to primarily somatic symptoms. This focus on cognitive and affective symptoms may stem from a tendency to "psychologize" what is in fact both a psychosocial and a physical process. Western cultures uphold a philosophical distinction between mind and body, and between physical and psychological distress, while non-Western cultures may not (Kirmayer, 1996; Kleinman, 1986). However, even among members of the majority culture, the rate of somatic presentation of major depression and anxiety is 84 percent (Kirmayer, Young, and Robbins, 1994).

Patients from all cultures may selectively attend to the somatic aspects of their distress due to cognitive, developmental, or cultural influences (Katon, Kleinman, and Rosen, 1982). For example, depression and other mental disorders may not be recognized as legitimate illnesses by the family or by the larger society (Finkler, 1985). Individuals suffering from depression and other mental disorders may have to manifest physical illness in order to receive care and treatment for their distress. In addition, mental illness may be strongly stigmatized, while physical illness is not, leading to help seeking for physical rather than emotional problems (Castillo,

Waitzin, and Escobar, 1994; Chun, Enomoto, and Sue, 1996; Canino and others, 1992; Katon, Kleinman, and Rosen, 1982). For example, in a recent review of the literature concerning Asian Americans and somatization, Chun, Enomoto, and Sue (1996) concluded that Asian Americans and whites experience somatic symptoms at a similar rate; however, due to discomfort with mental illness, Asian Americans experiencing psychological distress initially are more likely than whites to report exclusively somatic symptoms to practitioners and interviewers.

Indeed, other researchers have found that although most depressed and anxious patients present somatically, most also are willing to cite psychosocial distress as a possible source of their symptoms when asked directly (Kirmayer, Young, and Robbins, 1994). Patients may expect that physicians are interested in physical rather than psychological distress, and so may selectively report somatic symptoms (Cheung, 1982); similarly, physicians may fail to inquire about psychosocial distress (Kirmayer and Robbins, 1996). In other words, the phenomenon of somatization is often context dependent (Chun, Enomoto, and Sue, 1996, p. 358), a product of the health care system itself.

Thus, a major obstacle to effective detection and treatment of depression and anxiety in primary care is somatic presentation of the disorders by patients coupled with lack of awareness by physicians. Bridges and Goldberg (1985) found that primary care physicians detected only half of all psychiatric disorders that presented somatically. Underdetection may be compounded by cultural and linguistic barriers between physicians and patients. Badger and others (1994) found that physicians relied heavily on factors such as appearance and behavior in making their diagnosis of depression, rather than inquiring specifically about DSM criteria of depression. This reliance on observation may make cross-cultural detection of mental disorders particularly difficult.

## Somatization in Primary Care and Utilization of Mental Health Services

Because somatization involves medical help seeking, it is important to explore the relationship of somatizing individuals to the health care system. Depending on the exact criteria used, between

11.5 percent and 26.3 percent of the multiethnic primary care patient population Kirmayer and Robbins (1991) studied are judged to be somatizers. A study of primary care encounters showed that somatizing patients made 50 percent more office visits than their nonsomatizing counterparts (DeGruy, Columbia, and Dickinson, 1987). Similarly, Lin, Carter, and Kleinman (1985) found that 25 percent of visits to a health clinic by Asian immigrants and refugees were for "vague somatic symptoms," with those visits costing more on average than visits for diagnosed physical or mental disorders. These statistics represent a potential overutilization of primary care services by somatizing patients. However, given the high levels of distress experienced by these patients, perhaps the term *misutilization* is more appropriate. As we have seen, many somatizing patients are suffering from undiagnosed and untreated mental disorders.

Recent National Comorbidity Survey (NCS) data show that only 36 percent of subjects with major depression and only 25 percent of those with anxiety disorders received professional treatment, including that provided by general physicians (Kessler and others, 1996). One aspect of utilization that remains to be studied is the use of nonallopathic sources of health care such as traditional Chinese medicine by immigrant groups; these treatments are potentially useful for mind-body problems that otherwise would be treated by the medical and mental health care systems.

## Perspectives on Treatment

Several potential treatment approaches for somatization within the medical and mental health care systems have been proposed in the literature. One approach involves the detection of underlying mental disorders by primary care providers, since disorders such as anxiety or depression may contribute to somatic symptomatology in many patients. This approach, described by Chun, Enomoto, and Sue (1996) with respect to Asian Americans, could be useful for immigrant women patients of many ethnicities. Practitioners are encouraged to ask questions about psychological as well as physical symptoms when taking an initial patient history. They also should ascertain the patient's beliefs about the etiology and treatment of her symptoms in order to avoid misunderstandings and facilitate the patient's engagement in the therapeutic process. Furthermore, because patients may be unfamiliar with and wary of mental health services, the patient should be eased into mental health treatment (Chun, Enomoto, and Sue, 1996). This transition could be facilitated by a team relationship between primary care and mental health providers.

Unexplained somatic distress can cue the provider to inquire about psychosocial stressors such as domestic violence or hardships related to immigration as well as about psychiatric symptoms. If somatization is indeed functioning as an idiom of distress for a particular patient, such an inquiry gives the patient a forum to express her psychosocial concerns.

Another approach to the treatment of somatization addresses somatic symptoms more directly. For example, Barsky, Geringer, and Wool (1988) describe a cognitive-behavioral therapy group in which somatizing patients learn to attribute their symptoms to nonpathological causes and also are taught distraction and relaxation techniques. Griffith and Griffith (1994), who are family therapists, have used a narrative therapy approach with somatizing patients. They believe that some somatic symptoms occur as a result of "unspeakable dilemmas" (p. 45), where a powerful emotion is experienced but cannot be expressed. They encourage patients to talk about their somatic symptoms as emotional messages and to discover which emotions and situations trigger not only somatic symptoms, but also bodily experiences of peace and contentment. These approaches to somatization need not be the sole province of mental health providers. Primary care providers could, for example, educate patients about the benign etiologies of their symptoms and encourage them to learn and practice relaxation techniques. Finally, primary care providers also could help patients elucidate which emotions or situations trigger their symptoms, and which emotions or situations are experienced as calming and healing.

# Neurasthenia

*Pamela Yew Schwartz*

*Neurasthenia,* a term coined in the 1860s by an American neurologist, George M. Beard (1869), describes a cluster of physical symptoms associated with a weakened nervous system. The characteristic symptoms were profound physical and mental exhaustion, combined with other dysfunctions such as headaches, insomnia, vague pains, dyspepsia, palpitations, and flushing. Beard (1880) saw these diverse symptoms as resulting from excessive demands placed on the nervous system and expenditure of nervous energy. He also postulated neurasthenia to be a peculiarly American phenomenon, secondary to the psychological demands placed on individuals in a rapidly advancing modern society.

Many neurologists and psychiatrists in Europe and the United States wrote about neurasthenia between the late 1800s and early 1900s, espousing a variety of hypotheses regarding its etiology, usually emphasizing somatic, neurological, or psychological causative factors (Lin, 1992). In the 1940s and 1950s, American psychiatrists began to debate its usefulness given the multitude of symptoms, its indiscriminant use, and the nonspecific and ambiguous nature of the condition (Lee and Wong, 1995). Its popularity declined, and neurasthenia was eventually excluded from the third edition of the *Diagnostic and Statistical Manual of Mental Disorders* (DSM-III) (American Psychiatric Association, 1980), the official taxonomy of the American Psychiatric Association, where it had previously been listed as "neurasthenia neurosis" in the DSM-II (American Psychiatric Association, 1968).

More recently, there has been growing interest in a condition known as chronic fatigue syndrome (CFS), which is characterized by the experience of pervasive fatigue accompanied by a diffuse constellation of somatic, cognitive, and emotional symptoms (Ware and Kleinman, 1992b). Its etiology remains unclear. Hypotheses and research on CFS have entertained several linkages, including Epstein-Barr virus (Jones and others, 1985), other viruses, immunological factors, and psychiatric disorders, particularly depression (Straus, 1988; Youssef and others, 1988). The question of whether CFS is a contemporary revival of neurasthenia, and therefore neurasthenia may be subsumed under it, or whether they should continue to be considered as two separate if somewhat similar diagnostic entities has been raised in the psychiatric literature (Abbey and Garfinkel, 1991; S. Lee, 1994; Zheng and others, 1992).

Outside the United States, clinicians have continued to use the term *neurasthenia*. The ninth revision of the World Health Organization's *International Classification of Diseases* (ICD-9), published in 1978, defined *neurasthenia* as a neurotic disorder. The following edition, ICD-10, published in 1996, presented a set of well-defined inclusion and exclusion criteria for the diagnosis. The core symptoms were identified as mental or physical fatigue or both, accompanied by at least two of seven conditional symptoms: dizziness, dyspepsia, muscular aches or pains, tension headaches, inability to relax, irritability, and sleep disturbance. The illness duration needed to be persistent, and exclusion criteria included the presence of mood, panic, or generalized anxiety disorders.

## Neurasthenia in the Asian Context

The use of neurasthenia in Asia appeared to have followed a pattern similar to the one in Europe; it began with popular acclaim, was followed by critical assessment, and ended with transforming this condition into culturally meaningful diagnostic concepts.

In Japan, neurasthenia is known as *shinkeisuijaku,* meaning "nervousness or nervous disposition" (Lin, 1992). Initially it was seen as "a psychological reaction developed in a certain type of personality characterized by hypersensitivity, introversion, self-consciousness, perfectionism, and hypochondriacal disposition" (Lin, 1992). Morita therapy, the treatment of choice at that time, aimed at breaking the cycle of sensitivity and anxiety by assisting the patient to cope with the anxiety. Shoma Morita developed this traditional Zen Buddhism–based treatment modality at the turn of the century. It has been characterized by bed rest and isolation and by work therapy with the goal of helping the patient accept life's situation and assume a social role. More recently, neurasthenia has been used by both professionals and laypeople to "camouflage" more serious mental disorders such as schizophrenia and affective illnesses (Lin, 1992). This allows patients to assume a more socially acceptable sick role and the biologically focused Japanese psychiatric professionals to apply their treatments. Neurasthenia currently is considered a curable physical condition without the stigma of a psychiatric diagnosis (Machizawa, 1992). The treatments of choice include rest, good environment, and time.

The traditional Chinese construction of the person is grounded in a holistic, unitary system, integrating both the psychological and the physical; what happens to the mind affects the body, and vice versa. This basic Eastern tenet lends itself naturally to permitting the coexistence of depression and somatic complaints. The introduction of neurasthenia to China in the 1920s and 1930s coincided with a period of social upheaval (Lin, 1992). Lin (1985) hypothesized that the marked increase in use of neurasthenia during the early communist years was due to the severe tension between the country's social and political condition and the people's physical and psychological hardships. Medical clinics were reporting 80 percent to 90 percent incidence of neurasthenia. As Chinese people tend to express their distress physically and psychological symptoms could be interpreted as forbidden discontent with the government (Kleinman, 1986), neurasthenia became the safer and preferred expression of distress (Lin, 1992).

In the *Chinese-English Terminology of Traditional Chinese Medicine* (1983), the etiology of neurasthenia is given as a decrease in vital energy *(qi)*. Harmful factors, both exogenous and endogenous to the patient's body, reduce the functioning of the five internal organ systems (*wuzang*, heart, liver, spleen, lungs, kidneys), which leads to deficiency of vital energy *(qi)* and lower bodily resistance.

In 1983, Xu and Zhon established a more elaborate set of diagnostic criteria for neurasthenia, known as *shenjingshuairou* (weakness of nerves). Currently these are found in the Chinese Classification of Mental Disorders (CCMD-2) (Chinese Medical Association, 1989). Unlike the ICD-10, there is no dominant feature in this classification. Three of the following five conditional symptoms are required: (1) "weakness" symptom, (2) "emotional" symptom, (3) "excitement" symptom, (4) tension-induced pain, and (5) sleep disturbance. The duration of illness must be at least three months, and one of the following is required: (1) disruption of work, study, daily life, or social function; (2) significant distress caused by the illness; or 3) pursuit of treatment. Other clinical conditions that may produce similar symptoms must be absent.

Kleinman (1982, 1986) noted the striking difference in the epidemiology of psychiatric disorders in China compared to the West. He found a high prevalence of neurasthenia and a low prevalence of major depression in China, as depressed patients tended to avoid help due to the stigma of mental disorder. Kleinman (1982) did an empirical study of one hundred patients with the diagnosis of neurasthenia who attended the psychiatric outpatient clinic of the Hunan Medical College. The most significant finding was that of one hundred neurasthenic patients, ninety-three had clinical depression of one kind or another, eighty-seven met the diagnostic criteria of major depressive disorder, and sixty-nine suffered from anxiety states. In addition, 90 percent of the neurasthenia sample reported some form of pain, and 87 percent of those with major depressive disorder exhibited pain, findings similar to those reported in studies on pain and depression in the West.

All patients with the diagnosis of major depressive disorders were treated with antidepressants, and 87 percent were assessed as having subsequent symptomatic improvement. Kleinman (1986) saw these findings as supporting somatization in Chinese medical anthropology and cultural psychiatry. He concluded that neurasthenia was most beneficial clinically when it was regarded as a "biculturally patterned illness experience (a special form of somatization), related to either depression and other diseases, or to culturally sanctioned idioms of distress and psychosocial coping" (p. 115).

## Research on Neurasthenia in Chinese Populations

Until recently, most studies of neurasthenia in the Chinese population were conducted outside the United States. Xu and Zhon
(1983) reported a prevalence rate of 6.1 percent in Shanghai. Yan
(1989) found that after twenty years of treatment, 93 percent of
eighty-nine patients who were suffering from neurasthenia recovered without ever using antidepressant medication. When these
neurasthenic cases were reassessed with the DSM-III and the Present State Examination (PSE), 40 percent were found to be depressed, and they responded well to antidepressant medication.
Cheung (1991) reviewed research conducted in China during the
1980s and found low depression rates, but neurasthenia emerged
as the most common neurotic disorder. Similar rates for neurasthenia were found in Hong Kong and Taiwan (Draguns, 1996). A
more recent study of a Southeast Asian refugee sample (Chung
and Singer, 1995) in California used factor analysis of symptom
expressions and found one robust factor that was very similar to
the neurasthenia construct. These findings support the importance of retaining neurasthenia as a diagnosis, which clearly cannot easily be subsumed under the Western criteria of depression.

Over the past several years, there has been more interest in res-
urrecting the neurasthenia diagnosis for assessing Chinese Americans. Hong, Chan, Zheng, and Wang (1992) examined seventy-six
native Chinese university students in the United States and found
that those who had been diagnosed as neurasthenic frequently
had experienced symptoms of depression, as measured by the
Center for Epidemiological Studies–Depression Scale (CES-D).
Using data from the Chinese American Psychiatric Epidemiological Study, a five-year National Institute of Mental Health–funded
study involving 1,747 completed households in Los Angeles
County, Zheng and his colleagues (1997) found that 6.4 percent of
the participants met ICD-10 diagnostic criteria for neurasthenia
(compared to 3.6 percent who suffered from major depression).
Of those, 56.3 percent did not experience any current or lifetime
DSM-III-R diagnoses; they were "pure" sufferers of neurasthenia.
Again, this suggests the utility of retaining neurasthenia as a
distinct diagnosis in Chinese Americans, a conclusion drawn as
well by other researchers (Ware and Kleinman, 1992a; Yan, 1989;

Zheng and Lin, 1991; Zheng and others, 1992). Using the same data set, Takeuchi, Wang, and Chun (1996) found that less acculturated Chinese immigrants tended to express their distress through somatic and neurasthenic symptoms, whereas the expression of depression was similar for both the low and the highly acculturated.

## Evaluation and Treatment

As with depression, neurasthenia has been thought to be more prevalent in women than men (Beard, 1880; Chin and Chin, 1969), although no gender difference was found in the Chinese American Epidemiological Study (Zheng and others, 1997). Although this finding deserves further investigation, neurasthenia is likely to be a common diagnosis in Chinese immigrant women. A major reason that it has survived as a diagnostic category is that it is not viewed as a mental health problem, which often is stigmatized. Cheung (1987) has suggested that when they are asked directly, Chinese immigrant patients acknowledge both affective and somatic symptoms in their experience of depression and distress. In the intake evaluation process, inquiring about neurasthenic experiences may avert the stigma-ridden resistance that the term *depression* tends to invoke for this population. Rapport and therapeutic alliances may then be achieved more expeditiously. Cheung (1981, 1987) has further suggested that somatic complaints and medical assistance are more acceptable for more severe psychological difficulties.

Traditional therapy for neurasthenia has included diet, hygiene, massage, medication, the appropriate use of rest, adjustment of work, and change of lifestyle (Kleinman, 1986). The Chinese treatment of illnesses in general has been symptom driven. Cheung (1989) reported that herbal medicines, self-management methods such as rest and exercise, development and "change in personality and attitudes," using tonic medicines and special nutrient foods, as well as other methods aimed at symptom relief and increase in relaxation were used for lay treatment of neurasthenia. Antidepressant medications and psychological counseling have been the standard treatments of choice more recently and in medical settings.

## Conclusion

It is essential that mental health practitioners be able to understand, evaluate, and treat patients in a culturally appropriate manner. Given that the stigma of mental illness continues to play an important role in how Asian immigrants seek services, awareness of the neurasthenic condition in primary care and mental health settings may not only deter future costs but also promote physical and mental health and well-being.

# Culture-Bound Syndromes

*Anthony T. Ng*

*Culture-bound syndrome* is a term used to refer to a range of recurrent patterns of aberrant behaviors and experiences that are locality specific and outside the domain of conventional psychiatric diagnosis as described by the DSM-IV (American Psychiatric Association, 1994). Older terms to describe this syndrome have included *ethnic psychoses, ethnic neurosis, atypical culture-bound reactive syndromes,* and *exotic psychotic syndromes* (Gaw, 1993). Many of these culture-bound syndromes may resemble one or more DSM-IV or ICD-10 (World Health Organization, 1992) diagnoses. Unlike the diagnosis of schizophrenia or depression, which have fairly identifiable symptoms and universal courses, culture-bound syndromes usually are seen in only one or a few societies in the world.

Culture-bound syndromes are bound to specific cultures because they are linked in a cultural context different from the cultural expectations of the Western clinician. Certain behaviors seen in culture-bound syndromes may occur in various settings, and they may be experienced and interpreted differently in each culture. These behaviors also may be categorized differently. The common underlying theme is that understanding of these behaviors is influenced by region-specific views of the individuals, their values, their sense of vital essence, the presence of supernatural beings or power, sickness, and health.

While many of these culture-bound syndromes have a stronger predisposition in ethnic males, females from those cultures may be at risk for significant distress if their spouse or another male family member is afflicted. The relationship between the two may be strained, and the male may no longer be able to care for the family. The woman may attempt to do everything possible to confine the coping within the family, and she may feel a tremendous obligation to maintain the family unit. Failure to do so may bring shame to the family as well as the patient. This may overwhelm the woman's coping mechanisms, and emotional and physical impairments such as depression or somatization may follow. The family may be at risk for domestic violence or substance abuse. Reversal of the caretaker role may occur. Reversal of gender roles, however, may also be a precipitating factor for culture-bound disorders. In their home countries, some women are held at a lower status. Men are the primary decision makers for the family, and they provide the basic necessities for everyone, while women are expected to tend to the needs of the home. When the family immigrates, they realize that the economic survival of the family in their new home country may require the women to enter the workforce. Working outside the home may clash with traditional values about the roles of men and women and can cause significant distress in the family.

Despite the fact that culture-bound syndromes usually are associated with non-Westernized societies, the increased mobility of people, including surges in migration to the United States, Canada, and other developed countries, increases the likelihood that Western clinicians will encounter one or more of these disorders. Primary care clinicians, often the first point of contact for many disadvantaged ethnic and cultural groups, need to have a heightened awareness of culture-bound syndromes, especially since many symptoms of these disorders are somatic in nature. A brief and general description of some of the more commonly encountered culture-bound syndromes follows. Clinicians should search current literature on additional culture-bound disorders if they encounter ethnic individuals in whom the presence of these syndromes is suspected.

## *Koro*

*Koro*, also known as *Suk-yeong*, is a fairly well-studied syndrome that often is encountered in the Chinese culture. This condition is characterized by an individual's complaining of genital retraction, with the fear that it will lead to impending harm, including death. Age at onset usually is early adulthood through the thirties. Males are more often affected. A male may complain that his penis is retracting into his abdomen and that it will kill him. Although this disorder is much less common in women, women may present with the complaint that their breasts or labial folds are retracting, and this may harm them. *Koro* usually occurs in an acute panic like attack during such a state. Alone or with the help of others, an afflicted individual may attempt various methods, including the use of clamps, pins, or fellatio, to keep his or her genitals from retracting. The condition is self-limiting, but it can last from days to weeks.

There have been *koro* epidemics, especially in the Guangdong region of southern China, where five epidemics have been reported since World War II, the most recent in 1984 (Mo, 1992). In the West, cases usually are isolated and occur in overseas Chinese. Cases of *koro* also have been seen in other South Asians. Afflicted individuals have little formal education. Individuals with *koro* may have social, psychological, and occupational dysfunction. There may be accompanying depression and even suicidality. *Koro* is believed to be a disorder influenced by the interactions among cultural, social, and psychodynamic factors. Cultural fears about masturbation, sexual identity, or sexual intercourse also may be precipitating factors.

Although females have a much lower rate of *koro* than males, they may suffer significant distress if their spouse or a male family member is afflicted. The male may no longer be able to work and care for the family, and the woman will have to assume that responsibility. Their sexual relationship may be strained. The woman may feel obligated to help the male to overcome this illness; failure to do so may have serious consequences. For example, she may be forced to perform frequent fellatio on the man to alleviate his fears. If she refuses, she may be verbally or physically abused. Family structure may be disrupted if the man engages in extramarital affairs or feels his spouse was unable to help him. In addition to the emotional strain, a woman who is afflicted with *koro* may self-mutilate by using devices to stop her genitals from shrinking.

Psychiatric differential diagnosis of *koro* includes delusional disorder, schizophrenia, sexual disorders, and substance abuse.

Organic causes such as brain tumor, malaria, or epilepsy also need to be considered. Treatment for *koro* not due to medical causes may include psychotherapy and antipsychotic drugs. Family therapy may aid in helping the family to cope with this disorder. Electroconvulsive therapy is used occasionally.

## Amok

*Amok* is another culture-bound syndrome that has been seen in Asians, primarily Malays, although cases have been reported in Chinese individuals too. It typically affects young or middle-aged males who may have been living away from home and recently suffered some form of loss, including loss of face, as in insults. The individual may be of low socioeconomic class and is poorly educated. Individuals with *amok* have been described as isolative and withdrawn. They may have past histories of impulsivity, immaturity, emotional lability, or social irresponsibility (Gaw, 1993).

In this condition, an afflicted individual experiences a period of preoccupation and brooding, which is followed suddenly and without provocation by outbursts of violent, aggressive behavior that may include indiscriminately attacking and maiming any people or animals that are in their way (Carr and Tan, 1976). After an attack, which usually lasts a few hours, the individual has no recollection of the event and feels exhausted. Some may even commit suicide over what they had done. Perception of insult and a belief in magical possession by demons and evil spirits are thought to precipitate the attacks.

Due to their sudden occurrence and acuity, the spouse and other family members may be at risk of physical harm. It is important to differentiate *amok* from general medical conditions such as epilepsy, infections (malaria or syphilis), or the presence of brain lesions. Psychiatric conditions that have been associated with *amok* include schizophrenia, bipolar disorder, or major depression. Treatment for individuals during an attack consists primarily of physically and, if necessary, pharmacologically overpowering them and gaining control over them. Afterward, the individuals may require ongoing treatment for the psychosis and the presence of any depression.

# Hwa-Byung

*Hwa-byung* is a culture-bound syndrome that clinicians may encounter because of the increased migration of Koreans to the United States. It was first reported in the English literature in 1983 (Lin, 1983). This disorder frequently is seen in females in their forties and fifties, who are less educated, of lower socioeconomic status, and usually from rural areas.

In this disorder, the main complaint of an afflicted individual appears to be gastrointestinal in nature. The individual often reports epigastric pain, which is attributed to a mass in the throat or upper abdomen, and fears that this will lead to death. Additional physical symptoms are excessive fatigue, insomnia, indigestion, loss of appetite, anorexia, dyspnea, palpitations, headaches, dizziness, sexual dysfunction, blurred vision, heat sensation or an intolerance to heat, generalized pains and aches, and a sensation of pushing up in the chest. Emotional symptoms include depression, self-guilt, anxiety, anger, irritability, obsession-compulsion, destructive impulses, panic, and a fear of impending death. Patients often cite family stressors, typically with spouses, in-laws, or children. Alcoholism and domestic violence also may be present. Some DSM-IV diagnoses that have been associated with this disorder are major depression, dysthymia, anxiety disorder, phobic disorder, somatization disorder, obsessive-compulsive disorder, and panic disorder.

*Hwa-byung* translates into "anger illness" in English. The etiology of the disorder has been associated with the Korean understanding between fire and anger (Gaw, 1993). In the Korean culture, as in the Chinese culture, an individual's existence is based on a series of complicated interactions within the individual, as well as between the individual and the surrounding universe. The interactions involve five basic elements, one of which is fire. These elements represent certain emotions. When there is an excess or a deficiency in one of the elements, disharmony, which will affect one's emotions, occurs. Fire often is associated with the emotion of anger. It is believed that in *Hwa-byung,* an individual has excessive anger, which is expressed inwardly and not outwardly. For many of the Asian cultures, including the Korean, there is a cultural inclination to preserve harmony in social relationships by not openly expressing anger. Cultural norms dictate that one should suppress anger, which in turn leads to its accumulation. This is especially so for women, who often are forbidden to disagree with the man because any release of anger or frustration may lead to disharmony in the family, disrupting family cohesion. Another name for *Hwa-byung* is *wool hwa-byung* (*wool* means "pent-up").

## Ataque de Nervios

*Ataque de nervios* is a culture-bound syndrome that is seen in Latino cultures, especially in individuals from the Caribbean (Gaw, 1993). It is a dissociative condition characterized by a sense of loss of control. When an individual suffers an attack, one observes uncontrollable verbal outbursts, crying, faintinglike experiences, or seizurelike movements. Physical symptoms include chest palpitations, tight chest feeling, trembling, shortness of breath, a sensation of heat rising to the head, and occasionally striking out at others. Amnesia of the event may occur when the attack subsides.

A person with *ataque de nervios* may complain of being possessed by evil spirits. The stressor for this syndrome generally is an event related to the family such as the death of a family member, divorce or separation from a spouse, or conflicts between family members. Males are more often afflicted, although the disease is more common among women in Puerto Rico. This disorder has been viewed as a culturally recognized manner of expressing anger or the stress of one's inability to cope over a period of time. Although the symptoms observed in an episode of *ataque de nervios* closely resemble those seen in panic disorder, the presence of a clear precipitating factor and the absence of symptoms of acute fear or apprehension differentiate it from panic disorder.

## Susto

*Susto* is an illness commonly seen in many Latin and South American cultures, although it also has been reported elsewhere in the world. Local terms such as *espanto, lanti, pasmo, tripa ida, perdida del alma,* or *chibih* also have been used to describe this disorder. It is believed that the etiology of susto centers around the individual's being frightened or startled, and as a result, the soul leaves the person. Onset of illness may be from days to years after the stressor. Further, it may not necessarily be the individual who was exposed to the stressor initially. It may be his or her child (Klein, 1978). Characteristic symptoms of this disorder are appetite changes, sleep disturbances, depression, amotivation, and poor self-worth. Physical complaints may include diffuse aches and pains, headache, and gastrointestinal upset. Related DSM-IV diagnoses include major depression, posttraumatic stress disorder, and somatoform disorder. Treatment of susto focuses on cleansing the person to restore bodily and spiritual harmony.

## Brain Fag

Brain fag, which has been described in individuals from many parts of Africa, is a syndrome that consists of difficulties in concentration, memory, and thinking (Morakinyo, 1980). There may be problems with reading and understanding. The individual may complain of the brain and the body being "fatigued," as well as anxiety symptoms. Somatic symptoms may be present, centering around the head and neck. They may include pain, pressure or tightness, blurring of vision, or feelings of heat or burning. The feeling of worms crawling in the head also has been reported. Many of the complaints in brain fag appear to resemble those seen in some anxiety, depressive, and somatoform disorders.

## Falling-Out

Falling-out is a disorder that has been observed in some African Americans and African Caribbean Islanders (Bahamians and Haitians), mostly in the southeastern United States, and especially around the Miami, Florida, area. It is an episode associated with a sudden collapse precipitated by feelings of dizziness or "swimming" in the head. The individual may complain of an inability to see despite the eyes being open. He or she usually is able to hear and understand what is happening but is powerless to move (Weidman, 1979). Although this disorder is seizurelike, there is no convulsion, tongue biting, bladder or bowel incontinence, or other symptoms suggestive of a genuine seizure. It is believed that this falling-out is a response by the individual to some traumatic situations, although other stressors may be implicated. Differential diagnosis of falling-out may include conversion disorder and/ or a dissociative disorder.

## Conclusion

There is increasing interest in cultural diversity and the health and illness of ethnic individuals in the literature. It is important that clinicians develop greater insight into these relationships and understand how individuals interpret and cope according to their cultural determinants. Culture-bound syndromes are a clear illustration of such relationships. There is a constellation of aberrant symptoms that are culture specific. The continued increase of interest in and understanding of culture-bound syndromes will provide greater insight into the complex matrix of the relationship between culture and psychiatry.

# Part Four

# Meeting the Health Care Needs of Immigrant Women

## Model Programs and Tools

# Applications of Linguistic Strategies in Health Care Settings

*Sherry Riddick*

Chapter Three described the range of strategies available for serving limited-English-proficiency (LEP) populations. The focus here is on their use within specific health care settings: the various ways that health care organizations use bilingual staff, hire and deploy interpreters, train providers, and reach out to the community. Each institution has developed an approach, usually encompassing a combination of strategies, that fits its particular circumstances. The variations, as well as similarities, will be apparent from the discussion that follows. It is noteworthy that most organizations still are struggling to find the best approach for serving their LEP clients—one that combines high quality of service and access with efficiency and cost-effectiveness.

## Community Health Centers

Community health centers (CHCs) historically have focused on serving at-risk, underserved populations. Their community-oriented boards and staff have placed a high priority on hiring employees who reflect the communities they serve. CHCs have used a combination of approaches to serve their LEP patients:

- Hiring bilingual and bicultural provider staff as a top priority
- Hiring health aide and family health workers and other ancillary staff who are bilingual and bicultural and also function as interpreters
- Hiring interpreters
- Implementing special projects of outreach, education, and advocacy that train and employ bilingual community members

Although culturally and linguistically appropriate care has been a special attribute of CHCs, screening and training for language and interpreting skills of staff have varied. As in other health care settings, a lack of agreed-on interpretation standards, assessment tools, and training has been a barrier to the provision of optimal linguistic services.

Federal, state, local, and other grants often have subsidized the bilingual services offered by CHCs, but cuts in government funding and the implementation of Medicaid managed care may change the ways that services are provided. To minimize potential negative impacts of capitated rates, various strategies can be, and in some locales have been, initiated. These strategies include carving out interpretation services as a specialty that is excluded from the capitated rates and providing supplemental fees for special populations such as those who need interpretation.

The Providence Ambulatory Health Care Foundation has implemented the strategies described. This community health center was founded in 1967 in the inner city of Providence, Rhode Island, and now has five freestanding health centers with a total budget of $9.1 million in 1995 and over twenty-four thousand active registrants. About half of the clients are Latino, but a diversity of other language groups, including Cambodian, Lao, Hmong, Portuguese, and Cape Verdean, is represented.

Strategies for dealing with the LEP population have evolved over the years to meet changing client demographics. From its earliest roots, Providence has strived to hire bilingual and bicultural staff from the community it serves. This approach became problematic in the early 1980s with the influx of Southeast Asian refugees. Unlike the clinic's experience with other ethnic communities, there was no established community from which to draw interpreters and bilingual staff. Initially, staff from other community agencies, such as the voluntary agencies that sponsor refugees, provided bilingual staff to assist with their clients' medical appointments. Over time, Providence was able to hire its own bilingual staff as refugees with more developed English skills immigrated into the area. Currently, 50 to 60 percent of health aides in the clinics are bilingual and bicultural, and work directly with patients in their native tongue, as well as interpret for the medical providers. The clinics with high numbers of LEP patients employ several bilingual providers who speak the languages of their patients. As the patient population continues to diversify beyond the language capacity of staff, Providence has begun hiring freelance interpreters on an hourly basis for the smaller numbers of Armenian, Haitian, Vietnamese, Arabic, and other LEP patients.

In 1995, screening of the language skills of staff began by using an oral interview to evaluate bilingual experience and education and a written translation exercise to measure language skills and medical knowledge. Drawing on the expertise of Boston's more developed medical interpretation programs, interpreter training for staff was implemented. Future plans include developing a better assessment tool and providing more interpreter training for staff, if funding allows.

This community health center has been successful in meeting the needs of an LEP population because of its commitment to a wraparound bilingual-bicultural model, which has the following key components (M. Francis, Providence Ambulatory Health Care Foundation, Providence, R.I., personal communication, Aug. 1995):

- A board of directors that reflects the community served (56 percent are minority, and 19 percent speak English as a second language)
- An agency philosophy that emphasizes responsiveness to the community
- Policy statements that reflect the mission and include affirmative action, recruitment strategies, staffing patterns, and allocation of resources
- Client input with patient satisfaction surveys conducted in multiple languages and delivered verbally
- A shared staff and administration vision of cultural competency

- Vigilance for funding streams
- Consistent client advocacy in the legislative, health policy, and funding arenas

## Public Health Departments

Local health departments have historically been the first to meet the health needs of new immigrants in the United States, and this tradition is being continued as they seek to provide basic preventive health service assessment, assurance and policy development needs of linguistic and cultural minorities" (National Association of County Health Officials, 1992). The commitment of public health agencies to serve LEP populations has recently been demonstrated through the production of three different reports and surveys that examine how health departments can best respond to the linguistic and cultural differences of their populations. One report focuses on strategies for state health agencies; the other two look at strategies and model programs of local health departments (Association of State and Territorial Health Officials, 1992; National Association of County Health Officials, 1992; U.S. Conference of Mayors and U.S. Conference of Local Health Officers, 1993).

Although state public health agencies have primary responsibility to carry out assessment of needs, policy development, and assurance of public health measures at the state level, their actual programs vary considerably, with some providing direct services and others contracting with and supporting local health departments and community agencies (Association of State and Territorial Health Officials, 1992). Local health departments also operate many different types of programs in widely divergent environments. Thus, current practices of both state and local health departments in serving LEP populations vary significantly, depending on the type of public health services traditionally provided, the type of structural and financial arrangements within a jurisdiction, the diversity of languages spoken, and the local experience in providing health services to LEP or non-English-speaking persons (U.S. Conference of Mayors and U.S. Conference of Local Health Officers, 1993). The three reports cite these specific strategies that state and local health departments use:

- Providing translated health education and promotional materials and disseminating them through mainstream media, community organizations, and ethnic newspapers, radio, and television stations
- Hiring full-time or part-time interpreters
- Hiring bilingual and bicultural outreach workers or health aides and advocates
- Utilizing employee language banks
- Setting up special clinics where language services are provided, such as refugee screening clinics and migrant worker clinics
- Providing cultural training to staff
- Working with community advisory councils to help with needs assessment, problem solving, and planning

Attempts of public health agencies to improve access and quality of health care are hampered by several circumstances: lack of data and a lack of access to needs assessments for the LEP populations, uneven provision of services, insufficient funding for supplemental services, and difficulty recruiting bilingual and bicultural staff.

The Massachusetts Department of Public Health (DPH) is one state public health agency that has applied a multifaceted approach to improving health care access for its diverse population. The Office of Refugee and Immigrant Health (ORIH) in the DPH was established to improve access to and appropriateness of health services and health information for refugees and immigrants throughout the state of Massachusetts. ORIH promotes culturally and linguistically relevant health care and acts as a focal point for planning programs, training staff, developing policies, monitoring legislation, and developing health education strategies on refugee and immigrant health issues (Massachusetts Department of Public Health, 1995).

One factor in the success of the Massachusetts effort has been the implementation of public health needs assessments for the refugee and immigrant populations in the state. The ORIH has worked closely with the community, including groups such as the Refugee Health Advisory Committee and the Latino Health Council, to identify health needs of the LEP populations, assess public health programs, and develop strategies appropriate to the refugee and immigrant population.

Programs developed as a result of these processes have targeted specific health care areas. One example is a perinatal and pediatric care program that uses a community-based team of Southeast Asian staff to provide health education, case management, advocacy, and interpretation services for Southeast Asian women in Lowell, Massachusetts. Another program ensures that substance abuse education and treatment programs are accessible to all linguistic groups by training bilingual and bicultural human services providers in the area of substance abuse, arranging for interpreter services for treatment programs when needed, and conducting conference and site visits to educate treatment providers about cultural differences. Training on the subject of HIV and AIDS also is provided for bilingual and bicultural human service providers, and educational materials are developed in various languages.

To encourage utilization of health care services by the refugee population, the ORIH has offered courses on the U.S. health care system to bilingual and bicultural human service providers and collaborated on a handbook, *Newcomer's Guide to Health Care in Massachusetts,* which is available in several languages. ORIH also has produced fact sheets on the major cultural groups and distributed them to health and human services providers. To increase the pool of bilingual providers, ORIH has worked to facilitate the licensing of refugee and immigrant physicians. To ensure the availability of interpreters in hospitals, it has been active in promoting the inclusion of interpreter services in the determination of need process. When hospitals seek approval for new construction or equipment, they must undergo the determination of need, which attaches conditions requiring the provision of interpreter services.

To promote access, several departmental policies have been developed and adopted by the DPH: active recruiting, hiring, and supporting bilingual, bicultural personnel at all staffing levels; requiring that all contractors and vendors hire cultural and linguistic minorities for positions and provide interpreter services when necessary; and developing a standard translation procedure. A centralized interpreter and translator pool run by ORIH ensures quality translations and appropriateness of health education materials for the intended community and also provides interpreter services for specific programs. Program effectiveness is evaluated yearly, and translated materials are reviewed by community representatives who serve as members of language review committees.

## Hospitals

In the past, hospitals have relied heavily on the use of bilingual staff or patients' family and friends to bridge the language gap with LEP patients. Recently some hospitals have seen the need to go further to ensure that quality care is provided to all patients. A survey and report completed by the National Public Health and Hospital Institute (NPHHI) in 1995 provides an overview of the current status of interpretation services in teaching hospitals (Ginsberg and others, 1995). It found that hospitals' responses to meeting language needs depend on a combination of their language mix, bed size, number of LEP patients served, and linguistic abilities of their staff.

In this area, hospitals often use multiple resources and strategies—for example:

- Hiring bilingual staff, although few hospitals recruit or give preference to hiring bilingual staff.
- Using bilingual staff to interpret. Most hospitals identified staff as the most frequent providers of interpretation.
- Hiring interpreters. Hospitals with the greatest need for interpreters tend to hire and use paid staff interpreters as the predominant means of meeting language needs.
- Using contract services. Many hospitals have access to services, such as the AT&T Language Line, although frequency of use may be less than for other methods. The AT&T Language Line has a large network of interpreters who speak many languages. Providers can call a toll-free number to be connected with an interpreter in minutes or even seconds.
- Using volunteer interpreters. This is a frequent practice.
- Using family and friends to interpret. Although not reported as a common provider of interpretation, this category is most likely to be undocumented and underreported.

Interpreter services in hospitals are organized in various ways. About half of the surveyed hospitals have one department that administers all interpreter services. However, the designated department varies considerably from facility to facility and includes guest or patient relations, social services, volunteer services, human resources, and interpretation departments. Language banks usually are not centrally administered. Instead, each department is responsible for locating its own interpreters through the language bank list. The NPHHI report notes that when there is a large language mix, centralization of administration of interpretation services is useful.

Few hospitals provide training for either paid or volunteer interpreters, and the training that is provided varies in both definition and extent. About one-third of institutions do some type of evaluation of interpreter services, usually through auditing interpreted patient encounters or testing interpreters in their language ability. Although rarely done, evaluation of interpretation service should be included in a formal quality assurance plan. A centralized, consistent documentation of need is essential for tracking, monitoring, and assessing need but often is absent.

The Seattle area hospitals present the range of strategies undertaken by hospitals in one community. As a result of community and legal pressure on hospitals to hire qualified interpreters, a group of hospitals in Seattle, Washington, in the early 1980s implemented several mechanisms to provide bilingual services to their patients. Previously they had relied on the services of patients' friends and families, bilingual staff from community agencies, and unevaluated, untrained hospital staff (often newly arrived refugees working in entry-level housekeeping or kitchen positions). Complaints filed with the Office for Civil Rights, U.S. Department of Health and Human Services, on behalf of clients at three different hospitals ultimately brought about the hospitals' acknowledgment of their responsibility and obligation to provide qualified bilingual interpretation services free of charge to patients (Riddick, 1991).

Strategies subsequently developed by the hospitals included hiring their own full-time, part-time, or on-call interpreters and providing training to bilingual staff from various hospital departments to be used as interpreters when needed. However, the wide diversity of the languages spoken by the patients made it difficult for each hospital to provide adequate coverage for all languages. Thus, the idea of contracting collectively for a shared interpretation service was attractive and cost-effective. The result was the creation of the Hospital Interpretation Program (now called the Community Interpretation Services, or CIS) in 1982, whereby the hospitals' local association contracted with a nonprofit community clinic consortium that already had experience in providing interpreter services for community clinics. Since that time, CIS has been an essential component of the hospitals' strategies to meet the language needs of their patients, providing twenty-four-hour interpretation service through the use of on-call, hourly interpreters who carry pagers and respond to both emergency and prescheduled appointments. In 1994, CIS had almost eighteen thousand encounters, using over one hundred on-call interpreters for more than thirty languages.

In addition to the ready availability of interpreters who speak a wide range of languages, another benefit of using CIS has been the assurance that interpreters are screened, assessed, and trained. To be considered for hire, applicants to CIS must pass written and oral tests in English and the target language that evaluate their knowledge of medical terminology, understanding of interpreter role and ethics, and general language skills. Successful performance on the test results in an interview and reference checks. New interpreters with limited experience are mentored by experienced interpreters until their skills are established. All interpreters receive a three-hour orientation to rules, policies, and ethics, followed by a twelve-hour course, the Art of Interpreting, that covers ethics, roles, and standards for interpreters (Riddick, 1990, 1991). In combination with workshops on specific medical topics, this training has provided interpreters with the basic skills and information they need. However, a comprehensive, competency-based training for interpreters would further ensure the proficiency of the interpreters and has long been needed.

As a result of efforts by both OCR and a local legal advocacy group, health and social service agencies throughout the state of Washington are now well aware of their legal obligation to provide bilingual services to their clients. In comparison to other parts of the country, hospitals in the region have a relatively broad array of language services to choose from, both in-house and external, with CIS continuing to be a leading provider of interpreter services.

## Managed Care Organizations

Managed care organizations are a strong and growing force in most health care markets. Newly created managed care organizations often subsume or mesh with a variety of existing health care providers, including community health centers, hospitals, and health departments. The rapid expansion of Medicaid managed care is becoming an issue for managed care organizations, many of which had not previously considered the special needs of their LEP and other underserved populations. Some managed care organizations are finding that it is to their advantage to become more inclusive and reach out to underserved groups, a previously untapped market. For example, Greater Atlantic Health Service in Philadelphia has found that with its new commitment to diversify membership, Medicaid enrollment increased 76 percent over a three-year period (Manfiletto, 1995). A few managed care programs have begun to make significant contributions to serving the LEP population. One of them is the Minneapolis Metropolitan Health Plan (MHP).

Minneapolis MHP is an HMO developed in response to Minnesota's implementation of Medicaid managed care. Institutions participating in MHP include Hennepin County Medical Center, the Minneapolis Health Department, community clinics, and independent affiliate doctors. The majority of clients are Medicaid recipients, many of whom are limited English speaking. The largest LEP group speaks Spanish, but significant numbers also speak Cambodian, Hmong, Lao, Vietnamese, Russian, and a variety of other languages.

MHP aims to provide a comprehensive service program to the LEP population, starting with its marketing strategy. Bilingual and bicultural customer service representatives have been hired who speak Spanish, Hmong, Vietnamese, and Russian. These service representatives go into the community to provide education about the plan and how services are provided. Information about benefits also is provided by the bilingual representatives by telephone. In addition, an automated telephone system provides translated information about the plan to new members. As part of an early education project, members are asked at enrollment if they need interpreters. To make sure they understand the system and the need to select a primary provider, all new members are contacted by telephone by the customer representatives or by interpreters from the medical center.

Interpretation services are provided through several mechanisms:

- AT&T Language Line. This service has limited use, with ten to twenty-five calls per month in 1995. It is not used at all by the Hennepin County Medical Center.
- Location-specific interpretation programs. The Hennepin County Medical Center has its own interpretation service, with an interpreter coordinator, twelve staff interpreters, and fourteen on-call contract interpreters, who provided six thousand patient contacts per month in 1995. Telephone interpretation is provided by these interpreters for after-hour needs, with MHP subsidizing after-hour on-call interpreter pay and two interpreter positions at the medical center. The Minneapolis Health Department also has its own interpretation program.
- MHP-contracted interpreters. Freelance interpreters are contracted to fill the needs of the affiliated private providers who lack bilingual resources. This service is coordinated by an interpreter manager employed by MHP.
- Bilingual providers. Efforts are made to hire and affiliate with bilingual providers.
- Written translations. Plan information, correspondence, and brochures are translated into the languages of MHP's members.

Other efforts to provide efficient bilingual care to patients include the development of language-specific clinics at the medical center. For example, an afternoon of ten or so Russian-speaking prenatal clients enables the Russian interpreter to function more efficiently than when appointments are scattered throughout the day or week.

Training for interpreters employed through the different components of MHP has varied. Most have received basic orientation to ethics and role, but only a few have completed the comprehensive, competency-based interpreter training program at the University of Minnesota. Provider training geared toward working with interpreters has been conducted at some sites and is viewed as an important aspect of cross-cultural competency. Other factors identified as needing more attention include collaboration locally and nationally among institutions and with communities. Although it is too early to determine if the marketing and outreach efforts are cost-effective, enrollment appears to have been positively affected. MHP plans to continue efforts to expand services to the LEP community in the belief that improving access leads to early assessment and intervention and a healthier patient population (R. Schluter and E. Rau, Metropolitan Health Plan and Hennepin County Medical Center, Minneapolis, Minn., personal communication, Aug. 1995).

## Conclusion

The examples presented in this chapter are but a few of the exemplary programs that have sprung up around the country in an effort to improve services for the LEP populations. Although some cross-country collaboration has occurred, most programs have developed independently, often recreating similar systems from the ground up. All suffer from a lack of nationally established standards, policies, and protocols and would benefit from a mechanism for sharing. We need to work together to achieve this important end.

# Chapter Fifteen

# A Model Posttraumatic Stress Disorder Support Group for Cambodian Women

*Judith Shepherd*

Cambodian refugees are among the most severely traumatized of all recent refugee populations to enter the United States (Shepherd and Faust, 1993; Baughan and others, 1990; Mollica and others, 1987; Rozee and Van Boemel, 1990). They face extreme risk for health and mental health problems, especially posttraumatic stress disorder (PTSD). On average, Cambodians have been found to have worse health than other refugees (Mollica and others, 1987). An astounding 95 percent of the women patients treated at the Indo Chinese Psychiatry Clinic in Boston had been raped during Pol Pot's reign of terror between 1975 and 1978 (Mollica and others, 1987) but never disclosed these assaults until they had been in therapy for an average of three years. Rozee and Van Boemel (1990) linked suffering under the Pol Pot regime to psychogenic blindness in thirty middle-aged women who sought treatment at a southern California medical clinic.

In the late 1970s, when Cambodian and other Southeast Asia refugees began arriving in the San Francisco area, the Refugee

The author was director of the Immigrant and Public Health Grant Program for PTSD at the San Francisco General Hospital Refugee Clinic during the study period.

Clinic opened to provide federally mandated screening services to the new arrivals. The clinic became part of the Family Health Center at San Francisco General Hospital in 1982. Over the years, it expanded into a family practice center that served monolingual indigent refugees and immigrants from Mexico and Central America, as well as the former Soviet Union, Ethiopia, Eritrea, Cuba, Tibet, Haiti, the Middle East, and Bosnia. A staff of multilingual, bicultural health workers–interpreters who spoke approximately twelve languages and dialects served this diverse community.

The Refugee Clinic's interpreters served as culture brokers between Western health care providers and the patients' health belief systems; they interpreted cultural concepts and behaviors, and collaborated with physicians and nurses. Together the multilingual and multicultural health workers and providers discovered the challenges of serving refugees who had experienced extensive, prolonged torture during civil war. Merely providing health services, without also addressing the mental effects of torture, would not produce positive health outcomes for these refugee women.

In 1992, the San Francisco General Hospital Refugee Clinic began a PTSD assessment and treatment program for Cambodian women, Vietnamese men, and women from Mexico as well as Central and South America. The program's first priority was PTSD assessment and treatment of Cambodian women patients, who had some of the most serious chronic physical complaints of the clinic's immigrant and refugee patients. Complaints included constant back pain, headaches, dizziness, and exhaustion that accompanied quantifiable illnesses like tuberculosis, parasite-related gastrointestinal disorders, hypertension, and diabetes. Despite more frequent clinic visits than other refugee populations, neither standard Western medicines like analgesics nor traditional Asian remedies like cupping and coining (Aronson, 1983) resulted in significant improvement. In short, clinic providers had little or no success in mediating patients' suffering. The staff hypothesized, first, that the effects of multiple trauma, like enforced labor, torture, rape, and starvation, on Cambodian women during the Pol Pot regime prior to immigration to the United States could be correlated with their unremitting physical and somatic symptoms, and, second, that a low-cost public health program that addressed patient needs from a psychosocial viewpoint might be a positive link to existing medical services.

The weekly two-hour support group for Cambodian women patients who suffered from multiple trauma is relevant to other immigrant and refugee women who exhibit serious problems in health or mental health settings. With funds from the Federal Office of Refugee Resettlement, I devised a PTSD support group program that used social workers, bilingual health workers, and volunteers to address the suffering of Cambodian women and other patients. From the beginning, the support groups were designed to address PTSD symptoms through ego-supportive, psychoeducational, and behavioral interventions. The behavioral component stressed patients' ability to learn relaxation and desensitization techniques to interrupt and defuse persistent intrusive thoughts and their attendant unpleasant bodily sensations (Barsky, Geringer, and Wool, 1988). The underlying assumption was that PTSD was the natural outcome of extraordinarily unnatural events and that patients could learn and practice behaviors and techniques during the group and at home that would enable them to reduce the discomfort and effects of severe trauma.

## Support Group Referral, Assessment, and Treatment

Refugee clinic health providers referred long-term Cambodian women patients who frequently had used services with limited success to the social worker and Cambodian bilingual health worker for a PTSD assessment using the Harvard Trauma Scale and the Hopkins Short List Depression Inventory, both of which were found to be both valid and reliable for Cambodian patients at Boston's Indo-Chinese Psychiatry Clinic (Mollica and others, 1992). The Harvard Trauma Scale successfully measured multiple traumas in Cambodians who lived through the Pol Pot era. Indicators of trauma, such as combat and other near-death experiences, witnessing of others' unnatural deaths, starvation, isolation from family, and enforced labor, were correlated with varying degrees of anxiety, fear, avoidance, and depression that comprise PTSD. The depression inventory determined degree of suicidality, which was not assessed in the Harvard Trauma Scale.

Assessment, which took an average of an hour to complete, provided an opportunity for the patient to talk at length about multiple trauma. Since the Harvard Trauma Scale identifies more than twenty types of trauma, these data could be helpful in determining organic versus nonorganic causes of headaches and other physical complaints. Many of the patients had been routinely asked about medical problems but rarely about the horrific circumstances and feelings related to them. Although use of the Harvard Trauma Scale could and frequently did trigger traumatic memories, patients often were grateful for the opportunity to discuss in depth the multiple traumas they had experienced in Cambodia. One of the common themes in the assessment of the seventy or more Cambodian women patients was the horror of having their children die in their arms from malnutrition and disease. Although the same women also had experienced bodily injuries and forced labor, and had witnessed the executions and/or disease and starvation of spouses, parents, and siblings, their memories of the deaths of their infants and children far overshadowed their own struggles—and remained the source of survivor guilt and helplessness that may have underscored many physical complaints years after the deaths occurred.

One Cambodian patient's memories of her children's death—in this case, murder—was sufficiently traumatic to contribute to severe somatic problems after she immigrated to the United States.

L fled Cambodia on foot with her two teenage children in the late 1970s. Her husband had been killed previously, and she hoped to find safety in one of the Thai refugee camps on the Cambodia-Thailand border. She and her children were caught by soldiers just before they reached the Thai camp. The soldiers dragged L away and raped her. After the sexual assault, L realized her children were in danger, so she picked herself up and ran through the bush to look for them. She found her children lying on the ground dead, their legs severed from their bodies.

Years later, alone in San Francisco, L suffered blackouts on the bus and at home. She could no longer remember how to count. Calling an acquaintance or friend on the telephone was out of the question. It seemed impossible for her to learn even the most rudimentary English, although it was apparent that she was talented and bright.

L taught us the utility of inquiring about trauma regarding children in assessing health and mental health conditions of Cambodian women patients.

One of the volunteers, a nurse, spent extra time with L, helping her relearn or remember basic skills like counting. The support and love of other women patients also contributed to positive changes in L's behavior over time. A year after attending the support group, she was able to use the telephone and enjoy knitting and crocheting, activities with which she reconnected after six months of support from our volunteers and other group members.

Entry into the group was facilitated by the assessment. Offering women the opportunity to talk individually about their preimmigration experiences and the establishment of rapport between the patients and the worker contributed to the women's willingness to enter the group. The health worker's training in administration of the Harvard Trauma Scale and Depression Inventory, as well as the insight she gained about her own experiences and PTSD, helped her sublimate her own trauma to help the patients talk about theirs. The voluntary nature of the group and assurance of confidentiality also may have contributed to many of the women's decisions to join the support group. If the assessment instruments revealed suicidal feelings or severe depression, the social worker made additional immediate referrals to the patients' providers, who contacted psychiatric emergency services at the main hospital for further consultation.

## Induction into the Support Group

More than 90 percent of the Cambodian patients scored high on the PTSD and depression scales. Seventy-five to 80 percent of the patients accepted their referrals to the support group. More than seventy women were referred during the five-year period of operation. The women stayed an average of one year, with a range of six months to three years. Secondary migration and childbearing caused interruptions in attendance for some patients. All patients were exposed to education about PTSD and received handouts on how to attain regular sleep, since sleep disturbances are a hallmark of PTSD. Periodically they were given lectures on the nature of anxiety and depression, and their manifestations as natural effects of trauma. The social worker explained that each week for two hours, patients would be engaged in three highly structured activities, followed by homework several times a week, which they were to record in a workbook. This activity would help them reduce some of the adverse effects of trauma, like emotional numbing, intrusive thoughts, anxiety, and sleep disturbances.

The three structured activities—crocheting and knitting, interactive English as a Second Language (ESL), and desensitization and stress reduction exercises—were used to alter the patients' PTSD symptoms over time. The activities were based on the premise that changing behaviors could ultimately change emotional states, at least while patients were in the group each week, and possibly longer if they carried the activities over into their personal lives outside the group. By setting up an artificial situation in the group to reduce social isolation, a critical variable in nourishing intrusive thoughts and depression, we demonstrated how patients might shift their emotional states to more positive ones by being with others and altering or adding a few simple behaviors. We also hypothesized that the support the women gave one another in this safe, structured setting would have a positive impact if replicated outside the hospital in their homes and community. We explained that these changes would take time. If the patients were willing to stay in the group or with each other, patterns of fearfulness and anxiety that resulted from the remapping of the brain during the Pol Pot reign of terror might gradually be reworked to their baseline mental and emotional states.

The support group program relied heavily on volunteers and in-kind donations of materials, such as yarn and needles from the community. A grant proposal was submitted to the hospital to fund an adjunct children's group, so that the patients' preschool-age children would be cared for while their mothers obtained some respite. The social worker ensured the availability of competent and culturally sensitive knitting and crocheting teachers, credentialed ESL teachers, as well as individuals trained in yoga, massage, visualization, and meditation, along with Eastern methods of body work like *shin jon jitsu*, t'ai chi, and *chi qong*.

The first portion of each session was devoted to the practice of knitting or crocheting. These crafts enabled patients who had experienced severe emotional numbing and social isolation to do an activity with their hands that required some degree of concentration, the lack of which also is a hallmark of PTSD. The needed hand-eye coordination served to interrupt intrusive thoughts. These activities also provided individuals with an excuse not to talk with others until they felt comfortable or safe. The second activity, interactive ESL, took place during the middle forty minutes of the group. Some women appreciated the structure of loose, game-filled, music-driven activities that gave them a reason to talk to one another, albeit in a second or third language.

The last activity, a half hour of guided imagery, sometimes using relaxation tapes that were translated into Cambodian, clearly were the activities that we wanted patients to practice in both the group and at home as often as possible. To this end, half-hour Cambodian relaxation tapes and workbooks were given to each patient along with encouragement to reinforce her practice at home and note her progress during the week. The social worker or health worker periodically checked the workbooks during the group. Certificates of completion and small tokens of appreciation were given to patients every six months to a year.

The social worker and health worker kept weekly attendance sheets and a summary of individual and group dynamics. The hospital's Family Health Center provided funding for tea and cookies, audiotapes, workbooks, and other miscellaneous expenses. Nurses and physicians frequently were consulted when individual patients in the group revealed medical or psychological problems that might need special attention. Refugee Clinic providers made referrals to emergency psychiatric services, psychiatric evaluation, and prenatal care when women suffered from problems that were beyond the scope of the support group program. When requested, Refugee Clinic and Family Health Center providers also made presentations on topics like diabetes, menopause, and other health issues of concern to the support group's members.

## Social Contact and Crafts

Although it seemed logical to provide the stress-reduction portion of the program during the first forty minutes, the order of the activities was changed because patients preferred to talk with each other when they arrived. Starting with the knitting and crocheting portion gave patients time to establish social contact with others if they so chose. Initially they were so numb, depressed, emotionally flooded with memories from the past, or so involved in combating somatic and physical pain that they hardly spoke to one another.

The introduction of colorful, tactile yarns appeared to elicit no interest during the first few months. It was difficult to believe that the patients had any knitting or crocheting experience prior to migration. During this period, little or no pressure was exerted on patients to knit or crochet. Instead, the health worker encouraged the patients to talk about PTSD symptoms they experienced and also about concrete issues like housing, education, employment, and other concerns with which they needed help.

After about six months, one or two women began to "remember" how to crochet and knit again in the support group. This appeared to be a signal for other women to take the crocheting and knitting materials, which served as a means of interrupting intrusive thoughts by giving them something positive to do with their hands when they became anxious or depressed at home, whether they felt like talking or not. More important, they enabled women to fraternize freely in their own language while doing something that gave them a sense of mastery and a material accomplishment.

Nowhere was the healing power of simple conversation and knitting and crocheting more apparent than in the case of one patient who had witnessed the deaths of most of her immediate family and as a consequence may have developed psychogenic blindness. Our patient, K, would be escorted to the group by her husband. He and other patients helped her get comfortable at the conference table around which the group members sat. The social worker, health worker, and other patients treated K as though she were sighted. Often she would choose one color of yarn over another. K frequently allowed the other women to help her set up her crocheting. During the knitting period, patients would frequently pat K's hair or touch her face. K never spoke in the group. During the transition period, when patients were asked to move their chairs to begin the relaxation exercise portion of the session, K could be seen tracking the movements of the other women with her eyes. Then, inexplicably, at the end of the session, she would return to being blind again.

Eighteen months after the support group began, all but one or two patients participated fully in the craft portion of the class, and it became difficult to meet their demand for yarn and needles. Patients began to show one another what they now remembered about knitting and crocheting. They began to work closely with the volunteer teachers on how to construct elaborate designs for sweaters and gloves. At the end of five years, the core group of patients had incorporated the activity into their personal lives. They had an exhibit and sale of their wares, which reflected their continuous hard work on an emotional and physical level.

## English as a Second Language

The ESL teachers used humorous language games, including crossword puzzles and word bingo, to break down social isolation and elevate the patients' moods, and their efforts were successful. Even the most emotionally shutdown patients participated in the group exercises. Most patients still did not have an opportunity to study English formally in the United States because of their child-rearing responsibilities. The adjunct children's group allowed the women to study English while their preschool children were next door. The ESL teachers stressed many medical terms as well as basic English used in everyday life.

## Stress Reduction and Guided Meditation

The women over age forty may have been familiar with Buddhist meditation as practiced on the general culture before Pol Pot came to power in 1975; those younger than age forty did not have the same familiarity with indigenous religious practices. This segment began with the social worker's teaching patients to engage in yoga breathing exercises, followed by a guided visualization during which they lay on sheets on the floor. First, they listened to a new age music tape that consisted of water and forest sounds for ten minutes.

The social worker and health worker then asked the patients to go on a guided journey with them, in which each person was asked to see her breath as a warm ball of gold that would progressively relax all parts of her body. At the end of the session, patients were slowly brought out of the light trance state. While still relaxed and lying on the floor, they were reminded to practice the warm ball of gold exercise at home during the week. Certificates pasted in their workbooks while they were studying English served as reinforcement for this practice. In the fifth year of the program, we tried a relaxation tape that combined music and imagery, but patients preferred the live guided imagery. The light trance state that was induced may have been more successful when the stimuli of the health worker's and social worker's voices were employed.

Women in the group program also were given the opportunity to try yoga, *chi qong, shi jin jitsu,* and therapeutic massage at different intervals throughout the five years the program was in operation. Several practitioners of all of these arts volunteered to teach patients the fundamentals of these exercises. One skilled volunteer massage therapist brought her portable massage table to the group, and individual members would allow themselves to have a massage in a small room adjoining the meeting room during the ESL or craft portion of the class. Patients found this helped to alleviate headache, backaches, and fatigue. Considering the level of "bad touch" that our patients had experienced in Cambodia, either torture or sexual assault, their willingness to participate in these exercises suggested that body work could be a larger and more prominent part of future support group programs for refugee and immigrant women with multiple trauma. Body work and meditative exercise seemed to bring relief from PTSD symptoms.

## Outcomes

During the five years that the Cambodian women's group operated (1991–1996), those who remained in the group began to understand the chronic nature of the syndrome. Continuous weekly support lessened patients' panic when new traumatic events triggered the old and appeared to impart the understanding that at least some of their physically and psychologically undesirable conditions were periodic and time limited and thus need not be so strongly feared or reacted to so adversely.

Preliminary evaluation of the group after five years suggested that an understanding of PTSD and group-reinforced practice in abating PTSD symptoms made it possible for many Cambodian women patients to begin to separate some of their symptoms such as headaches and stomachaches, other pains, dizziness, and hyperventilation that were routinely treated unsuccessfully as physical illness from the unpleasant sensations or feelings that were engendered by memories of trauma. Unfortunately, there was no funding for an in-depth evaluation of the program. Therefore, the effectiveness of a group such as this needs to be substantiated by future empirical studies.

Over time, patients began to recognize that all the exercises—knitting, ESL, guided imagery, and meditation—could make them feel better mentally and physically, if only for the two-hour period the group met each week. Attendance generally was good. Even women with several children in elementary school and others at home attended the group regularly. For those with severe, protracted PTSD, a continuous ongoing support group program may be better than shorter, time-limited groups. Some of the structured learning that occurs during the operation of a support group for several or more years may serve to recondition women to less traumatic ways of thinking and feeling.

## Conclusion

The PTSD Assessment and Treatment Program for Immigrants and Refugees illustrates that ongoing structured support groups can be of value in improving the health of women suffering from serious multiple trauma. Our experience over five years revealed that in conjunction with primary care, Cambodian women patients could benefit from an opportunity to address the effects of PTSD and learning methods to alleviate their suffering. If they are truly to address the medical problems of refugee and immigrant women patients, medical professionals cannot ignore the impact of serious premigration trauma on these women (Shepherd, 1992a). Outpatient clinics that serve refugee and immigrant women can provide better and more efficient care to them when social support and psychoeducation for PTSD are included in comprehensive services.

# Chapter Sixteen

# An Educational Program for Families on Intergenerational Conflict

*Yu-Wen Ying*

This chapter addresses the development of intergenerational and intercultural conflict between migrant adults and their children, and introduces an intervention that may prevent or reduce this conflict and promote the well-being of migrant-headed families. Throughout the chapter, the term *migrant* refers to individuals who were not born in the United States, including immigrants and refugees. (A more detailed discussion of the intervention and findings may be found in Ying, 1998.)

## Intergenerational and Intercultural Conflict

Sluzki (1979) proposed that the development of intergenerational and intercultural conflict is normative in migrant families, typically young adults who are likely to be bearing or raising children (Parrillo, 1991). A generational and cultural gap develops when parents retain the values and behaviors that are normative in their culture of origin, while their children progressively adopt mainstream American values and behavior (Drachman, Kwon-Ahn, and Paulino, 1996; Parrillo, 1991; Yao, 1985; Ying and Chao, 1996). Ying (1994) found that second-generation Chinese American adults felt less understood by their immigrant mothers than either immigrant or third-generation Chinese Americans. This intergenerational difference in values and behavior may become a significant source of conflict between migrant adults and their children.

For migrants from non-Western cultures whose values vary significantly from those of mainstream European American society, the risk for intergenerational and intercultural conflict is even more pronounced. For example, the values of cooperation and interdependence of Latino and Asian immigrants and refugees are diametrically opposed to European American values of competition and independence. The virtue of obedience and adhering to prescribed rules at home may become a weakness in the classroom if the student is rewarded for creativity and critical thinking (Drachman, Kwon-Ahn, and Paulino, 1996; Garcia Coll, Meyer, and Brillon, 1995; Harrison and others, 1990).

The speedy acculturation of the children occurs partly because European American values are rewarded by teachers, peers, and other people who are viewed as competent and powerful in mainstream American contexts. As children of migrants gain increasing competence in American society, role reversal occurs: they assume adult responsibilities, and their parents are reduced to being children in their negotiations with mainstream American society. Conflict is likely to result when the children are pulled to acculturate and their parents try to keep them connected to their culture of origin and, indeed, to themselves.

An additional factor in the development of intergenerational and intercultural conflict is migrant parents' unavailability to their children. Economic survival is one of the first challenges they must face. Due to language differences and the inability to transfer past educational degrees and work experience, the majority of migrants are likely to hold jobs that are time- and labor-intensive but low-paying, at least initially (Ben-Porath, 1991; Grant, 1983), leaving them little opportunity to be with their children (Drachman, Kwon-Ahn, and Paulino, 1996). Over time, the children may become estranged, seeking support and understanding outside the family.

Compared to other often-cited risk factors migrants face, the experience of intergenerational and intercultural conflict may be an even more powerful risk factor for the development of mental health problems in migrant parents and their children. For example, racial and ethnic discrimination, which is perpetrated by an outsider (a nonfamily member), is certainly painful and likely to be associated with negative mental health consequences. However, the experience of rejection from an insider (such as one's child) is likely to be even more devastating.

The in-group versus out-group distinction defines proper interpersonal behavior for many migrants entering the United States (Triandis and others, 1988), especially for Latinos and Asians who come from a collectivistic society, where the rules of behavior vary significantly depending on whether one is interacting with a member of an in- or out-group. When migrants from collectivistic cultures experience discrimination at the hands of native-born Americans, the in-group versus out-group distinction and expected differential treatment may, ironically, soften the blow. Although the offending behavior may indeed be painful, there is no real attachment to the perpetrator nor necessarily any expectation of kindness and understanding, and its impact cannot be compared to that resulting from an affront from a family member. Intergenerational and intercultural conflict strikes individuals where they are most vulnerable.

Children not only are members of the in-group; they often are the very reason for migration. The hope that their children will enjoy a better future sustains migrants through their difficult adjustment process. Unlike European American parents, who expect their children to separate and individuate, in most non-Western societies the parent-child relationship is expected to persist, even when the child marries. For Latinos, the commitment to the family and familial obligation and respect, and for Asians, the value of filial piety and respect for elders are central (Garcia Coll, Meyer, and Brillon, 1995; Harrison and others, 1990). Children are not expected to leave their parents; instead, they continue to retain an important role in their lives. When they begin to express dissenting views, want greater separation, and make choices that are inconsistent with their parents' wishes, migrant parents feel dismayed and even betrayed (Drachman, Kwon-Ahn, and Paulino, 1996). In extreme cases, they feel they have lost their children to America (Ying and Chao, 1996).

Migrant parents are not the only ones who suffer. The children are caught between their parents and the larger society. When they start school, they are increasingly exposed to expectations and demands that may vary significantly from those at home. Particularly during adolescence, they may experience identity confusion; mainstream society views them as not quite American, while their parents and members of the ethnic culture view them as too American. They seem to be both and neither. Sadly, they receive little assistance in negotiating these differences. They are caught between two different worlds, and negotiating them can be quite difficult. For some, gangs take on the role of the family in providing protection, support, and guidance (Adler, Ovando, and Hocevar, 1984; Ying and Chao, 1996). Other studies have found that intergenerational and intercultural conflict predicts school problems, depression, and anxiety in children of immigrants (Aldwin and Greenberger, 1987; Hernandez-Guzman and Sanchez-Sosa, 1996; Yao, 1985). In sum, intergenerational and intercultural conflict is likely to occur in migrant families and to hold negative consequences for the well-being of both the parents and the children.

## The Strengthening of Intergenerational/Intercultural Ties in Immigrant Chinese American Families Curriculum

Primary and secondary prevention (intervening before the occurrence of the problem or at its early stages) are likely to reduce the severity of the problem and its negative consequences. In the case of Asian and Latino Americans, such an approach is particularly fitting because they may be reluctant to use existing services for reasons discussed earlier in the book. Other than Szapocznik and his colleagues' (1984, 1989) treatment program targeting Cuban American families with drug-abusing adolescents, few intervention programs are described in the literature. The Strengthening of Intergenerational/Intercultural Ties in Immigrant Chinese American Families (SITICAF) curriculum was developed to address this gap.

SITICAF aims to bridge the intergenerational and intercultural gap in Chinese American immigrant families by bringing the intergenerational and intercultural differences to the parents' awareness, promoting greater cross-cultural competence in the parents, improving parenting skills, particularly in the area of communication, and helping parents to cope better with the stresses of cross-cultural parenting. Because the attainment of these outcomes involves a fundamental shift in how parents experience the world (recognizing that they are cultural beings, with culture-bound values), the course uses a combination of the traditional lecture method, experiential exercises, and homework assignments to encourage infusion of the course content into the parents' daily interactions with their children. Homework assignments are discussed in the following class, and individual assignments are turned in and reviewed by the instructor, allowing for individual feedback to the parents. In the pilot program, parents with more than one child were asked to target their oldest child in completing all their homework assignments and the assessment questionnaires.

The program consists of eight weekly parenting classes, each two hours long, which are aimed at first-generation Chinese American parents with school-age children. The course is offered entirely in Mandarin Chinese, the parents' preferred language. Although the program was developed specifically for Chinese immigrant parents and their American-born children, its content may easily be adapted for use with other migrant populations.

## Class 1. Overview of the Course and Simulation of a Cross-Cultural Encounter

The primary objective of the first meeting is to provide the parents with an experience of a cross-cultural encounter. Intergenerational and intercultural conflict occurs because children experience more cross-cultural encounters and are more open to and shaped by them than their parents are. Migrant parents often may prefer to remain in a social world inhabited by members of their own culture group. Although they may be cognitively aware of the presence of cultural differences, if they migrated to the United States as adults, they are likely to be embedded in their culture of origin and to view it as superior. This varies significantly from the experiences of their children, who travel between two culturally different worlds, their home and the American classroom, and are concurrently influenced and shaped by both contexts. The simulation game Barnga (Thiagarajan, 1990) provides an affective (and effective) experience of cross-cultural encounter and promotes the parents' empathy for the challenges of cross-cultural living.

## Class 2. Learning About Cultural Differences

This class provides an overview of current theories and knowledge about ethnic identity formation in children and adolescents, and acculturation in adult immigrants. The possibility of differential outcome is highlighted—that immigrant parents may remain separated from the mainstream American society, but children may become bicultural or even assimilated, perhaps preferring the dominant culture over the ethnic one (Berry, Kim, Minde, and Mok, 1987). If parents are able to recognize potential culture-based differences between their parenting styles and expectations of their children and those of their child's teacher and the larger American society, they are more likely to be able to serve as a bridge for their children as they negotiate these different demands.

Child-rearing practices have been developed over generations to promote competencies that are most valued in a given cultural context (Garcia Coll, Meyer, and Brillon, 1995; Harkness and Super, 1995). Parents are helped to reflect on their parenting methods and to consider their appropriateness given the historical, social, and multicultural contexts in which their children live. To highlight cultural differences in general, and their application to the parent-child relationship in particular, the popular fairy tales of The Monkey King and Hansel and Gretel are used to demonstrate fundamental differences in the nature of Chinese and European American parent-child relationships, including whether it should be hierarchical or egalitarian, and whether adulthood is defined by veneration and obedience to or leaving and surpassing the previous generation. Parents are not encouraged to abandon their culture-bound values, but they are encouraged to ponder the dissonance of the two cultures and how they may help their children negotiate them.

## Class 3. Understanding Your Child

The objective of the third class is to provide both a cognitive understanding of child development and an affective experience of listening to the experiences of an American-born Chinese young adult growing up in the United States. The first is addressed by presenting an overview of major developmental milestones from birth to adolescence, and the concomitant challenges for parenting. Erik Erikson's (1963) psychosocial developmental model is presented, and parents are invited to reflect on potential differences in the standards they uphold to their children and what is normative in European American culture.

This more theoretical presentation is followed by an autobiographical account of a parent-child relationship from the perspective of an American-born Chinese young adult. The presenter discusses the challenges of growing up in an immigrant Chinese household and a non–Chinese American larger social context, identifying areas of conflict, such as cross-cultural differences in showing affection, the importance of academic achievement, the role of extracurricular activities, and rules about dating. She or he also addresses parenting methods she or he found helpful and not helpful, and provides suggestions to the parents about how to maintain a strong relationship with their children from the child's perspective. Along with Barnga, this experience of listening to the child's perspective is cited by parents as being one of the most memorable of the course.

## Class 4. Promoting Understanding

This and the two following classes are based on filial therapy, a clinical method developed by Bernard and Louise Guerney that uses parents as therapists for their children. Their research suggests the feasibility and effectiveness of this approach (Guerney, 1964, 1983). Each parenting technique is presented with a rationale, followed by an explanation of its use, a demonstration, in-class practice, and home practice (see Guerney, 1987, for details).

Filial therapy consists of a constellation of parenting methods that are grounded in European American culture. Immigrant parents are asked to assess their merits in various situations. In this class, teaching parents to listen actively, to identify the child's feelings, and to mirror his or her statement and feeling without commentary and judgment may be viewed as inconsistent with the traditional "parents talk and children listen" Chinese perspective. It is not suggested that the traditional perspective be abandoned; instead, it is proposed that at different times and contexts, one may be more appropriate than the other. Thus, if the objective is to decrease the communication gap between parents and children, active listening may be an appropriate and useful tool. In addition, methods for conveying the parents' message are presented, including identification of the parents' feelings, expressing the cause of this feeling (whether it is in response to a child's behavior), and not criticizing the child.

## Class 5. Establishing Structure and Rewarding the Child

This class presents the use of structure, rewards, and punishment (Guerney, 1987). The establishment of structure, as well the anticipation and effective removal of potential interference, are discussed and demonstrated through examples and classroom exercises. Similarly, the use of rewards and punishments is presented, demonstrated, and practiced.

## Class 6. Rules, Limits, and Special Time

The importance of setting rules and limits is presented, followed by a discussion of their uses. Rules are positive and limits are negative guidelines. Effective use of rules reduces the need to resort to limit setting. The successful implementation of rules and limits is discussed and demonstrated, and parents practice both in class and at home with their children for homework.

Introduction of the uses of "special time" represents the hallmark of these three classes (Guerney, 1987). It is time parents spend together with their children with the explicit task of building their relationship. The rules for special time closely resemble those of a psychodynamically oriented therapy session. Whether playing or talking, parents are instructed not to lead but to follow the child's desires, to listen and demonstrate understanding. Parents are instructed to set aside a special time, say, half an hour per week, to protect this time, and not to allow any interference.

## Class 7. Coping with Stress

Given the importance of special time, the first part of this class is devoted to discussing the experience of trying it at home and practicing it in class. Initially parents may find it difficult not to lead or respond to the child's questions, but to follow and demonstrate that they have heard what the child said and are interested in his or her thoughts. They are reassured that this is not a stance they may want to adopt at other times, and that it may be reserved only for special time. Parents are encouraged to continue practicing it after the end of the course.

The second half of the class is devoted to discussing the stresses of parenting, particularly in a culturally different context. For employed parents, balancing work and family responsibilities may be especially difficult. It is important for parents to cope with the stressors they face, not only for their own well-being but also for that of their children, because only happy parents will raise happy children. Parents are taught to recognize signs of distress, which may range from physical (loss of appetite and sleep disturbance) to psychological (irritability, depression, anxiety) manifestations. They are taught three methods of dealing with the distress: relaxation, doing pleasant activities, and developing and strengthening social networks. These cognitive-behavioral methods have been used in the prevention and treatment of depression, and are adapted from Munoz and Ying (1993).

## Class 8. Review and Integration

The last class is devoted to further discussion of special time and the stress-reduction techniques introduced the preceding week. This is followed by a general review of the entire course. In particular, the intergenerational tie is likely to be strengthened when, affectively, parents care about their child's view and feelings; cognitively, they understand that the context in which their child is growing up is different from that of their own childhood, and they are willing to learn about this new context; and behaviorally, they seek to reach out to their child and his or her world, especially by using understanding and special time. The remaining time is devoted to the completion of postclass assessment forms.

## Results of a Pilot Test of the SITICAF Program

The SITICAF program was pilot-tested with a group of fifteen Chinese American immigrant parents whose children attend a weekend Chinese language school in northern California (see also Ying, 1998). Of them, 80 percent were mothers. All were married. The mean age was 42 ($SD$ = 5.9). Their mean age at migration was 24.6 ($SD$ = 3.1). The parents were highly educated, with a mean education of 17.9 years ($SD$ = 2.4). All of their children, who ranged in age between 1 and 17, were born in the United States. All of the parents were fluent in English, but preferred to speak Chinese with their children. The social network of the parents consisted primarily of other immigrant Chinese (81.3 percent), with the remainder affiliating with American-born Chinese and/or other Asians.

Parents participated in the SITICAF program over an eight-week period. Immediately before the beginning of the course (pre), immediately after taking the course (post), and three months after its completion (three months follow-up), they completed assessment instruments that examined their attitude toward parenting (measured by the Parental Locus of Control Scale by Campis, Lyman, and Prentice-Dunn, 1986), the intergenerational relationship (measured by the Intergenerational Relationship in Immigrant Families–Chinese Parent Scale, Ying, unpublished), their child's esteem (measured by Coopersmith's [1967] Self-Esteem Inventory), and their own well-being (as measured by the Center for Epidemiological Studies Depression Scale by Radloff [1977]).

Using dependent $t$ tests (one-tailed tests), the pre scores were compared to the post and three-month follow-up scores. Parents reported an increased sense of efficacy from pre to post and three-months follow-up. They felt more responsible for their children's behavior at post than at pre, and less fatalistic about parenting from pre to three-months follow-up. There was a significant improvement in the quality of the intergenerational relationship from pre- to postassessment. The parents rated their child's esteem as having increased from pre- to post-follow-up. Finally, the parents reported significantly fewer depressive symptoms at post- than at preassessment.

The correlation of the intergenerational relationship with the child's esteem and parents' well-being was empirically tested. Closeness in the intergenerational relationship was found to be significantly associated with the child's esteem at post and three-months follow-up. The parent's well-being (depression level) was not statistically significantly associated with intergenerational relationship, although a negative correlation was found across all three assessment periods. Parental sense of control of their child's behavior was significantly associated with a positive intergenerational relationship at post and three months follow-up. Also, parents with children who controlled their lives were more depressed at all three assessment periods, supporting the importance of imparting skills to change that perception and reality in increasing the parents' well-being.

## Conclusion

As a pilot, the study did not use a randomized controlled design. As such, the confidence that the positive parent, child, and intergenerational outcomes are due solely to the class is compromised. Also, given the very small sample size, the power of the various statistical tests was greatly compromised and excluded the use of multivariate analyses. Nonetheless, the initial testing of the SITICAF with this small group of parents yielded encouraging results. It affirmed the association of the intergenerational relationship and child's esteem, parental control over their child's behavior and improved intergenerational relationship, and child's control over parents and parental depression.

SITICAF was tested with a middle-class Chinese American immigrant parent sample. Being well educated, these parents easily understood the more theoretical discussions and completed the weekly written assignments and assessment instruments. The class needs to be tested with a less well-educated group. It may be necessary to modify some of the classes, especially the more theoretical presentations, and to focus more on practical concerns. For a less educated group, it may also be important to include more coverage of other available community resources for immigrant families.

Notably, despite an average stay of eighteen years in the United States and their educational and professional achievement (itself associated with a certain degree of Westernization), these parents continued to affiliate primarily with other immigrant Chinese, to prefer speaking Chinese with their American-born children, and generally to maintain a strong tie to their culture of origin. This supports the relevance of a program such as SITICAF to encourage the parents' increased cross-cultural competence and to develop means to improve the potential cultural gap between them and their children.

Although SITICAF was developed specifically for immigrant Chinese American parents, it may be easily adapted for other groups. The culture-specific content (such as the use of the fairy tale, The Monkey King) can be changed to fit another culture. Essentially the intervention assumes that migrant parents are familiar with their culture-based parenting values and methods, but may not be consciously aware of their cultural relativity. This is demonstrated, and parents are introduced to European American values and parenting methods, with the aim of enriching rather than replacing their repertoire of parenting techniques. The emphasis on active listening and effective communication specifically targets the risk of intergenerational and intercultural conflict.

Some parents initially expressed discomfort with active listening, repeating the child's feelings without comment, and conducting special time because these were unfamiliar and inconsistent with their usual mode of interaction. However, after practicing them at home, parents returned to class astounded and delighted by their children's positive responses. One mother noted that her usually quiet adolescent daughter now had much to share with her. Another mother reported her child sought her out and requested more special time. These reports suggest that new and initially uncomfortable methods are likely to be adopted if they prove to be effective in increasing communication.

Intergenerational and intercultural conflict is very prevalent and perhaps even normative in migrant families; the time is right for the development and testing of prevention programs such as SITICAF. Community-based interventions are needed to inform and help immigrant and refugee groups to anticipate and successfully meet the challenge of intergenerational and intercultural conflict. Although SITICAF targets parents, a companion intervention may be developed for the children of migrant parents. Not only is prevention better than treatment when problems can be anticipated, it also effectively addresses the problem of stigma that may deter non–European American immigrants and refugees from seeking and obtaining mental health services.

# Chapter Seventeen

# The Korean Breast and Cervical Cancer Screening Demonstration

*Barbara A. Wismer,*
*Arthur M. Chen,*
*Stella Jun,*
*Soo H. Kang,*
*Rod Lew,*
*Katya Min,*
*Joel M. Moskowitz,*
*Thomas E. Novotny,*
*and Ira B. Tager*

The Korean Breast and Cervical Cancer Screening Project, Health Is Strength, is a collaboration between Asian Health Services (AHS) (see Chapter Eighteen) and the Center for Family and Community Health (CFCH), a prevention research center at the University of California at Berkeley's School of Public Health. The project, funded by the CDC, has three primary goals: to investigate the ability of a community intervention program to improve breast and cervical cancer screening among Korean American women in Alameda County, California; to conduct an assessment of the health status of Korean Americans in Alameda County; and to empower the community to take responsibility for their health in the long run. The Korean Community Advisory Board (KCAB), comprising members and leaders of the Korean American community in Alameda County, plays an active role in decision making, providing access to community resources, and ensuring cultural appropriateness in all phases of the project. Baseline and follow-up surveys were completed, and an intervention program was implemented. This first phase of the project ended in September 1998.

The 1994 Korean Health Survey was a baseline population-based telephone survey on health and community issues. Of the women who were interviewed, 97 percent were born outside the United States, 75 percent did not speak English well or fluently, and 91 percent completed the interview in Korean (Center for Family and Community Health, 1997). We estimated that only 55 percent of Korean American women from the two counties had had a Pap smear in the preceding three years (Wismer and others, 1998b) and only 24 percent performed breast self-examination at least monthly (Center for Family and Community Health, 1997). Of those age fifty and older, only 34 percent had had a mammogram and 32 percent a clinical breast examination in the two years prior to the study (Wismer and others, 1998a).

## Intervention Program Components

The community intervention program was launched in March 1996. Program planning was guided by principles of cultural appropriateness and long-term capacity building, other successful published programs, interviews with individuals involved with similar programs, census and baseline survey data, and community input on community infrastructure and individuals' knowledge and barriers to access. The several components of the program addressed the predisposing, enabling, and reinforcing factors that affect health-related behaviors (Green and Kreuter, 1991).

### Educational Materials

A brochure on women's health was developed, using focus groups to guide content and presentation. Topics included diet, physical activity, and stress management, as well as breast and cervical cancer and screening. Korean American staff felt that information about breast and cervical cancer screening would be more acceptable if it was presented after more general information about women's health. The brochure contained a list of medical providers and mammogram facilities in the county that provide low-cost screening or have Korean-language capabilities, or both. This list included information about the Federal Breast and Cervical Cancer Control Program and the State of California Breast Cancer Early Detection Program, which provide free screening to women who have low incomes and no health insurance. A workshop and slide show with content similar to the brochure were developed. All materials were written in Korean by Korean American staff at AHS with assistance from Korean community focus groups. Photographs of women in the community were used for the cover of the brochure and some of the slides.

The brochure and resource list were distributed at workshops, businesses (including Korean beauty salons and grocery stores), and medical providers offices, and they were mailed to Korean households in Alameda County that participated in the survey. The workshop was conducted in Korean churches and other organizations, elderly housing units, and women's homes.

## Korean Churches

The baseline survey revealed that 76 percent of Korean American women in the two counties attended religious activities monthly or more often (Center for Family and Community Health, 1997), and the KCAB and AHS Korean American staff felt that the church was an important social institution in the county. Further, because the Korean American population in the county was geographically dispersed, there was no single area where most women lived or met. It therefore was felt that the best way to reach women was through their churches.

Relationship building with the approximately forty Korean churches in Alameda County started several years before the intervention program began with periodic letters and telephone calls to ministers that introduced the project and provided updates. At a meeting, to which all Korean ministers in the county were invited, representatives from AHS, the CFCH, the KCAB, and the county health department made presentations about the project, its importance, and the health of the Korean American community. They acknowledged the importance of the Korean church in its community, and asked for the ministers' help and support in implementing the intervention program by recommending women to be health counselors (HCs), allowing workshops to be held in their churches, and making health a priority within the church.

After the meeting, telephone calls were made to recruit women as HCs and to arrange workshops and other meetings. Relationships with other organizations (such as the elderly association) and businesses (such as beauty salons) that could provide access to the community also were developed.

## Health Counselors

Korean American women, recruited from their churches and other organizations, were trained for four hours, using a curriculum developed for the project that was based on curricula from other community health adviser programs. Content included facts and resources about breast and cervical cancer screening; communication, organizational, and advocacy skills; confidentiality issues; and use of a tracking system. The HCs had the following responsibilities:

1. Organize activities at their organization.
2. Follow up with women who attended workshops to identify those who needed screening and those with barriers to screening.
3. Help women minimize barriers by assisting them in accessing Medicare or Medi-Cal (California's Medicaid); low-cost county screening services; Korean medical providers; mammogram facilities; and volunteers or AHS Korean American staff that would provide translation and transportation.
4. Act as a liaison between women and AHS.
5. Keep track of the screening status of women in their church.

Women were encouraged to explore the idea that health should and can be a priority within the church and to actualize that idea through formation of a health committee or designation of a person to identify and respond to the health needs of its members.

## Mammogram Facilities

Representatives of all mammogram facilities in the county were invited to a meeting at which AHS and CFCH staff presented information about the project. Proposals to decrease barriers (particularly cost, language, transportation, and wait) for Korean American women were solicited. Women were referred primarily to two facilities that were selected because of their low cost, translation capabilities, optimal location, short waiting time, or expanded hours.

## Medical Providers

Information about the project, the resource list, and current screening recommendations was sent to Korean American medical providers in the county and medical providers at AHS.

## Preliminary Results and Lessons Learned

During the intervention program, about fifty-one hundred brochures and resource lists were distributed; forty-nine workshops and small group meetings, attended by about a thousand women, were held; and thirty-seven HCs were recruited and trained. Questionnaires completed by 626 women before and after workshops revealed that breast and cervical cancer and knowledge about screening improved. Information on 577 women revealed that the HCs were reaching more Korean American women who were older or less fluent in English compared with the general population of Korean American women in the county, which numbers about four thousand.

Community-sensitive research principles have been followed throughout the project (Chen and others, 1997): ensuring cultural appropriateness in all activities, building infrastructure for sustainable community action, and responding to community health needs as defined not only by public health data but also by community perceptions. To realize these principles, the KCAB has been an equal partner with AHS and the CFCH in decision making, and AHS Korean American staff are an integral part of the project team. This kind of community involvement enables the program to be tailored to the unique cultural and social characteristics of the community and to better ensure long-lasting change.

The intervention program was culturally tailored to the Korean American community. For example, because of this population's holistic view about health and negative ideas about cancer, cancer facts and figures were described after a more general introduction in the brochure and workshop, thus framing breast and cervical cancer screening within the context of a healthy lifestyle. Since most women could read Korean, the brochure, resource list, and workshop were written or presented in Korean. Because of the more hierarchical and formal structure of the Korean social system, the ministers were approached by a series of letters and an elaborate meeting that included dinner, because sharing food is an important component of social interactions.

One of the important lessons learned during the intervention program is that strategic relationship building is key to the design and implementation of sustainable interventions. However, development of relationships with individuals and organizations, and building infrastructure within organizations and the community, are labor and time intensive. This ongoing process requires constant attention. Success requires working with community members who know the community's social structure and networks for planning and implementation. The process must remain flexible because development of relationships is not entirely predictable.

For example, the approach to building relationships with and implementing the program in churches required more time than originally planned, and the program had to be modified. The KCAB and AHS Korean American staff, which include two ministers' wives, felt that churches should be approached through the ministers in a gradual way through a series of letters to the ministers, and the legitimacy of the project emphasized through the meeting described. However, the ministers were busy and more difficult to reach than other church members, so more staff time was required by this approach.

Originally the team planned to recruit HCs based on the ministers' recommendations after the meeting. However, churches did not begin to be committed to the program until its legitimacy was established by conducting workshops on site. Consequently, recruitment and training of HCs occurred after workshops had been held, thus delaying this part of the program. Churches' interest and involvement was sustained only by periodic telephone calls and site visits, which consumed many additional hours of staff time.

The workshop presentation required modification as well. Most workshops were conducted after Sunday church services. Some husbands, who had to wait for their wives, decided to attend the workshops too. Many ministers, who were almost uniformly men, attended as well. The presentation included explicit descriptions and slides of female anatomy and cancer that were designed for a female audience. Remarkably, the content was acceptable to both women and men, including the ministers. However, the tone of the presentation was altered. It was felt that even though the discussion might be limited by the presence of men, their interest should be supported, especially because church involvement hinged on support from the ministers.

During the last year of the project, the intervention program is being evaluated through reassessment of breast and cervical cancer screening behaviors. The hope is that health will remain a priority within Korean churches and other organizations, with infrastructure (such as health committees or persons) in place to support their ability to identify and act on the health needs of their members. Since this capacity and infrastructure building has been the most difficult to plan and implement, the project team is applying for a grant to strengthen health as a priority in the Korean community through Korean churches and other community organizations.

## Programs That Serve Other Groups

There are other programs to improve breast and cervical cancer screening among populations comprising largely immigrant women. A community program to improve screening among older Cambodian American women in Minnesota was designed and implemented using input from focus groups (Kelly and others,

1996). An educational videotape was developed to improve knowledge and attitudes. To overcome English and technical language barriers, materials were developed in Cambodian with input from women from the community. Because of suspicion of authority figures, small group educational meetings were hosted by Cambodian American women to show the videotape. These meetings included time for socializing and eating. Group appointments were made, and women were accompanied by Cambodian American staff to address fears of large medical facilities and individual appointments. Transportation was provided to facilitate access. Because of the women's shyness with male providers, women providers performed screening. After the program, screening among women who were part of the health care system improved. A similar program targeting Vietnamese American women in the same area was modeled after this one (Tosomeen, Marquez, Panser, and Kottke, 1996).

A neighborhood-based program was implemented in the Vietnamese American community of the San Francisco Bay Area (McPhee and others, 1996). *Suc Khoe La Vang!* (Health Is Gold!) included small group educational sessions, written materials, and health fairs. Women in this community tend not to leave their neighborhoods and to obtain information from within their social networks. Community solidarity is strong, and neighbors cooperate. As a result, indigenous lay health workers helped develop and implement the program. Their roles and responsibilities evolved during the program, in part because of incongruity between program plans and cultural norms and community structure. For example, health workers were expected to conduct sessions without program staff present (Bird, Otero-Sabogal, Ha, and McPhee, 1996). However, because of fear of loss of face or credibility, difficulty thinking independently (rather than conforming to the group norm), and general feelings of insecurity related to the refugee experience, this was difficult to implement. Small group sessions were held in neighborhood homes; this promoted an atmosphere of trust and active participation. Because community residents lacked knowledge about and orientation to Western medicine and prevention, and had limited English proficiency, brochures, posters, and videotapes were developed in Vietnamese with input from focus groups, and the first phase of the program emphasized getting a regular checkup. This program is part of a larger project, Pathways to Cancer Screening for Four Ethnic Groups, which is investigating the similarities and differences of the pathways to appropriate breast and cervical cancer screening among different racial and ethnic groups, as well as the similarities and differences in design and implementation of programs to improve screening (Hiatt and others, 1996). Results of the evaluation are not yet available.

Latinas in the Bay Area are another target population for Pathways. *En Accion Contra el Cancer* (In Action Against Cancer) used mass media, educational materials, and community outreach (Perez-Stable, Otero-Sabogal, Sabogal, and Napoles-Springer, 1996). Program materials and implementation were tailored to certain Latina cultural values. Authorities are respected, and it is important to have positive interpersonal interactions. The needs of the family are more important than those of the individual. Finally, Latinas tend to have a fatalistic attitude about life.

The media campaign primarily used television and radio. There were paid commercials advertising the program, television pieces on screening and cancer, and radio talk shows featuring Latino health care professionals and patient testimonials. A Spanish-language booklet was developed. Presentations were made to community groups, especially health care organizations. Staff and volunteers conducted classes for Latinas to improve their skills for obtaining screening tests. Peer networkers distributed materials to women, community businesses and organizations, and at health fairs; shared information, including news about media events, with other women; and recruited other networkers. Some served as role models and gave testimonials for the media. *Promotoras* were recruited from among the networkers. These women found, educated, referred, and tracked women in the community. There was an advisory board of professionals, and outreach was coordinated with other state and federal programs. Although program evaluation results are not yet available, keys to its success have been identified: program staff at all levels were Latino; the association of the program with the University of California at San Francisco added prestige; and Spanish-language media were available.

In another innovative program, a randomized controlled study was implemented to evaluate the ability of a voucher to improve mammography use among Mexican American women attending migrant health clinics in Washington (Skaer, Robison, Sclar, and Harding, 1996). Cost had been identified as one of the major barriers to getting mammography. Use of the procedure improved significantly among the women who received vouchers, compared with those who did not receive them.

Substantive participation by community members as focus group members, lay health workers, program staff, or advisory board members in development and implementation of these programs is the common thread in all of these programs. This participation allows a better understanding of the unique cultural, social, individual, and structural characteristics of the community, so that the program framework and content can be tailored to unique strengths and needs. It also is key to promoting ownership and sustainable action in the community. Another common characteristic of the programs is that they are multifaceted, which allows many of the variables—individual and environmental characteristics of both the community and the health care system—that may affect screening to be addressed.

# Chapter Eighteen

# A Case Study of Asian Health Services

*Sherry M. Hirota*

Asian Health Services (AHS) was founded in 1973 by members of the Asian community in Oakland, California. These visionaries included students, health professionals, and community activists whose driving purpose was to advocate on behalf of the medically underserved Asian population, which was not getting access to the health care delivery system due to language differences, cultural incompetence, or lack of insurance. Since 1974, the health center has provided direct health care services to the limited- and non-English-speaking Asian population in Alameda County.

AHS has grown to become a comprehensive primary care clinic that provides medical care, health education and promotion, case management, and patient advocacy services to more than twelve thousand users and twenty-five hundred managed care members of all ages per year. All services are provided in eight Asian languages: Chinese (Mandarin and Cantonese), Korean, Vietnamese, Tagalog, Mien, Laotian, and Cambodian. Vietnamese, Cantonese, Mandarin, Korean, Cambodian, and Filipino are available within the provider pool alone.

I gratefully acknowledge Welmin Militante, Asian Health Services senior planner, for his assistance in data collection, and Kathy Lim Ko for her help in preparing the chapter.

Diagnostic laboratory, radiology, and pharmacy services are provided through written contractual arrangements with local providers. These contractors are able to meet the language needs of the patient population, and most are located within a one-block radius of the clinic. To address the translation and cultural needs, as well as the access issues, AHS continues arrangements with additional ancillary providers such as mammography for low-income women.

AHS's mission reflects its origins in advocating on behalf of the community for access to care, most notably in the areas of linguistic and culturally competent standards, immigrant policy, and the working uninsured. The center now has the capacity to provide forty thousand medical visits a year at its two new facilities. The typical AHS patient is a low-income, limited- or non-English-speaking individual who has been in the United States for fewer than five years.

All staff who have direct patient contact speak at least one Asian language and are bicultural. Many have the same immigration or refugee experiences as the patients and thus are aware of the various needs, values, and health practices patients might have. A wide variety of patient education materials, many of them developed in-house, are made available in the various Asian languages.

AHS's primary service area is Alameda County, California. Although AHS is located in the heart of Oakland's Chinatown neighborhood, its language-accessible and culturally competent services increasingly draw residents from nearby cities and Contra Costa, San Francisco, and Santa Clara counties. Those from other areas comprise 21 percent of the patient base.

Alameda is California's fifth largest county, with a population of 1.2 million and fourteen cities spanning 812 square miles. It is one of the most diverse communities in the nation: 50 percent white, 18 percent black, 17 percent API, and 15 percent Hispanic. The ethnic distribution among the county's APIs is even more diverse (see Table 18.1).

Indicative of the changing face of other metropolitan areas, a majority of the Asians in the area are foreign born. Often they have language, cultural, educational, and financial barriers that become additional stressors to the acculturation process.

**Table 18.1. Ethnic Distribution
in Alameda County, 1990.**

| Ethnicity | Number | Percentage of API Population |
|---|---|---|
| Chinese | 68,585 | 38.7 |
| Filipino | 52,535 | 29.6 |
| Japanese | 13,592 | 7.7 |
| Vietnamese | 13,374 | 7.5 |
| Korean | 9,537 | 5.4 |
| Pacific Islander | 7,995 | 4.5 |
| Cambodian | 3,538 | 2.0 |
| Other Asian | 4,420 | 2.5 |
| Laotian | 2,895 | 1.6 |
| Thai | 791 | Below 0.1 |
| Hmong | 10 | Below 0.0 |
| Total | 17,727 | 100.0 |

# User Population and Community Size

The Asian American population is the fastest-growing ethnic group both nationally and locally, doubling twice over the past two decades. From 1980 to 1990, California's API population increased by 117 percent (U.S. Bureau of the Census, 1993). APIs now account for nearly 10 percent of the state's population, up from 5 percent ten years prior. Of California's largest Asian ethnic groups, Filipinos, Chinese, Vietnamese, and Koreans have experienced growth rates of 100 percent or greater in the ten-year period. The Southeast Asian population, particularly Cambodian, Mien, and Vietnamese, is increasing most rapidly.

Roughly 40 percent of the total API immigrant population to the United States settle in California. Second only to the Los Angeles basin, the Bay Area is a favored destination for APIs, demonstrated by a sharp population increase of 124 percent from 1980 to 1990. Reflecting these exponential growth patterns, APIs are now the second largest ethnic minority group in Alameda County. Since the 1990 census, the API population has increased by 18.45 percent, from roughly 180,000 to 226,000, making it the fastest-growing ethnic minority population in the county.

## Emerging Communities

The continued growth among the newly arrived Southeast Asian communities of Alameda County has pointed to the inadequacies of the health care delivery system in its ability to provide medical access to this population group. AHS has been the sole entity that is capable of providing the services needed to meet the needs of the emerging Cambodian, Laotian, and Mien communities. As a result, intensive outreach to these communities is being conducted to allay community fears and distrust of Western medicine with which they are unfamiliar.

## English Proficiency and Education

APIs speak more than one hundred different languages and dialects. According to the 1990 federal census, of the API households in the service area, 50.4 percent are classified as "linguistically isolated" and can speak only limited English, if at all. In fact, 90 percent of the clients served at the AHS clinic speak a primary language other than English. For most of the clients served, language and cultural barriers are exacerbated by low educational levels completed in their own language. Nearly half of the clients (48 percent) have completed fewer than ten years of education.

## Income Level

The "myth of the model minority" has served to obscure factors that contribute to the APIs' economically disenfranchised status. In Oakland, 22.8 percent of APIs live below the poverty level. APIs have the second lowest per capita income in Oakland, at $10,285, compared to $8,537 for Latinos, $10,940 for African Americans, and $23,461 for Anglo-Americans. The poverty rate for API families in Alameda County in 1993 was 14 percent; for Anglo families it was 8 percent. These statistics mask the more severe poverty levels among specific Southeast Asian populations. Sixty-eight percent of Laotians, 66 percent of Hmong, 47 percent of Cambodians, and 35 percent of Vietnamese live at or below the poverty level. At AHS, 77 percent of patients have incomes below the federal poverty level. With such disadvantaged socioeconomic conditions, health risks abound.

## Unemployment and Underemployment

The unemployment rate for APIs in the Oakland Metropolitan Statistical Area is 8.1 percent for males and 7.0 percent for females. Although these rates are the second lowest of the ethnic groups, many newly arrived immigrants and refugees can secure jobs that earn only poverty-level wages. With limited English proficiency, many work in an underground cash economy that pays less than minimum wage. The plight of garment workers speaks to the employment conditions of many of the clients. Most of the patients work in low-paying jobs that offer no health insurance and may be at the borderline poverty level. However, they are precluded from receiving Medi-Cal (California's Medicaid program) benefits due to the extra margin of income they receive. The number of those without health insurance has grown enormously over the last few years.

## Medical Coverage

The proportion of uninsured in the target population historically has been high. The International Ladies Garment Workers Union indicates that 80 percent of workers in the Bay Area garment industry are Asian, and according to a survey of Asian Immigrant Women Advocates, 69 percent of these workers have no health insurance. According to *The State of Health Insurance in California* (Schauffler and others, 1998), uninsured figures for California reflect a disproportionate number of Hispanics and Asians in addition to African Americans. Of the 6.6 million people who are without health insurance, 36 percent are Hispanic, 23 percent are Asian, and 20 percent are African American. Although an estimated 16 percent of Alameda County's population is uninsured, 45 percent of AHS clients do not have coverage, amounting to over 3,760 indigent patients; the remainder are mainly indigent patients who are enrolled in Medi-Cal or Medicare. The uninsured have few options for receiving care, other traditional safety net providers have limited language interpretation staff, and private physicians provide very little uncompensated care.

Other factors that contribute to barriers to care for immigrant women and their families are eligibility for public entitlements, such as Medicaid and Medicare. The reluctance of immigrant families to apply for Medi-Cal results from fears that it would hurt their chances for citizenship or to reunite them with other members of their families. With on-site workers who are bilingual in an Asian language, AHS has managed to increase its third-party coverage for indigent patients. At AHS, 42 percent have Medi-Cal and 13 percent have Medicare.

Nearly half of the savings that were expected to come from welfare reform under the Personal Responsibility and Work Opportunity Reconciliation Act were due to restrictions on immigrant access to benefits. Clinics like AHS already have been hard pressed to assist patients in reconciling the difference between health services eligibility and Immigration and Naturalization Services (INS) policy. The newest developments of insurance for uninsured children, the Children's Health Initiative, has been deemed a federally means tested program and will leave many immigrant children virtually among the uninsured.

Having anticipated dire circumstances resulting from the passage of the Welfare Reform Act, AHS developed two tracks of addressing the growing number of uninsured health care consumers in its service area. An annual giving campaign, the AHS Community Care Fund, which began on January 1, 1998, will aim to raise additional monies from private sources—including individuals, foundations, and corporations—in order to continue to provide services to the very needy in the community. In conjunction, a community organizing effort will be undertaken to develop a medical insurance–type program for the working poor. The hope is that by approaching the issue from multiple perspectives, the most marginalized communities will have fewer barriers to gaining access to needed health care.

## Cultural Competency

Other than AHS, there are only a very few full-time equivalent Chinese-speaking primary care providers who accept indigent care patients. Language barriers are a problem for the majority of AHS clients; more than 90 percent have a primary language other than English or are limited-English or non-English speaking. The impact of these barriers is underscored by the observable clustering of high-risk factors in particular Asian subpopulations, such as those experienced in the Laotian-Mien community.

## Major Health Problems

The common health problems among APIs differ from those of the general population in the predominance of preventable conditions. APIs have high rates of morbidity and mortality from infectious and parasitic diseases such as tuberculosis, which is five times higher among APIs than the national average; hepatitis B, which has a 17 percent infection rate among APIs compared with 1 percent in the general U.S. population; and intestinal parasites, which are found in more than 50 percent of newly arrived Asians. In addition, thalassemia is carried in 10 percent of Chinese and up to 36 percent of Southeast Asian refugees.

APIs are at high risk for chronic conditions such as hypertension, diabetes, and tobacco use. Studies of tobacco use among Southeast Asian populations indicate that 91 percent of Laotian males smoke. Poor health status relative to immunizations, nutrition, exercise, high rates of smoking, and lack of knowledge of health risk behaviors contributes to a patient population at high risk and in great need of access to care.

## AHS Role in the Community

As the main community health center serving the API population in Alameda County, AHS is viewed as a leader in responsive and effective health care service delivery for the API population locally. And despite being a local health care provider, AHS's role has extended beyond local boundaries, to advising on statewide public and private policies regarding the distribution of resources for health care and in national-level discussions regarding the impact of welfare reform on AHS patients, immigration policies, and issues of cultural competence and language access to health care.

AHS shares its service delivery innovations and resources through several local, regional, and national networks. For example, it participates in the East Bay Asian Consortium, a group of twelve API-serving agencies based in Oakland that work together to eliminate service duplication, develop joint ventures, and advocate for API health needs.

AHS belongs to the Alameda Health Consortium, a community clinic association that shares technical assistance and advocates for community health needs with the county contract to provide services to medically indigent persons.

## Community Input and Involvement

Since AHS serves such a diversity of Asian communities, maintaining regular contact with its own patients, community groups, and other service providers is an essential part of its efforts to be responsive to community needs.

### Patient Input

Each year, AHS convenes a patient general meeting to inform clients of health care developments and seek their feedback on their satisfaction with AHS services and any service gaps that it should address. In past years, over three hundred patients attended these forums, where staff accommodated patient needs and addressed their concerns during exchanges that were simultaneously interpreted between English and the nine Asian languages. Patient input helps AHS determine service priorities for the year. Topics covered in recent years included President Clinton's proposed health care reform (1994), managed care (1995 and 1996), and welfare reform (1997).

### Community at Large

AHS engages leaders from the various Asian communities served in discussions about specific needs within their communities. This is particularly important for leaders from the growing Laotian and

Mien populations who are relative newcomers to the United States and are less aware of health resources available to them.

## Expansion of Scope of Services

With its enormous recent expansions, AHS's role in the community has become even more dynamic. With the high profile of owning a new building, it continues to receive numerous inquiries about ways of partnering with a wide variety of health care and social service organizations. Many of these inquiries represent opportunities to further agency priorities of creating a "one-stop shop" by offering a range of ancillary services, including a pharmacy on-site, and they have resulted in bringing a new vibrancy to the local community. In the coming years, it is seeking to integrate traditional Chinese medicine, including acupuncture, into its scope of services in order to address the needs of its consumer base further.

## Service Delivery Strategy and Model

Comprehensive primary health care services addressing the needs of the five major life cycles (perinatal, pediatric, adolescent, adult, and geriatric) are provided by a team of primary care physicians and midlevel practitioners in a culturally competent and linguistically appropriate manner. The clinical services program uses a family practice model, with all primary care services provided by the same clinician to all members of a family whenever possible.

With the opening of a second site, Adult Medical Services at Hotel Oakland (AMSHO), AHS has expanded the scope of services to serve better adult populations, particularly the elderly. That site offers centralized medical care for the retired and mobility-challenged community in the clinic's vicinity.

Translation services are an integral part of the clinical program. Translation capability in eight languages is available through in-house bilingual support services, providers, and health education staff and is incorporated into all aspects of clinical services. In addition, providers utilize the Language Cooperative Program's medical interpretation services to fill in any occasional gaps in translation needs.

In addressing the needs of each life cycle, the agency has accelerated its efforts to recruit providers, and with great success. In the past year, AHS has identified adolescent needs and has expanded teen health services to provide a broader scope of health education services.

Continuity of care remains central to AHS's overall clinical program. With the in-house on-call system, staff physicians are available to help enrolled patients around the clock. Linkages for secondary and tertiary care at local hospitals have been strengthened with increased admitting privileges for AHS physicians at Summit Hospital and Children's Hospital of Oakland, and pending at Alta Bates Medical Center. In emergencies, patients may be referred to Highland General Hospital, the county facility, or to one of the private hospitals.

AHS commitment to continuity of care is successful because of the strong leadership provided by its medical director. Through regularly scheduled provider meetings, clinicians participate in the decision-making process in the overall clinical practice. These monthly meetings provide clinicians with an opportunity to discuss programmatic concerns, advocacy issues, staffing concerns, implementation of policies and procedures, and updates from the executive leadership, management committee, and the board of directors.

## Program Revenues

AHS serves as a model for developing a strong financial base for operations while creatively generating new models for programs and the resources necessary to sustain them.

### Primary Care: Government Sources

In order to provide services to a patient population, nearly half of whom, and historically as high as 75 percent, are uninsured, government funds are critical.

Federal funding has been an important source of revenue to support primary care for indigent patients across the country. The Community Health Center program of the Bureau of Primary Health Care, Title 330 of the Public Health Service Act, is a major source of funds for care to the indigent and medically underserved.

State funds for indigent primary care have been much more limited and fragmented. Until recently, state-supported primary care was about $2 million per year. In the 1990s, with the advent of the state tobacco tax, expanded access to primary care (EAPC) was established as the first major state-supported primary care program with a budget of $15 million. However, this program is subject to the level of tobacco tax revenues and legislative re-authorization. Since its inception in 1989, the success of statewide tobacco use reduction programs and the number of clinics being funded by the EAPC program has decreased the total amount of funds available to each clinic site gradually.

Local county support beginning with revenue sharing in the early 1970s has been a consistent and major source of community clinic revenue. With the shift of many critical human services from the state to the counties in the 1980s, the counties have been a major provider of primary care and a major funding source for un-insured care. State law requires counties to be the provider of last resort; they cannot refuse to provide care. There was immediate and ongoing recognition on the part of local politicians and health officials that community health centers and clinics were able to reach and effectively serve the diverse ethnic and aging populations that their own institutions could not. As a result, in Alameda County, where AHS is located, there is a mix of providers, both county facilities and community clinics, which provide a closely co-ordinated and complementary network of primary care services.

## Categorical Programs

From time to time, certain special initiatives or programs are de-veloped by various levels of government or by foundations that provide funding for prevention, detection, and treatment of dis-ease. In the past, these initiatives have ranged from family plan-ning, perinatal services, hypertension, breast and cervical cancer screening, to immunizations. Often they come as a result of a wider public health concern about potential epidemics or through the advocacy work of health activists who bring special needs forward to the public or policymakers' attention. A particular feature of these sources of funds is that they have, in the main, been geared toward comprehensive, innovative programs for relatively low cost per participant. By reaching many different language groups and communities with similar programs, the cost-effectiveness is increased. AHS also has been able to work in collaboration with many community-based providers to provide comprehensive and innovative programs for Asian immigrant individuals and families.

Unfortunately, many of these initiatives are short-lived; some are as short as one year, and few are as long as three to five years. More often than not, just as a new program or initiative has begun to make an impact, the ongoing support is gone, and the patients are left with no place to secure these preventive, screening, or health promotion services.

Some programs have had longer lives. Prenatal care, funded through a variety of mechanisms over the years, has continued to be supported through a patchwork system of funds combining federal, state, and local dollars. AHS's early commitment (1988) to address HIV in the Asian community has propelled it to a position of leadership in the field. It is the only provider in the country that offers a comprehensive range of services (medical, psychosocial, practical, and death and dying issues) for HIV and AIDS that are accessible by language and culture for many API communities. In addition, AHS is a confidential test site contracted by Alameda County.

## Efforts to Go Beyond Base Funding for Indigent Care

Like many other community clinics and social service agencies that were founded in the 1960s and early 1970s as part of the civil rights and social movements addressing inequities and unmet social needs, AHS historically was underfunded and reliant on staff who were dedicated to the mission, despite the low pay. Because funding remained flat while the API population grew in unprecedented proportions, demand for services always exceeded capacity.

A number of successful strategies were employed to correct these shortfalls, including seeking core funding, getting a cost-based reimbursement status in recognition of the large degree of uncompensated care, and advocating for recognition of the health problems and size of the API population.

## Stabilization

Many nonprofit organizations began as small demonstration and pilot projects in the 1960s and early 1970s; they operated on bare-bones budgets and seed grants. After a decade of existence, those that did not find or establish a source of core funding found it increasingly difficult to sustain competent programs with a stable infrastructure of technical and management skills. After twenty years, AHS and the community clinic network in Alameda County had clearly established their effectiveness, becoming the major source of primary care to the underserved and indigent local community. In order to stabilize these essential providers of care, the county finally responded to a two-year campaign to provide stabilization grants to all contracting clinics. This brought their salaries to 85 percent of comparable county salaries. The average increase to each clinic was 20 percent of their primary care grant without a corresponding increase in patient visits. The effort also resulted in the adoption of a policy that ties the clinic contract cost-of-living adjustment to that of the county workers.

## Federally Qualified Health Centers

Strategies from the federal level included cost-based reimbursements to federally qualified health centers (FQHCs) that were adopted in 1990. In effect, this increased Medicaid and Medicare payments to community health centers in recognition of the disproportionate level of indigent care and more comprehensive scope of services they provide. This assurance of "full cost" reflected a significant difference in reimbursement. For example, in California, Medi-Cal generally was paying 35 percent of the full costs, or $35 for every $100 of cost. Now, Medi-Cal would be paying $100 for $100 of cost, although the balance of $65 would be in arrears and appear after a reconciliation audit.

These funds were strategically spent on expansion of care to the underserved, primarily to underwrite uninsured care, with a portion saved into a board-designated building fund.

## Community Base and Advocacy to Promote Access to Care

AHS's dual mission as an advocate and provider of quality accessible health care to the Asian community has contributed significantly to its success. It has given a focus to the organization's programming, remaining consistently rooted in the community's demonstrated need for accessible care. It avoids tendencies to develop programs just because funding is available. Instead, once the central needs of the community are identified, the organization concentrates its efforts on advocating for changes in policies and funding priorities that will respond to those needs.

Whether the issue is language accessibility or lack of health insurance, if the community determines the need, it is in a position to be organized and mobilized to articulate those needs. Harnessing that energy and experience can have a powerful, irrefutable effect on policy- and grantmakers because it is so concrete.

Taking those messages and issues to a national level depends on working with other organizations to network with broader coalitions of interested parties. Both the Asian Pacific Islander American Health Forum and the Association of Asian Pacific Community Health Organizations were spawned at AHS in the mid-1980s. These two national organizations have gone on to lead the work in educating policymakers on the health needs of Asian American and APIs, as well as the specific challenges faced by Asian-serving community health centers. Having both of these organizations involved at the state and federal levels has made the difference in having API concerns reflected in the Disadvantaged Minority Health Act of 1990 and in changing policies regarding medical research, programmatic funding, and the establishment of Asian-serving community health centers.

## Attempts to Level the Playing Field: Indicators Relevant to the Population

Funding clinical services is dependent on meeting a set of criteria that are established by the federal and state governments or by foundations. Those criteria generally are based on national data sets that most often miss or overlook health access problems and discrepancies in health status as they affect APIs. Until 1985, the U.S. DHHS had done little regarding minority health. That year, the *Report of the Secretary's Task Force on Black and Minority Health* (1985) finally documented excess mortality rates in at least five major areas for African Americans. These discrepancies in health status became significant indicators of need for programs and funding. The 1985 report, however, did not produce enough data on APIs in the United States; in particular, disaggregated data by ethnic and linguistic subgroup were not consistently collected to make any significant findings. In the absence of data that would reflect indicators of need among APIs, programs serving these populations remain at a disadvantage for funding.

## Adaptation to Changes in the Health Care Environment

Managed care has created the challenges of the next decade for health care providers. Along with the rise of for-profit HMOs, an extremely competitive financial environment has arrived within an environmental setting where all health care providers are required to play. Corporate consolidations, buyouts of one HMO by another, and the creation of new permutations of physician groups and intermediaries combine to leave individual practitioners, as well as individual community clinics, as dinosaurs in the making.

Negotiations can occur only if there are enough physicians and patient members at the table to have discussions. On the one hand, this brings with it a host of demands and responsibilities that rarely was the case for community clinics even ten years ago. On the other hand, these linkages provide new sources of revenue, and possibly even capital, to use to underwrite the primary mission of the clinic to serve the underserved.

Clinics that address the unique sociocultural needs of APIs are in a position to carve out a niche market for themselves. In California, Asians are seen as a growth market for health care. Clinics and other providers that historically have served these communities have become attractive as contracted physicians and major points of sale.

# An Attempt to Expand the Pie: Capital Assets

In recognizing the coming changes with managed care, and Medicaid managed care in particular in California, AHS undertook an ambitious capital development project in 1991. This consisted primarily of purchasing and renovating its own building and establishing donor relationships that would sustain the same amount of uninsured care into the next century.

The total project was valued at $9 million, $6.5 million of which was financed through tax-exempt bonds insured by the state of California, through its California Health Facilities Mortgage Insurance Program (Cal-Mortgage). The balance was raised through donations. Of the total $2.5 million capital campaign, receipts came from the following sources: 20 percent board-designated AHS retained earnings; 10 percent, corporations; 35 percent, foundations; and 35 percent, private individuals.

Although the building and the medical equipment are capital assets that can be used as collateral in the future, the capital campaign had many intangible and invaluable outcomes beyond these tangible assets. The donor program established by the fundraising campaign is now targeted to raise about $200,000 a year for uninsured care and other expenses not otherwise covered. This resulted from the donors of the capital campaign having known AHS and its work. The annual fundraising dinner raises about $60,000 to $80,000. These sources will become increasingly important as health care financing continues to be transformed.

The relationship established with corporations and major foundations also was a new step for AHS. Historically funded primarily through government grants, AHS had never before sought foundations as a regular source of revenue. Now, with the relationships developed, there are more—and more creative—ways for AHS to develop programs through private philanthropy.

Managing debt also is a new source of cash. Options considered include lines of credit, secured with collateral or not, as well as commercial loans, as an alternative to the tax-exempt bond financing. Learning to manage these debts while maintaining operational funds has been a new stage of organizational development.

# Conclusion

Despite the tremendous changes in the health care and political environments, the key to stability for AHS has been its dual mission. While striving for excellence in its services delivery systems, it has helped to shape an agenda built on the philosophy that health care is a right, not a privilege. It has worked closely with other clinics, national advocacy organizations, and national clinic organizations to have policymakers understand the needs in serving patients who otherwise have no access to care. As the AHS motto states, the ultimate test is "not only in the number of patients we serve, but also how fully our community understands and asserts its right to quality health care."

# Chapter Nineteen

# A Cultural Competence Curriculum

*Elizabeth J. Kramer and*
*William B. Bateman*

All health care providers and health care workers should be culturally competent in dealing with patients whose cultures are different from their own, especially since by the year 2000, 40 percent of the U.S. population will be new immigrants or first-generation Americans (Barker, 1992). Several groups have developed cultural competence curricula for specific population groups (Garza-Trevino, Ruiz, and Venegas-Samuels, 1997; Like, Steiner, and Rubel, 1996; Stein, 1994; Spielvogel, 1995; Thompson, 1996).

Ideally, cultural competence training should begin in the first year of medical school and continue through the end of residency. Although it does not identify specific issues related to cross-cultural medicine and diversity, the Accreditation Council for Graduate Medical Education has made a general requirement that primary care specialties include the teaching of psychosocial and cultural issues in their curricula (Accreditation Council for Graduate Medical Education, 1998). Both medical schools and residency programs have limited time for teaching this material, but with a concerted effort, much of it can be integrated into existing course blocks and rotations.

This chapter addresses the important knowledge, skills, and attitudes that future physicians should acquire over the course of training, provides specific behavioral objectives for one or two areas, and discusses how the material can be taught and integrated into the total learning experience of health care providers in training. Integration of this material with the clinical curriculum is much easier in areas where the patient base is multiethnic. Focusing on the attitudes, values, and social norms, as well as the historical background and cultural and ethnic heritage of each group served is vital. It is essential to build a sense of appreciation, curiosity, and respect for other cultures while instilling the attitudes and skills needed to avoid stereotyping ethnic-specific groups that are different from the health care provider and the dominant culture.

## Teaching Approaches

A number of teaching approaches can be employed: integrating cross-cultural information into a single unit within a given course, using a course or continuing education program to cover culturally relevant material, offering a series of courses that are extensions of one another, and integrating cultural concepts into every unit, course, and continuing education program (Millon-Underwood, 1992). To be relevant for house staff and medical students, these approaches must be integrated into both ambulatory and inpatient settings. The firm conference or small group teaching sessions (such as morning reports, team meetings, and house staff conferences) are good places to conduct "anthropology rounds" in both inpatient and outpatient settings.

Learners can gain a great deal from each other by exploring one another's cultural differences. This tends to provide a readily available and safe opportunity to see how much culture-driven beliefs rather than science influence individual judgment.

To ensure that institutional change is made, diversity and cross-cultural information can be mainstreamed into grand rounds, major medical conferences, and continuing medical education programs. Interdisciplinary faculty development training within the academic institution, hospital, or clinic is critical to achieving permanent institutional changes in attitude.

Specific teaching models, such as LEARN (listen, explain, acknowledge, recommend, negotiate), may serve as reference guides for improving cross-cultural communication in the clinical encounter (Berlin and Fowkes, 1983). The best training combines a multidimensional approach (cognitive, affective, and behavioral goals with culture-specific and culture-general content) and uses experiential and intellectual approaches targeted to the trainee's level of ethnosensitivity.

One of the most challenging and important teaching approaches is to immerse learners in an environment dominated by cultural norms that are different from their own. This is especially important for those who come from dominant cultural backgrounds, as ethnic minorities experience this regularly. However, well-designed learning-objective-driven immersion activities for all learners are fundamental to successful cross-cultural learning.

## Educational Objectives

In this section, we define the core contents of a cultural competence curriculum. The educational objectives are divided into three categories: knowledge, skills, and attitudes.

## Knowledge

It would be ideal if all major population groups in the United States could be included in the curriculum, but the reality is that there probably will not be adequate time for this to occur. Therefore, learners should become knowledgeable about the following aspects of each population they will be serving:

• The historical roots and backgrounds of the major subgroups who reside in their area. For example, for Hispanics this would mean learning about Mexican Americans, Puerto Ricans, Cuban Americans, Dominicans, or Salvadorans, depending upon where one is located. In New York, the emphasis would be on learning about Dominicans and Puerto Ricans; in Miami, focus would be on Cubans; and southern California teaching efforts would be directed toward Mexican Americans.

• Migration patterns and experiences, and their impact on health and mental health.

• The socioeconomic and cultural factors that affect health and mental health.

- Religious affiliations and spiritual beliefs.
- The role of the family in medical decision making, diagnosis, and treatment.
- Normative behavior of the culture and the impact of inter-generational confrontations.
- Gender role perceptions and expectations.
- Ways of expressing caring and respect and, conversely, offen-sive behaviors.
- Communication and behavioral patterns (such as use of body language and how emotions are expressed).
- Epidemiology of prevalent diseases, especially those that relate to the Department of Health and Human Services' health pro-motion and disease prevention objectives and those with high rates of morbidity and mortality.
- Explanatory belief systems related to the etiology of disease.
- Health-related behaviors, such as diet and beliefs about how to stay healthy.
- Folk healing remedies and practices and use of traditional practitioners.
- Medical problems and life stressors relating to the stage of the individual and family life cycles and major life events (preg-nancy, birth, marriage, death).
- The special medical and psychological problems of women from the culture.
- Health problems linked to culture shock from migration, in-tergenerational value orientation conflicts, and acculturation and assimilation processes.
- Signs, symptoms, and cumulative effects of trauma, such as incest, rape, and battering.
- Awareness of the potential ethnic differences in relation to pharmacogenetics, pharmacokinetics, and pharmaco-dynamics.
- Classic patterns of cultural expression for first-, second-, and third-generation immigrants in relation to their country of origin.
- Limits to the acceptance of cultural differences and an under-standing of how to determine this. For example, in some countries wife beating may be culturally acceptable; in the United States, it is illegal.

## Skills

At the end of the module, learners will be able to perform the following skills:

- Elicit a medical and psychosocial history and perform a physical examination in a culturally appropriate manner.
- Integrate cultural knowledge into the assessment of the patient.
- Develop a differential diagnosis based on knowledge of the epidemiology of diseases in a given culture.
- Be aware of their own cultural and ethnic backgrounds and the way that they may affect their practices.
- Be aware of any personal feelings that could be culturally biased.
- Demonstrate competence in eliciting a complete and accurate sexual and reproductive history.
- Obtain information about traumatic events common to women's lives, such as domestic violence, sexual abuse, sexual assault, and harassment.
- As part of a continuity of care experience, form and maintain a therapeutic alliance with at least three patients with different cultural backgrounds.
- Recognize and appropriately respond to verbal and nonverbal communication.
- Use the negotiated approach to clinical care, for example, Berlin and Fowkes's LEARN model (1983).
- Appropriately use family members, community gatekeepers, translators and interpreters, and other community resources to deliver culturally competent services.
- Work collaboratively with other health care professionals in a culturally competent manner.
- When ethically and legally appropriate, work with alternative or otherwise complementary medicine practitioners and indigenous, lay, or folk healers.
- Identify how one's own cultural values, assumptions, and beliefs affect patient care and clinical decision making.

## Attitudes

- Demonstrate an awareness of the impact of sociocultural factors on patients, practitioners, the clinical encounter, and interpersonal relationships.
- Accept one's individual responsibility to understand the cultural dimensions of health and illness as a core clinical task in the care of all patients.
- Appreciate the heterogeneity that exists within and across cultural groups and the importance of avoiding overgeneralization and negative stereotyping.
- Recognize one's own personal biases and reactions to individuals from different ethnic and sociocultural backgrounds.
- Appreciate how one's personal cultural values, assumptions, and beliefs influence the provision of care.
- Be willing to understand and explain those values, assumptions, and beliefs and to examine how they affect the care provided to patients who share and do not share a similar perspective.
- Express respect and tolerance for cultural and social class differences and their value in a pluralistic society

## Learning Experiences

Every student and resident should have a clinical experience, preferably a continuity experience, in caring for immigrant or transcultural patients. The undergraduate medical student experience might begin in the first year, with the student following a family from another culture throughout the four years of medical school. As the student acquires clinical skills, he or she might take on an additional patient or two (at minimum) to follow through the ambulatory care experience. In multicultural communities, students should acquire patients from various cultures so that experiences can be compared and contrasted.

Residents should acquire patients whom they can follow as part of their continuity experience throughout their training. In addition, they should follow inpatients during acute episodes. Again, cross-cultural comparisons are very important.

Seminars and case presentations led by experienced faculty should be offered to broaden the clinical experience. They should cover the topics required for knowledge acquisition, the clarification of learners' attitudes and beliefs, and the acquisition of skills required to deliver care competently. These activities can be supplemented with videotapes, interactive computer exercises, and the presentation of standardized cases. These activities are particularly important in areas where learners might be less likely to have frequent clinical experiences with patients from other cultures.

Evaluation should cover knowledge, attitudes, and skills and be linked to the instructional objectives. Paper-and-pencil tests of cognitive knowledge should be supplemented by direct observation of learners' taking care of patients or the use of simulated patients. Participation in discussions and expressions of thoughts and feelings can be part of the evaluation. The following set of objectives on domestic violence and their evaluation mechanism will illustrate the process.

At the end of the module, the learner will be able to do the following:

1. State the prevalence of domestic violence in the reference population.
2. Describe the most frequent methods of assault and resulting patterns of injury.
3. Recognize the constellation of symptoms and behaviors that should alert a clinician to include domestic violence in the differential diagnosis.
4. Isolate the patient from her spouse or any other family members who may accompany her.
5. In a nonjudgmental manner, elicit a thorough history, including a social and sexual history, with competence and sensitivity to the patient's cultural boundaries.
6. Explain the physical examination and any necessary laboratory procedures to the patient, and ascertain that she understands their purpose.
7. Perform the examination competently.
8. Counsel the patient about reporting requirements, if any, and

her right to protection, including asylum, and available community resources (such as safe houses or shelters).
9. Initiate and complete a social service referral.

In meeting these objectives, the learner will demonstrate a nonjudgmental attitude and the ability to confront and effectively manage his or her own feelings, attitudes, and beliefs about the subject matter, and the situation at hand.

# Chapter Twenty

# Cultural Competence Assessment of Practices, Clinics, and Health Care Facilities

*Dennis P. Andrulis*

Organizations that apply self-assessment tools have the opportunity to assess their cultural competence status, measure their progress, and compare themselves with other organizations. And yet, to date, attention to cultural competence has tended to focus more narrowly on limited areas within organizations, perhaps in reaction to a situation that arises or from a sense of a need to do something. For example, a number of institutions have developed training in which staff attend sessions—so-called workforce diversity training. These sessions may focus on respect for the individual, on how individual characteristics affect interactions and behavior, and on how to recognize one's own cultural assumptions. Similarly, addressing interpretation issues between providers and patients has garnered significant attention. In other situations, a single individual or program has been successful in developing special services or opening a clinic in an area where an ethnic or cultural community resides. These types of activities, however, may function successfully at only a very limited level, if at all, for two major reasons: they tend to work in isolation, divorced from any overall active administration incorporation and commitment, and they operate without a broader context that takes into account and involves ethnic and cultural perspectives within both the organization and the community. In both cases, there is a failure to recognize how these perspectives create and influence cultural norms, mores, and behavior within the organization. Instead, the health care organization must recognize the interdependence of community, management, employees, and patients and integrate these perspectives to be effective in caring for diverse populations.

The National Public Health and Hospital Institute, in conjunction with Beth Israel Hospital, Boston, and Harvard Medical School have undertaken an initiative to develop a design by which health care systems can assess the effectiveness of their efforts to address the health care needs of ethnically and culturally diverse communities. A team consisting of health care professionals, specialists in cultural issues, human resource experts, and researchers created and reviewed existing information and developed a site visit instrument. After discussions with health care professionals, the team selected hospital systems in six cities to review the instrument content and protocol.

## Objectives of the Assessment

This paper-and-pencil self-assessment tool is intended to do the following:

- Assist in determining provider knowledge and effectiveness in meeting patients' health care needs.
- Document the characteristics of provider relationships with their patients and their communities.
- Assess workforce, administration, and management roles and the status of efforts regarding cultural diversity.
- Assist in reviewing the current status of an organization's diversity activities.
- Document positive actions currently under way within the settings.
- Identify areas for improvement within the organization.
- Provide a framework for measuring progress in achieving desired process and outcome objectives.

This protocol is designed around the four cornerstones of cultural diversity in health care: the organization's relationship with its community, policies and actions of administration and management as they affect staff, intrastaff experience at all levels of the workforce, and the patient-provider relationship. The assessment tool can assist health care organizations in determining where they fall on a continuum of cultural competence. This continuum, or spectrum of cultural competence, is a five-point scale that identifies progressively more advanced levels of cultural activities and initiatives within that organization. The scale is a continuous representation of activities and involvement in cultural diversity.

## Stage Zero: Inaction

At this stage, an organization has undertaken little activity in the area of cultural diversity. There may be a nascent recognition or an understanding by individuals at any number of levels throughout the organization that it is an important issue, but there is no cohesive plan or consistent activity that addresses cultural competence. Rather, there is a randomness or undirected level of activity.

## Stage One: Symbolic Action and Initial Organization

Health care systems at this stage most likely have taken some action to recognize diversity within their staffs and their patient populations. Often there is a growing belief among staff that this issue is important and needs to be addressed. Actions to date, however, tend to have been relatively minor and symbolic in their expression. For example, organizations may choose to feature certain ethnic foods in their cafeterias, or they may organize internally to offer cultural diversity days to celebrate the ethnicity of their staff or the race and ethnic composition of their community. More frequently, these activities do not extend far beyond this symbolic level of recognition. Moreover, the staff's interests, from administration on down, although evident in terms of the importance of cultural competence, is not likely to extend much further than informal discussions and unorganized actions. Nonetheless, there tends to be a general understanding that this is an issue that needs to be addressed within the health care system.

## Stage Two: Formalized Internal Action

Stage Two organizations have consciously recognized the need to undertake cultural competence training to address diversity, especially as it relates internally to their health care settings. Often this need for recognition may have occurred as a result of a reaction to something in the environment (for example, a grievance, complaint, or lawsuit that is racially or ethnically motivated). This complaint leads an organization to concentrate resources and efforts on workforce diversity training. Staff at a number of levels will be either required or strongly encouraged to attend diversity training sessions. In contrast, the external activities related to the community and patient populations may still be relatively minimal. There may be actions that proceed beyond the Stage One level, such as encouraging certain initiatives to address a population's needs. However, in general, these external or patient-related activities remain fairly unformed. The general belief among administration and staff is that there is a strong need for the organization to look at cultural diversity and consider its current status. However, energies are devoted primarily to getting their own house in order.

## Stage Three: Patient and Staff Cultural Diversity Initiatives

During this stage, organizations have developed a more advanced commitment to cultural competence and may have taken a series of formal initiatives internally and externally. The internal activities may involve workforce diversity training, mentoring, recruitment, hiring, or other promotion activities. Externally, there may be a number of efforts to create a more effective approach to improving the health care of certain groups, such as targeted interventions, more formalized interpretation and translation services, and direct efforts to meet with community members. At the administration and staff levels, there may be a growing recognition of the importance of diversity and cultural competence and a sense that resources of time and effort should be devoted to it. However, full integration and measurement of cultural diversity and cultural competence within the organization tend to be missing.

## Stage Four: The Culturally Diverse Learning Organization

The health care organization that has reached Stage Four has taken cultural diversity and the objectives of cultural competence into the fabric of the organization. Issues of culture perfuse the way in which business is conducted in the organization. Cultural diversity no longer stands out but is part of the day-to-day life of the organization.

This integrated approach is manifest in the way that the community is brought into the decision-making process, the linkage of any kinds of internal diversity training and education programs to the health care objectives of the organization in relation to a culturally diverse population, and in monitoring and measurement of the effectiveness of any initiatives. Thus, for example, any training of staff and diversity issues that occurs may very well be accompanied by a pre- and postassessment of the effects and value of such training relative not only to attitudes but to improvement on the job in terms of addressing the needs of the population of concern. Ultimately, an effective organization at this level considers the impact of its initiatives on processes and outcomes of care related to the target populations.

## Potential Implications of the Cultural Competence Protocol

The cultural competence protocol must be seen in a broader context of community need, patient priorities, workforce concerns, and mission—both corporate and altruistic—of the organization itself. To that end, it is intended to integrate these important perspectives and the related objectives into a full review that benefits both the business objectives and the service and community objectives. The cultural competence protocol should provide an opportunity for organizations to understand and learn about their activities and their directions. To that end, it should work to achieve the following six objectives:

1. Provide an audit of the organization's diversity initiatives.
2. Measure the impact of the initiative on diversity throughout the organization.

3. Identify diversity strengths in areas requiring more attention.
4. Provide a framework for comparing diversity progress with other organizations.
5. Serve as an educational or informational tool and process for involving students, community representatives, board members, health care staff, other staff, and administration in improving and understanding diversity.
6. Provide a framework for developing diversity guidelines for health care organizations.

# Epilogue

*Elizabeth Kramer,*
*Susan L. Ivey, and*
*Yu-Wen Ying*

Immigrant health care and even immigrant women's health care is far too broad a topic to cover in a single book. We have barely scratched the surface here. Many fine programs could not be included, and for every one that is mentioned, there are at least a dozen, and probably more, that we have missed. A few of these are especially worthy of note.

The *New York Task Force on Immigrant Health* is a network of health care providers, social scientists, and community advocates who provide public health programs, technical assistance, conferences, and training services to immigrant and refugee communities in New York City. Its activities include a community tuberculosis prevention program, which addresses gaps in tuberculosis control in recent immigrant populations; development of a blueprint for interpreter services in New York based on a model analysis of interpreter programs in other parts of the country; development and implementation of a training course in medical interpreting; and partnerships with immigrant community–based organizations on public health concerns such as antitobacco and injury prevention. The task force, which is housed at the New York University School of Medicine, also sponsors national and regional symposia and provides technical assistance on immigrant health to several New York health care facilities.

*Opening Doors: Reducing Sociocultural Barriers to Health Care* is a nationwide grant initiative sponsored by the Robert Wood Johnson Foundation and the Henry J. Kaiser Family Foundation. Established in 1993, the program supports and encourages efforts to reduce social and cultural barriers to health care, particularly in maternal, child, and reproductive health services. Opening Doors has funded twenty-three projects, many of which serve immigrants and refugees, in eleven states, and has made significant inroads into the complex and multifaceted issues of sociocultural barriers to health care. The program has expanded the knowledge base of strategies being used in community and hospital settings to reduce these barriers and increased the capacity of individuals to incorporate these issues into their day-to-day work. More important, there is a greater awareness of the issues, a significant first step in addressing them.

In Seattle, the University of Washington Health Services Library has teamed up with Harborview Medical Center's Community House Calls program, an Opening Doors grantee, to create EthnoMed *(http://www.hslib.washington.edu/clinical/ethnomed)*, an electronic database that offers providers direct access to information on culture, language, health, illness, and community resources. EthnoMed currently contains information relating to the culture, language, health beliefs, and family structure of the Amharic, Cambodian, Eritrean, Oromo, Somali, Tigreinian, and Vietnamese ethnic groups. The information was collected with the help of community members through the Community House Calls program, which serves these groups in their homes.

Finally, *Shasta Community Health Center* in rural Redding, California, has initiated a relationship with a local shaman, the spiritual leader for the local Southeast Asian immigrant community, which is composed primarily of Laotians.

In this book, one of our acknowledged shortcomings is the failure to have addressed the issue of program evaluation. Over the years, there have been many innovative experiments in the delivery of immigrant health care, most of them operated solely as health services delivery programs, often on shoestring budgets that do not include funding for rigorous scientific evaluation of the programs. The time is long overdue for systematic evaluation of who uses each program, why, for how long, at what cost, and at what benefit.

The many minority groups that comprise the American population are fast becoming the majority, and the United States has indeed moved beyond the melting pot. The Census Bureau projects that in 2000, 71.8 percent of the U.S. population will be non-Hispanic white, 12.2 percent African American, 11.4 percent Hispanics of all races, and 3.9 percent APIs. By 2030, the respective proportions will be 60.5 percent white, 13.1 percent black, 18.9 percent Hispanic, and 6.6 percent API; and by 2050, non-Hispanic whites will comprise only 52.8 percent of the population, while African Americans will be 13.6 percent, Hispanics will make up 24.5 percent, and APIs, the fastest growing group, will comprise 8.2 percent. There is a pressing need to develop cultural competence in health care workers so that they can deliver optimal care to all patients regardless of language, race, creed, or country of origin. This training must include the unique needs of immigrant women as patients, caregivers, and health care decision makers for their families.

A key element in training culturally competent providers is recognition that the separation of body and mind is unique to Western medicine. In Africa, Asia, and Latin America, where large numbers of immigrants and refugees originate, physical health is inseparable from mental health and spiritual well-being. Therefore, culturally competent service providers need to consider nonorganically based contributions to their patients' symptoms. Although it may be unrealistic for health care providers to be knowledgeable about all possible explanatory models, they must learn how to inquire about how their patients understand the source of their disease and the remedies they prefer. When treating patients from non-Western cultures, culturally competent providers should learn to feel comfortable consulting with non-medical indigenous healers.

Managed care has made medical care be more and more protocol driven. The Agency for Health Care Policy and Research and a number of medical specialty societies and academic researchers have been focusing their efforts on the development of practice guidelines. Further, evidence-based medicine, which is predicated on epidemiology, is contributing more and more to clinicians' decision making. As biomedical science has advanced, we have learned that there are biological differences among groups that must be taken into account when treating patients. The dearth of data on the demographic variables, distribution of diseases, responses to treatment, acculturation variables, and cultural uniqueness of immigrants must be redressed if we are to provide high-quality, compassionate care and optimal health and disease information to the newest Americans. It is imperative that we address these issues.

Hospitals and health care facilities should be able and willing to collect data on country of origin and length of residence in the United States and should reassure patients that this information is being collected for statistical purposes only. The census that will be conducted in 2000 presents a unique window of opportunity for collecting data on country of origin and length of residence in the United States, as well as educational attainment, employment status, and language spoken in the home. Subsamples of specific ethnic groups are needed in order to calculate the prevalence of certain diseases within given populations and conduct small area analyses of the impact of environmental factors on health. It would be ideal to break out data by the legality of immigration status, but in the current political climate this probably is an unattainable goal.

Health care organizations are resistant to change, and medical organizations and providers have their own cultures. Although provider-patient relationships have become more collegial, immigrant patients may not always receive the same standard of consideration and care. Health care providers must recognize the need to be humble about the fact that all patients come to the health care encounter with their own cultural frameworks. By understanding a patient's culture, we will attain better health outcomes, better adherence, and a more satisfied patient, and we will gain a new sense of empowerment in caring for immigrant women.

It also is important that health care organizations employ bicultural and bilingual personnel as translators, culture brokers, and clinical providers and that health professions schools open their doors to the growing numbers of individuals from increasingly diverse backgrounds. This will help us to achieve the goal of a workforce that is more reflective of the general population, while gaining workers with language skills and bicultural frameworks.

Despite a need to decide on border policies, it is possible to have a rational immigrant policy without racism, ethnic bashing, and anti-immigrant sentiments. Migrant workers constitute a unique category of foreign-born individuals who regularly enter the United States, whether legally or illegally, to work here. In most cases, their employers do not provide health benefits for them, although they are working and paying their own way.

The 1996 welfare and immigration reforms displayed little concern for the people who immigrate for reasons of severe economic deprivation in their own countries, focusing instead on specific groups who seek asylum for political reasons. The goals of immigration policy reform (such as border control and allocation of temporary work visas for seasonal farmworkers) should be separate from U.S. immigrant policy (provision of health care, housing, and food benefits for workers and their families). This is the case in many countries that have universal or near-universal health care coverage. Immigration to the United States is at the highest level since the early part of the century (U.S. Bureau of the Census, 1993), and it is unlikely that the number of new immigrants who require medical care will shrink in the near future.

Rational allocation of resources for preventive and safety net services ultimately protects all Americans. Current federal health policy continues to favor acute care over preventive care, short-term savings over possible longer-term benefits of better overall societal health, and concealed subsidies for uncompensated medical care (using disproportionate share payments to hospitals) and cost shifting rather than more explicit federal programs that fund basic preventive care and early detection and treatment.

The 105th Congress has made multiple efforts to repeal the most onerous results of the 1996 Welfare and Immigration Reforms. Specific attempts include efforts to protect legal immigrant children under the new Children's Health Initiative Program (CHIP); to restore Supplemental Security Insurance (SSI) to those over sixty-five, the blind and disabled, and those with no other means of support who had been receiving benefits; and to protect immigrant women who are victims of domestic violence. In addition, attempts were made to ensure that funds would be available for states and localities that incur costs related to the delivery of emergency services to immigrants.

As of September 1, 1998, all of these bills are currently in committee. In the interim, President Clinton has issued executive orders mandating the restoration of food stamps and Supplemental Security benefits to those who otherwise would have been eligible.

It is too soon to get a real sense of what the states will do for immigrants as a result of the 1996 federal legislation. There are no federal penalties for those that choose to provide benefits to legal immigrants, and some states (for example, New York, Massachusetts, and Florida) are continuing to provide services. It seems absurd to us to deny prenatal care to pregnant immigrants whose children will be born U.S. citizens and who will perhaps start their lives with low birth weights and neonatal intensive care unit costs averaging between $31,000 and $71,000 per incident, when the average national cost for professional services associated with prenatal care is approximately $400 per pregnancy (Flowers-Bowie, 1997).

We believe that federal policy should ensure access to a minimum benefit package of primary care and preventive services, including prenatal care and delivery, immunizations, treatment of communicable diseases, and at least a minimum set of mental health services without fear of reprisal, for all individuals on American soil regardless of their country of origin. This inequity must be addressed by fair allocation of funds to states for strong public health infrastructures, which include the direct delivery of services as well as disease surveillance and enforcement of public health and safety laws.

# References

Abbey, S. E., and Garfinkel, P. E. "Neurasthenia and Chronic Fatigue Syndrome: The Role of Culture in the Making of a Diagnosis." *American Journal of Psychiatry,* 1991, *48*(12), 1638–1646.

Abbott, J., and others. "Domestic Violence Against Women: Incidence and Prevalence in an Emergency Department Population." *Journal of the American Medical Association,* 1995, *273,* 1763–1767.

Abraham, M. "Ethnicity, Gender, and Marital Violence: South Asian Women's Organizations in the United States." *Gender and Society,* 1995, *9*(4), 450–468.

Abueg, F. R., and Chun, K. M. "Traumatized Asian and Asian American Populations." In A. Marsella, M. Friedman, E. Gerrity, and R. Scurfield (eds.), *Ethnocultural Approaches to Understanding Post-Traumatic Stress Disorder: Issues, Research, and Clinical Applications.* Washington, D.C.: American Psychological Association, 1996.

Accreditation Council for Graduate Medical Education. *Graduate Medical Education Directory, 1998–99.* Chicago: APIA, 1998.

Acierno, R., Resnick, H., and Kilpatrick, D. "Health Impact of Interpersonal Violence 1: Prevalence Rates, Case Identification, and Risk Factors for Sexual Assault, Physical Assault, and Domestic Violence in Men and Women." *Behavioral Medicine,* 1997, *23,* 53–64.

Ackerman, L. K. "Health Problems of Refugees." *Journal of the American Board of Family Practice,* 1997, *10*(5), 337–348.

Acosta, F., Yamamoto, J., and Evans, L. *Effective Psychotherapy for Low-Income and Minority Patients.* New York: Plenum Press, 1982.

Acosta, F., Yamamoto, J., Evans, L., and Skilbeck, W. "Preparing Low-Income Hispanic, Black, and White Patients for Psychotherapy: Evaluation of a New Orientation Program." *Journal of Clinical Psychology,* 1983, *39*(6), 872–877.

Adams, C. *Nutritive Value of American Foods in Common Units.* Agriculture Handbook no. 465. Washington, D.C.: U.S. Department of Agriculture, Agriculture Research Service, 1975.

Aday, L., and Andersen, R. "Equity of Access to Medical Care: A Conceptual and Empirical Overview." *Medical Care,* 1981, *19*(12), 4–27.

344 REFERENCES

Adler, P., Ovando, C., and Hocevar, D. "Familiar Correlates of Gang Membership: An Exploratory Study." *Hispanic Journal of Behavioral Sciences,* 1984, *6,* 65–76.

Adrien, A., and others. "Many Voices: HIV/AIDS in the Context of Culture—A National Study." Paper presented at the International Conference on AIDS in Yokohama, Japan. Abstract in the conference syllabus, 1996, *11,* 172 (abstract no. MO-D-1690).

Advisory Committee on Immunization Practices. *American Academy of Family Physicians Bulletin.* Kansas City: American Association of Family Physicians, 1998.

Africa Watch Women's Rights Project. *Seeking Refuge, Finding Terror: The Widespread Rape of Somali Women Refugees in North Eastern Kenya.* New York: Human Rights Watch, 1993.

Agger, I. *The Blue Room.* London, N.J.: Zed Books, 1992.

Agger, I., and Jensen, S. B. "Testimony as Ritual and Evidence in Psychotherapy for Political Refugees." *Journal of Traumatic Stress,* 1990, *3*(1), 115–130.

Ahern, M., and McCoy, H. V. "Emergency Department Admissions: Changes During the Financial Tightening of the 1980s." *Inquiry,* 1992, *29*(Spring), 67–79.

Ahluwallia, K., and Gupta, R. *Circle of Light.* New York: HarperCollins, 1997.

Aitchison, R. "Reluctant Witnesses: The Sexual Abuse of Refugee Women in Djibouti." *Cultural Survival Quarterly,* 1984, *8*(2), 26–27.

Akutsu, P., Snowden, L., and Organista, K. "Referral Patterns in Ethnic-Specific and Mainstream Programs for Ethnic Minorities and Whites." *Journal of Counseling Psychology,* 1996, *43*(1), 56–64.

Aldwin, C., and Greenberger, E. "Cultural Differences in the Predictors of Depression." *American Journal of Community Psychology,* 1987, *15*(6), 789–813.

Almstrom, B. "Immigrants Receive Information About HIV/AIDS in Their Mother Tongue." Paper presented at the International Conference on AIDS in Berlin, Germany. Abstract in the conference syllabus, 1993, *9,* 813 (abstract no. PO-DO5–3570).

Amaro, H. "Women in the Mexican-American Community: Religion, Culture, and Reproductive Attitudes and Experiences." *Journal of Community Psychology,* 1988, *16,* 6–20.

Amaro, H., Russo, N., and Johnson, J. "Hispanic Women and Mental Health." *Psychology of Women Quarterly,* 1987, *11,* 393–407.

American College of Emergency Physicians. *Policy Statement on Emergency Medicine and Domestic Violence.* Dallas: American College of Emergency Physicians, Sept. 1994.

American College of Emergency Physicians. *Policy Statement on Mandatory Reporting of Domestic Violence to Law Enforcement and Criminal Justice Agencies.* Dallas: American College of Emergency Physicians, 1995.

American Medical Association. *Diagnostic and Treatment Guidelines on Mental Health Effects of Family Violence.* Chicago: American Medical Association, 1992a.

American Medical Association. Council on Ethical and Judicial Affairs. "Physicians and Domestic Violence: Ethical Considerations." *Journal of the American Medical Association,* 1992b, *267*(23), 3190–3193.

American Medical Association. Council on Scientific Affairs. "Violence Against Women: Relevance for Medical Practitioners." *Journal of the American Medical Association,* 1992c, *267*(23), 3184–3189.

American Medical Women's Association. *AMWA CHD in Women Curriculum.* Alexandria, Va.: American Medical Women's Association, 1996.

American Psychiatric Association. *Diagnostic Statistical Manual of Mental Disorders.* (2nd ed.) Washington, D.C.: American Psychiatric Association, 1968.

American Psychiatric Association. *Diagnostic and Statistical Manual of Mental Disorders.* (3rd ed.) Washington, D.C.: American Psychiatric Association, 1980.

American Psychiatric Association. *Diagnostic and Statistical Manual of Mental Disorders.* (4th ed.) Washington, D.C.: American Psychiatric Association, 1994.

American Thoracic Society/Centers for Disease Control. Consensus statement. "Treatment of Tuberculosis and Tuberculosis Infection in Adults and Children." *American Journal of Respiratory Critical Care Medicine,* 1994, *149,* 1359–1374.

Amering, M., and Katschnig, H. "Panic Attacks and Panic Disorder in Cross-Cultural Perspective." *Psychiatric Annals,* 1990, *20*(9), 511–516.

Andersen, R., Kochanek, K., and Murphy, S. "Report of Final Mortality Statistics, 1995." *Monthly Vital Statistics Report, 45*(11, suppl. 2), 1997.

Andersen, R., and others. "Exploring Dimensions of Access to Medical Care." *Health Services Research,* 1983, *18*(1), 49–74.

Anderson, J., and others. "Living with Chronic Illness: Chinese Canadian and Euro-Canadian Women with Diabetes—Exploring Factors That Influence Management." *Social Science and Medicine,* 1995, *41,* 181–195.

Andrulis, D. "The Public Sector in the Emerging Health Care Environment: Evolution or Dissolution?" A report for the Robert Wood Johnson Foundation conference called "What is Happening to the Safety Net?" Washington, D.C., Jan. 9–10, 1997.

Angel, R., and Guarnaccia, P. J. "Mind, Body, and Culture: Somatization Among Hispanics." *Social Science and Medicine,* 1989, *28,* 1229–1238.

Antonovsky, A. *Health, Stress, and Coping.* San Francisco: Jossey-Bass, 1979.

Appleby, J. "A Hospital in Martinez to Shut Down and a State Reviews Two Deaths After Transfer from Kaiser Center." *Oakland Tribune,* Mar. 14, 1997, p. 1A.

Applewhite, S. L. "Curanderismo: Demystifying the Health Beliefs and Practices of Elderly Mexican Americans." *Health & Social Work,* 1995, *20*(4), 247–253.

Aronow, W. S. "Prevalence of Atherothrombotic Brain Infarction, Coronary Artery Disease and Peripheral Arterial Disease in Elderly Blacks, Hispanics, and Whites." *American Journal of Cardiology,* 1992, *70,* 1212–1213.

Aronson, L. "Traditional Cambodian Health Beliefs and Practices." *Rhode Island Medical Journal,* 1983, *70,* 73–78.

Asch, S., Leake, B., and Gelberg, L. "Does Fear of Immigration Authorities Deter Tuberculosis Patients from Seeking Care?" *Western Journal of Medicine,* 1994, *161,* 373–376.

Association of State and Territorial Health Officials. *ASTHO Bilingual Health Initiative, Report and Recommendations: State Health Agency Strategies to Develop Linguistically Relevant Public Health Systems.* Washington, D.C.: Association of State and Territorial Health Officials, 1992.

Atkinson, D. R., Morten, G., and Sue, D. W. (eds.). *Counseling American Minorities: A Cross-Cultural Perspective.* (3rd ed.) Dubuque, Iowa: W. C. Brown, 1989.

Austin, J. E. "The Perilous Journey of Nutritional Evaluation." *American Journal of Clinical Nutrition,* 1978, *72*(5), 497–501.

Bachman, R., and Saltzman, L. E. *Violence Against Women: Estimates from the Redesigned Survey.* U.S. Department of Justice Special Report, NCJ–154348. Washington, D.C.: U.S. Government Printing Office, 1994.

Badger, L. W., and others. "Patient Presentation, Interview Content, and the Detection of Depression by Primary Care Physicians." *Psychosomatic Medicine,* 1994, *56,* 128–135.

Bagley, C. "Mental Health and Social Adjustment of Elderly Chinese Immigrants in Canada." *Canada's Mental Health,* 1993, *41*(3), 6–10.

Bailey, R. L., Arullendran, P., Whittle, H. C., Mabey, D.C.W. "Randomised Controlled Trial of Single-Dose Azithromycin in Treatment of Trachoma." *Lancet,* 1993, *342,* 453–456.

Baker, D., Stevens, C., and Brook, R. "Regular Source of Ambulatory Care and Medical Care Utilization by Patients Presenting to a Public Hospital Emergency Department." *Journal of the American Medical Association*, 1994, *271*(24), 1909–1912.

Baker, D., Stevens, C., and Brook, R. "Determinants of Emergency Department Use: Are Race and Ethnicity Important?" *Annals of Emergency Medicine*, 1996, *28*(6), 677–682.

Bakris, G., and White, D. "Effects of an ACE Inhibitor Combined with a Calcium Channel Blocker on Progression of Diabetic Nephropathy." *Journal of Human Hypertension*, 1997, *11*, 35–38.

Bamford, K. "Bilingual Issues in Mental Health Assessment and Treatment." *Latino Journal of Behavioral Sciences*, 1991, *13*, 377–390.

Bandura, A. "Exercise of Personal and Collective Efficacy in Changing Societies." In A. Bandura (ed.), *Self-Efficacy in Changing Societies* (pp. 1–45). New York: Cambridge University Press, 1995.

Barker, J. "Cross-Cultural Medicine: A Decade Later." *Western Journal of Medicine*, 1992, *157*, 248–374.

Barnett, O., and Fagan, R. "Alcohol Use in Male Spouse Abusers and Their Female Partners." *Journal of Family Violence*, 1993, *8*(1), 1–25.

Barsky, A. J., Geringer, E., and Wool, C. A. "A Cognitive-Educational Treatment for Hypochondriasis." *General Hospital Psychiatry*, 1988, *10*, 322–327.

Baughan, D. M., and others. "Primary Care Needs of Cambodian Refugees." *Journal of Family Practice*, 1990, *30*(5), 565–568.

Beard, G. M. *American Nervousness.* New York: Putnam's, 1869.

Beard, G. M. *A Practical Treatise on Nervous Exhaustion (Neurasthenia): Its Symptoms, Nature, Sequences, Treatment.* (2nd ed.) New York: William Wood and Company, 1880.

Becerra, J., Hogue, C., Atrash, K., and Perez, N. "Infant Mortality Among Hispanics." *Journal of the American Medical Asociation*, 1991, *265*(2), 217–221.

Becerra, R. M., and Iglehart, A. P. "Folk Medicine Use: Diverse Populations in a Metropolitan Area." *Social Work in Health Care*, 1995, *21*(4), 37–51.

Beiser, M. "Mental Health of Refugees in Resettlement Countries." In W. H. Holtzman and T. H. Bornemann (eds.), *Mental Health of Immigrants and Refugees.* Austin, Tex.: Hogg Foundation for Mental Health, 1990.

Bemak, F., Chung, R. C-Y., and Bornemann, T. H. "Counseling and Psychotherapy with Refugees." In P. B. Pedersen, J. G. Draguns, W. J. Lonner, and J. E. Trimble (eds.), *Counseling Across Cultures* (pp. 243–265). Thousand Oaks, Calif.: Sage, 1996.

Ben-Porath, E., and others. "Hepatitis B Virus Infection and Liver Disease in Ethiopian Immigrants to Israel." *Hepatology,* 1986, *6,* 662–666.

Ben-Porath, Y. S. "The Psycho-Social Adjustment." In J. Westermeyer, C. L. Williams, and A. N. Nguyen (eds.), *Mental Health Services for Refugees* (pp. 1–23). DHHS Publication No. ADM 91–1824. Washington, D.C.: U.S. Government Printing Office, 1991.

Bentwich, Z., and others. "TH2 Activation and Pathogenesis of African AIDS." Paper presented at the International Conference on AIDS in Berlin, Germany. Abstract in the conference syllabus, 1993, *9,* 200 (abstract no. PO-A19-0392).

Berger, L. "When Custom Looks Like Abuse." *Los Angeles Times,* Aug. 24, 1994.

Berk, M., Albers, L., and Schur, C. "The Growth in the U.S. Uninsured Population: Trends in Hispanic Sub-Groups: 1977–1992." *American Journal of Public Health,* 1996, *86*(4), 572–576.

Berlin, E. A., and Fowkes, E. G. "A Teaching Framework for Cross-Cultural Health Care: Application in Family Practice." *Western Journal of Medicine,* Dec. 1983, *139,* 934–938.

Berry, J. W., Kim, U., and Boski, P. "Psychological Acculturation of Immigrants." In Y. Y. Kim and W. B. Gudykunst (eds.), *Cross-Cultural Adaptation: Current Approaches* (pp. 62–89). Thousand Oaks, Calif.: Sage, 1987.

Berry, J. W., Kim, U., Minde, T., and Mok, D. "Comparative Studies of Acculturative Stress." *International Migration Review,* 1987, *21,* 491–511.

Berry, J. W., Poortinga, Y. H., Segall, M. H., and Dasen, P. R. *Cross-Cultural Psychology: Research and Applications.* New York: Cambridge University Press, 1992.

Bindman, A., and others. "Preventable Hospitalizations and Access to Health Care." *Journal of the American Medical Association,* 1995, *274*(4), 305–311.

Bindman, A., and others. "Primary Care and Receipt of Preventive Services." *Journal of General Internal Medicine,* 1996, *11*(5), 269–276.

Binkin, N. J., and others. "Overseas Screening for Tuberculosis in Immigrants and Refugees to the United States: Current Status." *Clinical Infectious Diseases,* 1996, *23,* 1226–1232.

Bird, J. A., Otero-Sabogal, R., Ha, N-T., and McPhee, S. J. "Tailoring Lay Health Worker Interventions for Diverse Cultures: Lessons Learned from Vietnamese and Latina Communities." *Health Education Quarterly,* 1996, *23,* S105–S122.

Block, G., Coyle, L., Smucker, R., and Harlan, L. C. "Health Habits and History Questionnaire, Diet History and Other Risk Factors," Personal Computer System Documentation. Bethesda, Md.: National Cancer Institute, 1995.

Bogen, E. *Immigration in New York.* New York: Praeger, 1987.

Boyd, M. "Family and Personal Networks in International Migration: Recent Developments and New Agendas." *International Migration Review,* 1989, *23*(3), 638–670.

Boyd-Franklin, N., and Garcia-Preto, N. "Family Therapy: A Closer Look at African American and Hispanic Women." In L. Comas-Diaz and B. Greene (eds.), *Women of Color: Integrating Ethnic and Gender Identities in Psychotherapy* (pp. 239–264). New York: Guilford Press, 1994.

Bradshaw, C. K. "Asian and Asian American Women: Historical and Political Considerations in Psychotherapy." In L. Comas-Diaz and B. Greene (eds.), *Women of Color: Integrating Ethnic and Gender Identities in Psychotherapy* (pp. 72–113). New York: Guilford Press, 1994.

Breslau, N. "Stressors: Continuous and Discontinuous." *Journal of Applied Social Psychology,* 1990, *20*(2), 1666–1673.

Breslau, N., Davis, G. C., Andreski, P., and Peterson, E. "Traumatic Events and Posttraumatic Stress Disorder in an Urban Population of Young Adults." *Archives of General Psychiatry,* 1991, *48*(3), 216–222.

Bridges, K. W., and Goldberg, D. P. "Somatic Presentation of DSM III Disorders in Primary Care." *Journal of Psychosomatic Research,* 1985, *29*, 563–569.

Browne, A. "Violence Against Women by Male Partners: Prevalence, Outcomes, and Policy Implications." *American Psychologist,* 1993, *48*, 1077–1087.

Browne, A., and Bassuk, S. "Intimate Violence in the Lives of Homeless and Poor Housed Women: Prevalence and Patterns in an Ethnically Diverse Sample." *American Journal of Orthopsychiatry,* 1997, *67*(2), 261–278.

Brownmiller, S. *Against Our Will: Men, Women, and Rape.* New York: Simon & Schuster, 1975.

Brownmiller, S. "Making Female Bodies the Battlefield." In A. Stiglmayer (ed.), *Mass Rape: The War Against Women in Bosnia-Herzegovina.* Lincoln: University of Nebraska Press, 1994.

Burdman, P. "Parents Blame Prop. 187 Fear in Son's Death." *San Francisco Chronicle,* Nov. 24, 1994a.

Burdman, P. "Woman Who Feared Prop. 187 Deportation Dies at SF General." *San Francisco Chronicle,* Nov. 26, 1994b.

Bureau of Primary Health Care. "Data on Federally Qualified Health Centers." [http://www.bphc.hrsa.dhhs.gov]. May 1998.

Burk, M., Wieser, P., and Keegan, L. "Cultural Beliefs and Health Behaviors of Pregnant Mexican-American Women: Implications for Primary Care." *Advances in Nursing Science,* 1995, *17*(4), 37–52.

Burt, V. L., and others. "Prevalence of Hypertension in the U.S. Adult Population: Results from the Third National Health and Nutrition Examination Survey, 1988–1991." *Hypertension,* 1995, *25,* 305–331.

California. *Economic Report of the Governor, 1991.* Sacramento: Office of the Governor, 1991.

California. *California Ballot Pamphlet: General Election.* Sacramento: Secretary of State, Nov. 8, 1994.

California. *Economic Report of the Governor, 1997.* Sacramento: Office of the Governor, 1997.

California Association of Public Hospitals and Health Systems. "Medi-Cal SB 855 DSH Payment Adjustment." Memorandum. Summer 1996.

Campbell, J. C., and Campbell, D. W. "Cultural Competence in the Care of Abused Women." *Journal of Nurse-Midwifery,* 1996, *41*(6), 457–462.

Campis, L. K., Lyman, R. D., and Prentice-Dunn, S. "The Parental Locus of Control Scale: Development and Validation." *Journal of Clinical Child Psychology,* 1986, *15*(3), 260–267.

Camus-Jacques, G. "Refugee Women: The Forgotten Majority." In Loescher and Monahan (eds.), *Refugees and International Relations.* New York: Oxford University Press, 1989.

Canda, E. R., and Phaobtong, T. "Buddhism as a Support System for Southeast Asian Refugees." *Social Work,* 1992, *37*(1), 61–67.

Canino, G., and others. "Sex Differences and Depression in Puerto Rico." *Psychology of Women Quarterly,* 1987, *11,* 443–450.

Canino, I. A., and others. "Functional Somatic Symptoms: A Cross-Ethnic Comparison." *American Journal of Orthopsychiatry,* 1992, *62,* 605–612.

Canino, J. "The Hispanic Woman: Sociocultural Influences on Diagnosis and Treatment." In R. Bercero, M. Karno, and J. Escobar (eds.), *Mental Health and Hispanic Americans* (pp. 117–138). New York: Gruen, 1982.

Cannistra, L. B., and Balady, G. L. "Comparison of Outcome of Cardiac Rehabilitation in Black Women and White Women." *American Journal of Cardiology,* 1995, *75,* 890–893.

Cantwell, M. F., Snider, D. E., Jr., Cauthen, G. M., and Onorato, I. M. "Epidemiology of Tuberculosis in the United States, 1985 Through 1992." *Journal of the American Medical Association,* 1994, *272,* 535–539.

Carlson, E. B., and Rosser-Hogan, R. "Trauma Experiences, Post Traumatic Stress, Dissociation and Depression in Cambodian Refugees." *American Journal of Psychiatry,* 1991, *148,* 1548–1551.

Carpenter, C.C.J., and others. "Antiretroviral Therapy for HIV Infection in 1997." *Journal of the American Medical Association,* 1997, *277,* 1962–1969.

Carr, J. E., and Tan, E. K. "In Search of the True *Amok: Amok* as Viewed Within the Malay Culture." *American Journal of Psychiatry,* 1976, *133,* 1295–1299.

Cascardi, M., and O'Leary, K. D. "Depressive Symptomology, Self-Esteem and Self-Blame in Battered Women." *Journal of Family Violence,* 1992, *7,* 249–259.

Castel, J. R. "Rape, Sexual Assault, and the Meaning of Persecution." *International Journal of Refugee Law,* 1992, *4*(1), 39–56.

Castillo, R., Waitzkin, H., and Escobar, J. "Somatic Symptoms and Mental Health Disorders in Immigrant and Refugee Populations." In J. Miranda, A. A. Hohmann, C. C. Attkinsson, and D. B. Larson (eds.), *Mental Disorders in Primary Care.* San Francisco: Jossey-Bass, 1994.

Castro de Alvarez, V. "AIDS Prevention for Puerto Rican Women." *PR Health Science Journal,* 1990, *9,* 37–41.

Center for Family and Community Health. *1994 Korean American Community Health Survey: Alameda and Santa Clara Counties, CA.* Berkeley: University of California, 1997.

Centers for Disease Control. "Use of BCG Vaccines in the Control of Tuberculosis: A Joint Statement by the ACIP and the Advisory Committee for the Elimination of Tuberculosis." *Mortality and Morbidity Weekly Review,* 1988, *37,* 663–664, 669–675.

Centers for Disease Control. "Tuberculosis Among Foreign-Born Persons Entering the United States: Recommendations of the Advisory Committee for Elimination of Tuberculosis." *Morbidity and Mortality Weekly Report,* 1990a, *39*(RR–18), 1–21.

Centers for Disease Control. "The Use of Preventive Therapy for Tuberculous Infection in the United States: Recommendations of the Advisory Committee for Elimination of Tuberculosis." *Mortality and Morbidity Weekly Review,* 1990b, 39(RR–8), 9–12.

Centers for Disease Control. *Core Curriculum on Tuberculosis.* Washington, D.C.: U.S. Department of Health and Human Services, 1991.

Centers for Disease Control. "Behavioral Risk Factor Survey of Vietnamese-California, 1991." *Morbidity and Mortality Weekly Review,* 1992a, *41*(5), 69–72.

Centers for Disease Control. "Cigarette Smoking Among Southeast Asian Immigrants—Washington State, 1989." *Morbidity and Mortality Weekly Review,* 1992b, *41,* 854–861.

Centers for Disease Control. *Chronic Disease in Minority Populations: 1994.* Atlanta, Ga.: Centers for Disease Control, 1994a.

Centers for Disease Control. *Community Health Advisors: An Annotated Bibliography.* 2 vols. Atlanta, Ga.: U.S. Department of Health and Human Services, Sept. 1994b.

Centers for Disease Control. "Surveillance for Selected Tobacco-Use Behaviors—United States, 1900–1994." *Morbidity and Mortality Weekly Review,* 1994c, *43*(SS–3), 1–43.

Centers for Disease Control. *Health Information for International Travel.* Washington, D.C.: U.S. Department of Health and Human Services, 1996–1997.

Centers for Disease Control. "Demographic Characteristics of Persons Without a Regular Source of Medical Care—Selected States, 1995." *Mortality and Morbidity Weekly Review,* 1998a, *47*(14), 277–279.

Centers for Disease Control. "1998 Guidelines for Treatment of Sexually Transmitted Diseases." *Mortality and Morbidity Weekly Review,* 1998b, *47*(RR–1), 1–111.

Centers for Disease Control. *Prevention Research Centers: Investing in the Nation's Health at a Glance.* Atlanta, Ga.: Centers for Disease Control, 1998c.

Centers for Disease Control. "Immunization of Adolescents." *Journal of the American Medical Association,* 1997, *227,* 203–205.

Cervantes, R. C., Salgado de Snyder, V. N., and Padilla, A. M. "Posttraumatic Stress in Immigrants from Central America and Mexico." *Hospital and Community Psychiatry,* 1989, *40,* 615–619.

Chan, C. "Asian-American Women: Psychological Responses to Sexual Exploitation and Cultural Stereotypes." *Women and Therapy,* 1988, *6*(4), 33–38.

Chan, T. C., Krishel, S. J., Bramwell, K. J., and Clark, R. F. "Survey of Illegal Immigrants Seen in an Emergency Department." *Western Journal of Medicine,* 1996, *164*(3), 212–216.

Chavez, L., Cornelius, W., and Jones, O. "Mexican Immigrants and the Utilization of U.S. Health Services: The Case of San Diego." *Social Science and Medicine,* 1985, *21*(1), 93–102.

Chemtov, D., and Rosen, C. *Be "Gobez" for the Sake of Your Health.* Jerusalem: Multi-Agency Committee for Education and Information on HIV Infection and Related Diseases, 1992.

Chemtov, D., and Rosen, H. "Epidemiological and Cultural Factors in the Case of Hepatitis B Virus Infection Among Ethiopian Adolescents in Israel." *International Journal of Adolescent Medical Health,* 1993, *6,* 95–111.

Chen, A. M., and others. "Health Is Strength: A Research Collaboration Involving Korean Americans in Alameda County." *American Journal of Preventive Medicine,* 1997, *13*(2), 93–100.

Chen, M. S. "Cardiovascular Health Among Asian Americans/Pacific Islanders: An Examination of Health Status and Intervention Approaches." *American Journal of Health Promotion,* 1993, 7(3), 199–207.

Cheung, F. M. "Mental Health and Recreational Activities in a Chinese Commune." In R. P. Lee and S. K. Lau (eds.), *The People's Commune and Rural Development.* Hong Kong: Chinese University Press, 1981. [In Chinese]

Cheung, F. M. "Psychological Symptoms Among Chinese in Urban Hong Kong." *Social Science and Medicine,* 1982, *16,* 1339–1344.

Cheung, F. M. "Conceptualization of Psychiatric Illness and Help-Seeking Behavior Among Chinese." *Culture, Medicine, and Psychiatry,* 1987, *11*(1), 97–106.

Cheung, F. M. "The Indigenization of Neurasthenia in Hong Kong." *Culture, Medicine and Psychiatry,* 1989, *13,* 227–241.

Cheung, P. "Adult Psychiatric Epidemiology in China in the 80s." *Culture, Medicine and Psychiatry,* 1991, *15,* 479–496.

Chicago Department of Public Health. *Prevalence of Domestic Violence Among Women Attending Chicago Department of Public Health Clinics: Epidemiology Program Publication* (pp. 1–12). Chicago: Chicago Department of Public Health, 1995.

*Children's Mental Health Organizations.* Boston: Technical Assistance Center for the Evaluation of Children's Mental Health Systems at the Judge Baker Children's Center, 1996.

Chin, K. "Out of Town Brides: International Marriage and Wife Abuse Among Chinese Immigrants." *Journal of Comparative Family Studies,* 1994, *25,* 53–69.

Chin, R., and Chin, A. L. *Psychological Research in Communist China, 1949–1966.* Cambridge, Mass.: MIT Press, 1969.

*Chinese-English Terminology of Traditional Chinese Medicine.* Changsha, China: Hunan Science and Technology Press, 1983.

Chinese Medical Association. Division of Neuropsychiatry. *Chinese Classification of Mental Disorders.* (2nd ed.) Changsha, China: Hunan University Press, 1989.

Chittick, J. B. "Cross-Cultural Experiences in Promoting Effective Prevention Among Youth in Developing Countries and as New Immigrants." Paper presented at the International Conference on AIDS in Yokohama, Japan. Abstract in the conference syllabus, 1996, *11,* 246 (abstract no. TU-C-334).

Chohan, S. "Evaluation of Community-Based Interventions with Non-English Speaking Asian Women." Paper presented at the International Conference on AIDS in Yokohama, Japan. Abstract in the conference syllabus, 1996, *11,* 206 (abstract no. MO-D-1903).

Chow, E. "The Influence of Sex-Role Identity and Occupational Attainment on the Psychological Well-Being of Asian American Women." *Psychology of Women Quarterly,* 1987, *11,* 69–81.

Chrischilles, E. A., Butler, C. D., Davis, C. S., and Wallace, R. B. "A Model of Lifetime Osteoporosis Impact." *Archives of Internal Medicine,* 1991, *151,* 2026–2032.

Chun, C. A., Enomoto, K., and Sue, S. "Health Care Issues Among Asian Americans: Implications of Somatization." In P. M. Kato and T. Mann (eds.), *Handbook of Diversity Issues in Health Psychology* (pp. 358–361). New York: Plenum Press, 1996.

Chun, K. M., Eastman, K., Wang, G., and Sue, S. "Psychopathology Among Asian Americans." In L. Lee and N.W.S. Zane (eds.), *Handbook of Asian American Psychology* (pp. 457–483). Thousand Oaks, Calif.: Sage, 1998.

Chung, R. C., and Kagawa-Singer, M. "Predictors of Psychological Distress Among Southeast Asian Refugees." *Social Science and Medicine,* 1993, *36*(5), 631–639.

Chung, R. C., and Lin, K. M. "Help-Seeking Behavior Among Southeast Asian Refugees." *Journal of Community Psychology,* 1994, *22*(2), 109–120.

Chung, R. C., and Singer, M. K. "Interpretation of Symptom Presentation and Distress: A Southeast Asian Refugee Example." *Journal of Nervous and Mental Disease,* 1995, *183*(10), 639–648.

Clarkson, T., and others. "The Potential of Soybean Phytoestrogens for Postmenopausal Replacement Therapy." *Proceedings of the Society for Experimental Biology and Medicine,* 1998, *217*(3), 365–368.

Cockram, C., and others. "The Prevalence of DM and IGT Among Hong Kong Chinese Adults of Working Age." *Diabetes Research and Clinical Practice,* 1993, *21,* 67–73.

Cole, E., and Ruthblum, E. (eds.). "Refugee Women and Their Mental Health: Shattered Societies, Shattered Lives." *Women and Therapy* (special issue), 1992, *13,* 1–2.

Coll, C. G., and Magnuson, K. "Cultural Differences in Beliefs and Practices About Pregnancy and Childbearing." *Medicine and Health/ Rhode Island,* 1996, *79*(7), 257–260.

Comas-Diaz, L. "Mainland Puerto Rican Women: A Sociocultural Approach." *Journal of Community Psychology,* 1988, *16,* 21–31.

Comas-Diaz, L. "Culturally Relevant Issues and Treatment Implications for Hispanics." In D. R. Koslow and E. Salett (eds.), *Crossing Cultures in Mental Health* (pp. 31–48). Washington, D.C.: Society for International Education and Training Research, 1989.

Comas-Diaz, L., and Greene, B. *Women of Color: Integrating Ethnic and Gender Identities in Psychotherapy.* New York: Guilford Press, 1994.

Compton, K. *The Strength to Travel Together: Eritrean Experiences of Violence, Displacement, and Nationalism in a Global Network.* Unpublished doctoral dissertation, Harvard University, 1998.

Connor, E. M., and others. "Reduction of Maternal-Infant Transmission of Human Immunodeficiency Virus Type 1 with Zidovudine Treatment." *New England Journal of Medicine,* 1994, *331,* 1173–1180.

Consensus Development Conference. "Prophylaxis and Treatment of Osteoporosis." *American Journal of Medicine,* 1991, *90,* 107–110.

*Consolidated Omnibus Budget Reconciliation Act* (42 U.S.C. 1395 §dd), now referred to as the Emergency Medical Treatment and Active Labor Act of 1986.

Coopersmith, S. *The Antecedents of Self-Esteem.* New York: Freeman, 1967.

Cornelius, L. "Ethnic Minorities and Access to Medical Care: Where Do They Stand?" *Journal of the Association for Academic Minority Physicians,* 1993, *4*(1), 16–25.

Corr, J. E., and Vitaliano, P. "The Theoretical Implications of Converging Research on Depression and the Culture-Bound Syndromes." In A. Kleinman and B. Good (eds.), *Culture and Depression: Studies in the Anthropology and Cross Cultural Psychology of Affect and Disorder* (pp. 244–266). Berkeley: University of California Press, 1985.

Council on Scientific Affairs. "Hispanic Health in the United States." *Journal of the American Medical Association,* 1991, *265,* 2448–2452.

Creamer, M., Burgess, P., and Pattison, P. "Reaction to Trauma: A Cognitive Processing Model." *Journal of Abnormal Psychology,* 1992, *101*(3), 452–459.

Crespo, C. J., Loria, C. M., and Burt, V. L. "Hypertension and Other Cardiovascular Disease Risk Factors Among Mexican Americans, Cuban Americans, and Puerto Ricans from the Hispanic Health and Nutrition Survey." *Public Health Reports,* 1996, *111*(suppl. 2), 7–10.

Crites, L. L. "Wife Abuse: The Judicial Record." In L. L. Crites and W. L. Hepperle (eds.), *Women, the Courts, and Equality.* Thousand Oaks, Calif.: Sage, 1987.

Crites, L. L. "Cross-Cultural Counseling in Wife Battering Cases." *Response to the Victimization of Women and Children,* 1991, *13*(4), 8–12.

Cross, L. "Pressure on the Emergency Department: The Expanding Right to Medical Care." *Annals of Emergency Medicine,* 1992, *21*(10), 1266–1272.

Cross, T. L., Bazron, B. J., Dennis, K. W., and Isaacs, M. R. *Towards a Culturally Competent System of Care.* Washington, D.C.: CASSP Technical Assistance Center, Georgetown University Child Development Center, 1989.

Cross, W. E., Jr. "The Negro-to-Black Conversion Experience." *Black World,* 1971, *20,* 13–27.

Cunningham, P., Clancy, C., Cohen, J., and Wilets, M. "The Use of Hospital Emergency Departments for Non-Urgent Health Problems: A National Perspective." *Medical Care Research and Review,* 1995, *52*(4), 453–474.

Dahl, S., Mutapcic, A., and Schei, B. "Traumatic Events and Predictive Factors for Posttraumatic Syndromes in Displaced Bosnian Women in a War Zone." *Journal of Traumatic Stress,* 1998, *11*(1), 137–145.

Daly, A. Jennings, J., Beckett, J. O., and Leashore, B. R. "Effective Coping Strategies of African Americans," *Social Work,* 1995, *40*(2), 240–248.

Dana, R. *Multicultural Assessment Perspectives for Professional Psychology.* Needham Heights, Mass.: Allyn & Bacon, 1993.

Das, V. *Language and Body: Transactions in the Construction of Pain.* In A. Kleinman, V. Das, and M. Lock (eds.), *Social Suffering.* Berkeley: University of California Press, 1997.

Dasgupta, S. D., and Warrier, S. "In the Footsteps of Arundhati." *Violence Against Women,* 1996, *2*(3), 238–259.

D'Avanzo, C., Frye, B., and Froman, R. "Culture, Stress, and Substance Use in Cambodian Refugee Women." *Journal of Studies on Alcohol,* 1994, *55,* 420–426.

Davidson, J.R.T., Hughes, D., Blazer, P., and George, L. K. "Post Traumatic Stress Disorder in the Community: An Epidemiological Study." *Psychological Medicine,* 1991, *21*(3), 1–9.

Davis, B. D. "Utilization of Screening Mammography, 1987–1994." In C. R. Morris and W. E. Wright (eds.), *Breast Cancer in California.* Sacramento, Calif.: California Department of Health Services, Cancer Surveillance Section, Mar. 1996.

Davis, C. E., and others. "Natural Menopause and Cardiovascular Disease Risk Factors: The Poland and U.S. Collaborative Study on Cardiovascular Disease Epidemiology." *Annals of Epidemiology,* 1994, *4*(6), 445–448.

DeGruy, F., Columbia, L., and Dickinson, P. "Somatization Disorder in a Family Practice." *Journal of Family Practice,* 1987, *25,* 45–51.

DeLay, P., and Faust, S. "Depression in Southeast Asian Refugees." *American Family Physician,* 1987, *36*(4), 179–184.

Delmas, P. D., and others. "Effects of Raloxifene on Bone Mineral Density, Serum Cholesterol Concentrations, and Uterine Endometrium in Postmenopausal Women." *New England Journal of Medicine,* 1997, *337,* 1641–1647.

Dempster, D. W., and Lindsay, R. "Pathogenesis of Osteoporosis." *Lancet,* 1993, *341,* 797–801.

Desjarlais and others (eds.). *World Mental Health: Problems and Priorities in Low-Income Countries.* New York: Oxford University Press, 1995.

Dion, K. L., Dion, K. K., and Pak, A. W. "Personality-Based Hardiness as a Buffer for Discrimination-Related Stress in Members of Toronto's Chinese Community." *Canadian Journal of Behavioural Science,* 1992, *24*(4), 517–536.

Doherty, W. J., and Campbell, T. L. *Families and Health.* Thousand Oaks, Calif.: Sage, 1988.

Dorkenoo, E. *Cutting the Rose: Female Genital Mutilation—The Practice and Its Prevention.* London: Minority Rights Group, 1994.

Drachman, D. "A Stage-of-Migration Framework for Service to Immigrant Populations." *Social Work,* 1992, *36*(1), 68–72.

Drachman, D., Kwon-Ahn, Y. H., and Paulino, A. "Migration and Resettlement Experiences of Dominican and Korean Families." *Families in Society: The Journal of Contemporary Human Services,* Dec. 1996, 626–638.

Draguns, J. G. "Abnormal Behaviour in Chinese Societies: Clinical, Epidemiological, and Comparative Studies." In M. H. Bond (ed.), *The Handbook of Chinese Psychology* (pp. 412–428). New York: Oxford University Press, 1996.

Duncan, L., and Simmons, M. "Health Practices Among Russian and Ukrainian Immigrants." *Journal of Community Health Nursing,* 1996, *13*(2), 129–137.

Dunham, N., and Leetch, L. *The Health Care Components of Domestic Violence and Abuse: Implications for Wisconsin Providers and Health Care Systems.* Madison: Wisconsin Network for Health Policy Research, Jan. 1996.

Dutton, M., Mitchell, B., and Haywood, Y. "The Emergency Department as a Violence Prevention Center." *Journal of the American Medical Women's Association,* 1996, *51*(3), 92–95.

Dwairy, M. "Addressing the Repressed Needs of the Arabic Client." *Cultural Diversity and Mental Health,* 1997, *3*(1), 1–12.

Dworkin, R. J., and Adams, G. I. "Retention of Hispanics in Public Sector Mental Health Services." *Community Mental Health Journal,* 1987, *23*(3), 204–216.

Echeverry, J. "Treatment Barriers: Accessing and Accepting Professional Help." In J. G. Garcia and M. C. Zea (eds.), *Psychological Interventions and Research with Latino Populations* (pp. 94–107). Needham Heights, Mass.: Allyn & Bacon, 1997.

Eisenberg, D. M. "Advising Patients Who Seek Alternative Medical Therapies." *Annals of Internal Medicine,* 1997, *127,* 61–69.

Eisenbruch, M. "From Post Traumatic Stress Disorder to Cultural Bereavement: Diagnosis of Southeast Asian Refugees." *Social Science and Medicine,* 1991, *33*(6), 673–680.

Enas, E., and others. "Coronary Heart Disease and Its Risk Factors in First-Generation Immigrant Asian Indians to the United States of America." *Indian Heart Journal,* 1996, *48,* 343–353.

Erikson, E. H. *Childhood and Society.* New York: Norton, 1963.

Escobar, J. I. "Psychiatric Epidemiology." In A. C. Gaw (ed.), *Culture, Ethnicity and Mental Illness* (pp. 43–73). Washington, D.C.: American Psychiatric Association, 1992.

Escobar, J. I., and others. "Somatic Symptom Index (SSI): A New and Abridged Somatization Construct." *Journal of Nervous and Mental Disease,* 1989, *17,* 140–146.

Espin, O. "Psychological Impact of Migration on Latinas: Implications for Psychotherapeutic Practice." *Psychology of Women Quarterly,* 1987, *11,* 489–503.

Faust, S. "Providing Inclusive Healthcare Across Cultures." In Hickey, J. V., Ouimette, R. M., Venegoni, S. L. (eds.), *Advanced Practice Nursing.* Philadelphia: Lippincott, 1996.

Fenton, C. R., and Hargreaves, W. "Effect of Proposition 187 on Mental Health Service Use in California: A Case Study." *Health Affairs,* Spring 1996, *15*(1), 182–190.

Fenton, J. J., Catalano, R., and Hargreaves, W. A. "Effect of Proposition 187 on Mental Health Service Use in California: A Case Study." *Health Affairs,* 1996, *15*(1), 182–190.

Fenton, J. J., Moss, N., Khalil, H. G., and Asch, S. "Effect of California's Proposition 187 on the Use of Primary Care Clinics." *Western Journal of Medicine,* 1997, *166,* 16–20.

Fernandez, M. "Domestic Violence by Extended Family Members in India: Interplay of Gender and Generation." *Journal of Interpersonal Violence,* 1997, *12*(3), 433–455.

Ferran, E. "Workplace Diversity: A Manager's Journal." *Journal of Child and Family Studies,* 1994, *3,* 1, 15.

Fieldhouse, P. *Food and Nutrition: Customs and Culture.* London: Croom Helm, 1986.

Finkler, K. "Symptomatic Differences Between the Sexes in Rural Mexico." *Culture, Medicine, and Psychiatry,* 1985, *9,* 27–57.

Flaskerud, J. "The Effects of Culture-Compatible Intervention on the Utilization of Mental Health Services by Minority Clients." *Community Mental Health Journal,* 1986, *22*(2), 127–141.

Flaskerud, J., and Uman, G. "Acculturation and Its Effects on Self-Esteem Among Immigrant Latina Women." *Behavioral Medicine,* 1996, *22,* 123–133.

Flowers-Bowie, L. "Funding Prenatal Care for Unauthorized Immigrants." Denver: National Conference of State Legislatures, May 1997.

Forbes, K., and Wegner, E. "Compliance by Samoans in Hawaii with Service Norms in Pediatric Primary Care." *Public Health Reports,* 1987, *102*(5), 508–511.

Fourcroy, J. *"L'Eternal Couteau:* Review of Female Circumcision." *Urology,* 1983, *22*(4).

Frankl, V. *Man's Search for Meaning.* New York: Simon & Schuster, 1959.

Franks, F., and Faux, S. A. "Depression, Stress, Mastery, and Social Resources in Four Ethnocultural Women's Groups." *Research in Nursing and Health,* 1990, *13,* 283–292.

Freeman, H., and Corey, C. "Insurance Status and Access to Health Services Among Poor Persons." *Health Services Research,* 1993, *28*(5), 531–541.

Freudenberg, N., Jacalyn, L., and Silver D. "How Black and Latino Community Organizations Respond to the AIDS Epidemic: A Case Study in One New York City Neighborhood." *AIDS Education and Prevention,* 1989, *1,* 12–21.

Friedman, A. "Rape and Domestic Violence: The Experience of Refugee Women." *Women and Therapy,* 1992, *13*(4), 65–78.

Friedson, E. *Patients' Views of Medical Practice.* New York: Russell Sage Foundation, 1961.

Frisancho, A. R. *Anthropometric Standards for the Assessment of Growth and Nutritional Status.* Ann Arbor: University of Michigan Press, 1990.

Fruchter, R. G., and others. "Screening for Cervical and Breast Cancer Among Caribbean Immigrants." *Journal of Community Health,* 1985, *10,* 121–135.

Fruchter, R. G., and others. "Cervix and Breast Cancer Incidence in Immigrant Caribbean Women." *American Journal of Public Health,* 1990, *80,* 722–724.

Frye, B. A. "Cultural Themes in Health Care Decision-Making Among Cambodian Refugee Women." *Journal of Community Health Nursing,* 1991, *2*(1), 33–44.

Frye, B. A., and D'Avanzo, C. D. "Cultural Themes in Family Stress and Violence Among Cambodian Refugee Women in the Inner City." *Advances in Nursing Science,* 1994, *16*(3), 64–77.

Fujino, D., Okazaki, S., and Young, K. "Asian-American Women in the Mental Health System: An Examination of Ethnic and Gender Match Between Therapist and Client." *Journal of Community Psychology,* 1994, *22*(2), 164–176.

Fujomoto, W., and others. "Susceptibility to Development of Central Adiposity Among Populations." *Obesity Research,* 1995, *3*(Suppl.), 179s–186s.

Fulton, J. *Canada's Health System: Bordering on the Possible.* New York: Faulkner & Gray, 1993.

Furbee, P., Sikora, R., Williams, J., and Derk, S. "Comparison of Domestic Violence Screening Methods: A Pilot Study." *Annals of Emergency Medicine,* 1998, *31*(4), 495–501.

Furnham, A., and Bochner, S. *Culture Shock: Psychological Reactions to Unfamiliar Environments.* New York: Routledge, 1990.

Galli, N., Greenberg, J. S., and Tobin, F. "Health Education and Sensitivity to Cultural, Religious, and Ethnic Beliefs." *Journal of School Health,* 1987, *57*(5), 177–179.

Gany, F., and Ebin, V. "Somatization in an Immigrant Senegalese Population in New York: The Value of Understanding Our Patients." *Language of Distress.* Forthcoming.

Gany, F., and Thiel-deBocanegra, H. "Overcoming Barriers to Improving the Health of Immigrant Women." *Journal of the American Medical Women's Association,* 1996, *51*(4), 155–160.

Garcia, J. G., and Zea, M. C. *Psychological Interventions and Research with Latino Populations.* Needham Heights, Mass.: Allyn & Bacon, 1997.

Garcia, N., and Warren, B. "Eating for Healthy Tomorrows." Minority Health Issues for an Emerging Majority, Proceedings of the Fourth National Forum on Cardiovascular Health, Pulmonary Disorders, and Blood Resources, June 26–27, 1992.

Garcia Coll, C. T., Meyer, E. C., and Brillon, L. "Ethnic and Minority Parenting." In M. H. Bornstein (ed.), *Handbook of Parenting: Biology and Ecology of Parenting* (pp. 189–209). Hillsdale, N.J.: Erlbaum, 1995.

Garza-Trevino, E., Ruiz, P., and Venegas-Samuels, K. "A Psychiatric Curriculum Directed to the Care of the Hispanic Patient." *Academic Psychiatry,* 1997, *21*(1), 1–10.

Gaviria, M., Stern, G., and Schensul, S. L. "Sociocultural Factors and Perinatal Health in a Mexican-American Community." *Journal of the National Medical Association,* 1982, *74,* 983–989.

Gaw, A. *Culture, Ethnicity, and Mental Illness.* Washington, D.C.: American Psychiatric Press, 1993.

Gelles, R. J., and Cornell, C. P. *Intimate Violence in Families.* Thousand Oaks, Calif.: Sage, 1990.

Ghaffarian, S. "The Acculturation of Iranians in the United States." *Journal of Social Psychology,* 1987, *127*(6), 565–571.

Giatras, I., Lau, J., and Levey, A. S., for the Angiotensin-Converting Enzyme Inhibition and Progressive Renal Disease Study Group. "Effect of Angiotensin-Converting Enzyme Inhibitors on the Progression of Nondiabetic Renal Disease: A Meta-Analysis of Randomized Trials." *Annals of Internal Medicine,* 1997, *127,* 337–345.

Gil, R. M. "Cultural Attitudes Toward Mental Illness Among Puerto Rican Migrant Women." In R. E. Zambrana (ed.), *Work, Family and Health: Latin Women in Transition.* New York: Fordham University, 1982.

Gilligan, C. *In a Different Voice: Psychological Theory and Women's Development.* Cambridge, Mass.: Harvard University Press, 1982.

Gillum, R., and Liu, F. "CHD Mortality in U.S. Blacks—1940–1978: Trends and Unanswered Questions." *American Heart Journal,* 1984, *108,* 728–732.

Gin, N., and others. "Prevalence of Domestic Violence Among Patients in Three Ambulatory Internal Medicine Clinics." *Journal of General Internal Medicine.* 1991, *6,* 317–322.

Ginsberg, C., and others. *Interpretation and Translation Services in Health Care: A Survey of US Public and Private Teaching Hospitals.* Washington, D.C.: National Public Health and Hospital Institute, 1995.

Ginzberg, E. "Access to Healthcare for Hispanics." *Journal of the American Medical Association,* 1991, *265,* 238–241.

Gjerdingen, D., and Lor, V. "Hepatitis B Status of Hmong Patients." *Journal of the American Board of Family Practice,* 1997, *10*(5), 322–328.

Goff, D. C., and others. "Acute Myocardial Infarction and Coronary Heart Disease Mortality Among Mexican Americans and Non-Hispanic Whites in Texas, 1980 Through 1989." *Ethnicity and Disease,* 1993a, *3*(1), 64–69.

Goff, D. C., and others. "Mortality After Hospitalization for Myocardial Infarction Among Mexican-Americans and Non-Hispanic Whites: The Corpus Christi Heart Project." *Ethnicity and Disease,* 1993b, *3*(1), 55–63.

Goldberg, K., and others. "Racial and Community Factors Influencing Coronary Artery Bypass Graft Surgery Rates for All 1986 Medicare

Patients." *Journal of the American Medical Association,* 1992, *267*(11), 1473–1477.

Goldstein, E. *Ego Psychology and Social Work Practice.* (2nd ed.) New York: Free Press, 1995.

Goletti, D., and others. "Effect of *Mycobacterium tuberculosis* on HIV Replication: Role of Immune Activation." *Journal of Immunology,* 1996, *157,* 1271–1278.

Gonzalez-Swafford, M., and Gutierrez, M. "Ethno-Medical Beliefs and Practices of Mexican Americans." *Nurse Practitioner,* 1983, *8,* 29–30.

Good, B., and DelVecchio, A. "The Meaning of Symptoms: A Cultural Hermeneutic Model for Clinical Practice. In L. Eisenberg and A. Kleinman (eds.), *The Relevance of Social Science for Medicine* (pp. 165–196). Boston: D. Reidel, 1980.

Gooding, S. S., Smith, D. B., and Peyrot, M. "Insurance Coverage and the Appropriate Utilization of Emergency Departments." *Journal of Public Policy and Marketing,* 1996, *15*(1), 76–86.

Gordon, S. "Hispanic Cultural Health Beliefs and Folk Remedies." *Journal of Holistic Nursing,* 1994, *12*(3), 307–322.

Gove, S., and Slutkin, G. "Infectious Diseases of Travelers and Immigrants." *Emergency Medical Clinics of North America,* 1984, *2,* 587–622.

Grant, G. "Impact of Immigration on the Family and Children." In M. Frank (ed.), *Newcomers to the United States: Children and Families* (pp. 27–37). Binghamton, N.Y.: Haworth Press, 1983.

Gray, E., and Cosgrove, J. "Ethnocentric Perception of Childrearing Practices in Protective Services." *Child Abuse and Neglect,* 1985, *9,* 389–396.

Gray, R. J., and others. "Adverse Five–Year Outcome After Coronary Artery Bypass Surgery in Blacks." *Archives of Internal Medicine,* 1996, *156,* 769–773.

Green, L. W., and Kreuter, M. W. *Health Promotion Planning: An Educational and Environmental Approach.* Mountain View, Calif.: Mayfield, 1991.

Griffith, J. L., and Griffith, M. E. *The Body Speaks: Therapeutic Dialogues for Mind-Body Problems.* New York: Basic Books, 1994.

Grinberg, L., and Grinberg, R. *Psychoanalytic Perspectives on Migration and Exile.* New Haven, Conn.: Yale University Press, 1989.

Guendelman, S., and Abrams, B. "Dietary, Alcohol, and Tobacco Intake Among Mexican-American Women of Childbearing Age: Results from HHANES Data." *American Journal of Health Promotion,* 1994, *8*(5), 363–72.

Guendelman, S., Gould, J., Hudes, M., and Eskenazi, B. "Generational Differences in Perinatal Health Among the Mexican Origin Population in Hispanic HHANES." *American Journal of Public Health,* 1990, *79,* 1263–1267.

Guendelman, S., and Schwalbe, J. "Medical Care Utilization by Hispanic Children: How Does It Differ from Black and White Peers?" *Medical Care*, 1986, *24*(10), 925–937.

Guerney, B. G., Jr. "Filial Therapy: Description and Rationale." *Journal of Consulting Psychology*, 1964, *28*(4), 303–310.

Guerney, L. "Introduction to Filial Therapy." In P. Keller and L. Ritt (eds.), *Innovations in Clinical Practice: A Source Book* (Vol. 3, pp. 26–39). Sarasota, Fla.: Professional Resource Exchange, 1983.

Guerney, L. *The Parenting Skills Manual: Leader's Manual.* State College, Pa.: IDEALS, 1987.

Guillermo, T. "Categorizing Asian Minorities May Lead to Wasted Time, Effort for All." Minority Health Issues for an Emerging Majority, Fourth National Forum on Cardiovascular Health, Pulmonary Disorders, and Blood Resources, June 26–27, 1992.

Gurin, P. "Women's Gender Consciousness." *Public Opinion Quarterly,* 1985, *49*(2), 143–163.

Gutierrez, L. M. "Working with Women of Color: An Empowerment Perspective." *Social Work,* 1990, *35*(2), 149–153.

Hahn, R. A. "The State of Federal Health Statistics on Racial and Ethnic Groups." *Journal of the American Medical Association,* 1992, *267,* 268–271.

Hahn, R. A., Mulinare, J., and Teutsch, S. "Inconsistencies in Coding of Race and Ethnicity Between Birth and Death of U.S. Infants: A New Look at Infant Mortality, 1983–85." *Journal of the American Medical Association,* 1992, *267,* 1467–1472.

Haines, D. W. "Kinship in Vietnamese Refugee Resettlement: A Review of the U.S. Experience." *Journal of Comparative Family Studies,* 1988, *19*(1), 1–16.

Hall, Cross, and Freedle. "A Five Step Paradigm for the Development of Racial Identity." 1972.

Hames, C. G., and Greenlund, K. J. "Ethnicity and Cardiovascular Disease: The Evans County Heart Study." *American Journal of the Medical Sciences,* 1996, *311*(3), 130–134.

Harkness, S., and Super, C. "Culture and Parenting." In M. H. Bornstein (ed.), *Handbook of Parenting: Biology and Ecology of Parenting* (Vol. 2, pp. 211–234). Hillsdale, N.J.: Erlbaum, 1995.

Harris, R., and Leininger, L. "Clinical Strategies for Breast Cancer Screening: Weighing and Using the Evidence." *Annals of Internal Medicine,* 1995, *122,* 539–547.

Harrison, A. O., and others. "Family Ecologies of Ethnic Minority Children." *Child Development,* 1990, *61,* 347–362.

Hart, B. J. "Battered Women and the Criminal Justice System." *American Behavioral Scientist,* 1993, *33,* 394–424.

364  REFERENCES

Harwood, A. "The Hot-Cold Theory of Disease: Implications for Treatment of Puerto Rican Patients." *Journal of the American Medical Association,* 1971, *216,* 1153–1158.

Harwood, A. *Ethnicity and Medical Care.* Cambridge, Mass.: Harvard University Press, 1981.

Havas, S., and Sherwin, R. "Putting It All Together: Summary of the NHLBI Workshop on the Epidemiology of Hypertension in Hispanic American, Native American, Asian/Pacific Islander American Populations." *Public Health Reports,* 1996, *111*(Suppl. 2), 77–79.

Hawaii. State Department of Health. *Hawaii's Health Risk Behaviors, 1993.* Hawaii: Hawaii Department of Health Services, May 1996.

Haywood, L. J. "Hypertension in Minority Populations: Access to Care." *American Journal of Medicine,* 1990, *88*(Suppl. 3b), 17s–20s.

Hazuda, H. P. "Hypertension in the San Antonio Heart Study and the Mexico City Diabetes Study: Sociocultural Correlates." *Public Health Reports,* 1996, *111*(Suppl. 2), 18–21.

He, J., and Whelton, P. K. "Epidemiology and Prevention of Hypertension." *Medical Clinics of North America,* 1997, *81,* 1077–1097.

Health Care Advisory Board. *Redefining the Emergency Department: Five Strategies for Reducing Unnecessary Visits.* Washington, D.C.: Advisory Board Company, 1993.

Heaney, R. "The Role of Nutrition in Prevention and Management of Osteoporosis." *Clinical Obstetrics and Gynecology,* 1987, *50,* 833–846.

Heise, L. *Violence Against Women: The Hidden Health Burden.* World Bank Discussion Papers. Washington, D.C.: World Bank, 1994.

Helzer, J. E., Robins, L. N., and McEnvoy, L. "Post-Traumatic Stress Disorder in the General Population: Findings of the Epidemiological Catchment Area Survey." *New England Journal of Medicine,* Dec. 24, 1987, pp. 1630–1634.

Henderson, S. M., and Brown, J. S. "Infant Feeding Practices of Vietnamese Immigrants to the Northwest United States." *Scholarly Inquiry for Nursing Practice,* 1987, *1*(2), 153–169.

Herbst, P. R. "From Helpless Victim to Empowered Survivor: Oral History as a Treatment for Survivors of Torture." Special Issue: Refugee Women and Their Mental Health: Shattered Societies, Shattered Lives: I. *Women and Therapy,* 1992, *13*(1–2), 141–154.

Herman, J. L. *Trauma and Recovery.* New York: Basic Books, 1993.

Hernandez-Guzman, L., and Sanchez-Sosa, J. J. "Parent-Child Interactions Predict Anxiety in Mexican Adolescents." *Adolescence,* 1996, *31*(124), 953–963.

Hiatt, R. A., and others. "Pathways to Early Cancer Detection in the Multiethnic Population of the San Francisco Bay Area." *Health Education Quarterly,* 1996, *23*(Suppl.), S10–S27.

Higginbotham, J. C., Trevino, F. M., and Ray, L. A. "Utilization of Curanderos by Mexican Americans: Prevalence and Predictors Findings from HHANES 1982–84." *American Journal of Public Health,* Dec. 1990, *80*(Suppl.), 32–35.

Ho, M. K. *Family Therapy with Ethnic Minorities.* Thousand Oaks, Calif.: Sage, 1987.

Hoang, G., and Erickson, R. "Cultural Barriers to Effective Medical Care Among Indochinese Patients." *Annual Review of Medicine,* 1985, *36,* 229–239.

Hodes, R. M. "Pattern of Heart Disease in Ethiopia as Seen in a Cardiology Referral Clinic." *Cardiology (Basel),* 1988, *75,* 458–464.

Hodes, R. M. "Cross-Cultural Medicine and Diverse Health Beliefs: Ethiopians Abroad." *Western Journal of Medicine,* 1997, *166,* 29–36.

Hodes, R. M., and Azbite, M. *Tuberculosis.* In H. Kloos and Z. Ahmed (eds.), *The Ecology of Health and Disease in Ethiopia* (pp. 265–284). Boulder, Colo.: Westview Press, 1993.

Hogeland, C., and Rosen, K. *Dreams Lost, Dreams Found: Undocumented Women in the Land of Opportunity.* San Francisco: Coalition for Immigrants and Refugee Rights and Services, 1990.

Hong, W., Chan, L., Zheng, D. C., and Wang, C. "Neurasthenia in Chinese Students at UCLA." *Psychiatric Annuals,* 1992, *22*(4), 199–201.

Hornstein, L., and others. "Persistent *Schistosoma Mansoni* Infection in Yemeni Immigrants to Israel." *Israel Journal of Medical Science,* 1990, *26,* 386–389.

Horowitz, M. J. *Stress Response Syndromes.* (2nd ed.) Northvale, N.J.: Aronson, 1986.

Hough, R. L., and others. "Utilization of Health and Mental Health Services by Los Angeles Mexican Americans and Non-Hispanic Whites." *Archives of General Psychiatry,* 1987, *44,* 702–709.

Houskamp, B. M., and Foy, D. W. "The Assessment of Post-Traumatic Stress Disorder in Battered Women." *Journal of Interpersonal Violence,* 1991, *6,* 367–375.

Howard, K., and others. "Patterns of Mental Health Service Utilization." *Archives of General Psychiatry,* 1996, *53,* 696–703.

Hoyert, D., and Kung, H. "Asian or Pacific Islander Mortality, Selected States, 1992." *Monthly Vital Statistics Report,* Aug. 14, 1997 (Suppl. 1).

Hsu, J. "Asian Family Interaction Patterns and Their Therapeutic Implications." In P. Pichot, P. Berner, R. Wolf, and K. Thau (eds.), *Psychiatry: The State of Art* (Vol. 8, pp. 599–606). New York: Plenum Press, 1985.

Hu, T., Snowden, L., Jerrell, J., and Nguyen, T. "Ethnic Populations in Public Mental Health: Services Choice and Level of Use." *American Journal of Public Health,* 1991, *81,* 1429–1434.

Hubbell, F. A., Chavez, L. R., Mishra, S. I., and Valdez, R. B. "Beliefs About Sexual Behavior and Other Predictors of Papanicolaou Smear Screening Among Latinas and Anglo Women." *Archives of Internal Medicine,* 1996a, *156,* 2353–2358.

Hubbell, F. A., Chavez, L. R., Mishra, S. I., and Valdez, R. B. "Differing Beliefs About Breast Cancer Among Latinas and Anglo Women." *Western Journal of Medicine,* 1996b, *164,* 405–409.

Hubbell, F. A., and others. "Access to Medical Care for Documented and Undocumented Latinos in a Southern California County." *Western Journal of Medicine,* 1991, *154*(4), 414–417.

Hui, K. K., and Pasic, J. "Outcome of Hypertension Management in Asian Americans." *Archives of Internal Medicine,* 1997, *157,* 1345–1348.

Hulme, P. A. "Somatization in Hispanics." *Journal of Psychosocial Nursing,* 1996, 34, 33–36.

Human Rights Watch/Africa. *Shattered Lives: Sexual Violence During the Rwandan Genocide and Its Aftermath.* New York: Human Rights Watch, 1996.

Hyman, A., Schillinger, D., and Lo, B. "Laws Mandating Reporting of Domestic Violence: Do They Promote Patient Well-Being?" *Health Law and Ethics,* 1995, *273*(22), 1781–1787.

*Illegal Immigration Reform and Immigrant Responsibility Act of 1996.* Public Law 104–208, 1996.

Institute of Medicine. *Access to Health Care in America.* M. Millman (ed.). Washington, D.C.: National Academy Press, 1993.

Institute of Medicine. *Violence in Families: Assisting Prevention and Treatment Programs.* Washington, D.C.: National Academy Press, 1998.

Ishisaka, H., Nguyen, Q., and Okimoto, J. "The Role of Culture in the Mental Health Treatment of Indochinese Refugees." In T. Owan (ed.), *Southeast Asian Mental Health: Treatment, Prevention, Services, Training, and Research* (pp. 41–63). Washington, D.C.: U.S. Department of Health and Human Services, 1985.

Ivey, S., and Kramer, E. "Immigrant Women and the Emergency Department: The Juncture with Welfare and Immigration Reform." *Journal of the American Medical Women's Association,* 1998, *53*(2), 94–95, 107.

Jamerson, K., and DeQuattro, V. "The Impact of Ethnicity on Response to Antihypertensive Therapy." *American Journal of Medicine,* 1996, *101*(Suppl. 3a), 22s–32s.

James, S. "Racial and Ethnic Differences in Infant Mortality and Low Birth Weight." *Annals of Epidemiology,* 1993, *3*(2), 130–136.

Janoff-Bulman, R. *Shattered Assumptions: Towards a New Psychology of Trauma.* New York: Free Press, 1992.

Jayakar, K. "Women of the Indian Subcontinent." In L. Comas-Diaz and B. Greene (eds.), *Women of Color: Integrating Ethnic and Gender Identities in Psychotherapy* (pp. 161–181). New York: Guilford Press, 1994.

Jenkins, C., and others. "Health Care Access and Preventive Care Among Vietnamese Immigrants: Do Traditional Beliefs and Practices Pose Barriers?" *Social Science and Medicine,* 1996, *43*(7), 1049–1056.

John Snow Public Health Group. *Common Health Beliefs and Practices of Puerto Ricans, Haitians and Low Income Blacks Living in the New York/New Jersey Area.* Washington, D.C.: John Snow Public Health Group.

Johnson, T., Hardt, E., and Kleinman, A. "Cultural Factors in the Medical Interview." In M. Lipkin, S. Putnam, and A. Lazare (eds.), *The Medical Interview.* New York: Springer-Verlag, 1995.

Jones, E. F., and Forrest, J. D. "Contraceptive Failure in the United States: Revised Estimates from the 1982 National Survey of Family Growth." *Family Planning Perspectives,* 1989, *21*(3), 103–109.

Jones, J. F., and others. "Evidence for Active Epstein-Barr Virus Infection in Patients with Persistent Unexplained Illnesses: Elevated Anti-Early Antigen Antibodies." *Annals of Internal Medicine,* 1985, *102,* 1–7.

Jones, P., Jones, S., and Yoder, L. "Hospital Location as a Determinant of Emergency Room Utilization Patterns." *Public Health Reports,* 1982, *97*(5), 445–451.

Jones, W., and others. "Female Genital Mutilation/Female Circumcision: Who Is at Risk in the United States?" *Public Health Reports,* 1997, *112*(5), 368–377.

Juarbe, T. "Access to Health Care for Hispanic Women: A Primary Health Care Perspective." *Nursing Outlook,* 1995, *43*(1), 23–28.

Kagan, A., and others. "Epidemiologic Studies of CHD and Stroke in Japanese Men Living in Japan, Hawaii, and California: Demographic, Physical, Dietary, and Biochemical Characteristics." *Journal of Chronic Diseases,* 1974, *27,* 345–363.

Kaiser Family Foundation. *Future of Medicaid.* Menlo Park, Calif.: Kaiser Family Foundation, 1995.

Kamya, H. A. "African Immigrants in the United States: The Challenge for Research and Practice." *Social Work,* 1997, *42*(2), 154–165.

Kang, S. H., and others. "Behavioral Risk Factor Survey of Korean Americans in Alameda County, California, 1994." *Morbidity and Mortality Weekly Report,* 1997, *46,* 774–777.

Kanis, J. A., and others. "The Diagnosis of Osteoporosis." *Journal of Bone and Mineral Research,* 1994, *9,* 1137–1141.

Kanuha, V. "Compounding the Triple Jeopardy: Battering in Lesbian of Color Relationships." *Women and Therapy,* 1990, *9*(1–2), 169–184.

Kanuha, V. "Women of Color in Battering Relationships." In L. Comas-Diaz and B. Greene (eds.), *Women of Color: Integrating Ethnic and Gender Identities in Psychotherapy* (pp. 428–454). New York: Guilford Press, 1994.

Kaptchuk, T. J. *The Web That Has No Weaver.* Chicago: Congdon and Weed, 1983.

Karno, M., and others. "Lifetime Prevalence of Specific Psychiatric Disorders Among Mexican Americans and Non-Hispanic Whites in Los Angeles." *Archives of General Psychiatry,* 1987, *44,* 695–701.

Kassebaum, D., and Anderson, M. B. "Proceedings of the AAMC's Conference on the Education of Medical Students About Family Violence and Abuse." *Academic Medicine,* 1995, *70*(11), 961–1001.

Katon, W., Kleinman, A., and Rosen, G. "Depression and Somatization: A Review, Part I." *American Journal of Medicine,* 1982, *72,* 127–135.

Katon, W., and others. "Somatization: A Spectrum of Severity." *American Journal of Psychiatry,* 1991, *148,* 34–40.

Katz, S. S. "Uvulectomy: A Common Ethnosurgical Procedure in Africa." *Medical Anthropology Quarterly,* 1989, *3*(1), 62–69.

Keane, V. P., and others. "Prevalence of Tuberculosis in Vietnamese Migrants: The Experience of the Orderly Departure Program." *Southeast Asian Journal of Tropical Medicine and Public Health,* 1995, *26,* 642–647.

Keenan, N. L., Murray, E. T., and Truman, B. I. "Hispanic Americans." In U.S. Department of Health and Human Services, *Chronic Disease in Minority Populations.* Atlanta, Ga.: Centers for Disease Control and Prevention, 1994.

Keil, J. E., Sutherland, S., Knapp, R., and Tyroler, H. "Does Equal Socioeconomic Status in Black and White Men Mean Equal Risk of Mortality?" *American Journal of Public Health,* 1992, *82*(8), 1133–1136.

Keil, J. E., and others. "Mortality Rates and Risk Factors for Coronary Disease in Black as Compared with White Men and Women." *New England Journal of Medicine,* 1993, *329*(2), 73–78.

Kelly, A. W., and others. "A Program to Increase Breast and Cervical Cancer Screening for Cambodian Women in a Midwestern Community." *Mayo Clinic Proceedings,* 1996, *71,* 437–444.

Kelly, N. "Political Rape as Persecution: A Legal Perspective." *Journal of the American Medical Women's Association,* 1997, *52*(4), 188–190.

Kelsey, J. L. "Breast Cancer Epidemiology: Summary and Future Directions." *Epidemiologic Reviews,* 1993, *15,* 256–264.

Kelsey, J. L., and Horn-Ross, P. L. "Breast Cancer: Magnitude of the Problem and Descriptive Epidemiology." *Epidemiologic Reviews,* 1993, *15,* 7–16.

Kessler, R. C. "The Effects of Stressful Life Events on Depression." *Annual Review of Psychology,* 1997, *48,* 191–214.

Kessler, R. C., and others. "Lifetime and Twelve-Month Prevalence of DSM-III-R Psychiatric Disorders in the United States." *Archives of General Psychiatry,* 1994, *51,* 8–19.

Kessler, R. C., and others. "Posttraumatic Stress Disorder in the National Comorbidity Study." *Archives of General Psychiatry,* 1995, *141*(5), 645–650.

Kessler, R. C., and others. "The Epidemiology of Co-Occurring Addictive and Mental Disorders: Implications for Prevention and Service Utilization." *American Journal of Orthopsychiatry,* 1996, *66,* 17–31.

Key, F. "Female Circumcision/Female Genital Mutilation in the United States: Legislation and Its Implications for Health Providers." *Journal of the American Women's Medical Association,* 1997, *52*(4).

Khazoyan, C. M., and Anderson, N.L.R. "Latinas' Expectations for Their Partners During Childbirth." *Maternal and Child Nursing,* July–Aug. 1994, 226–229.

Kilpatrick, D., Resnick, H., and Acierno, R. "Health Impact of Interpersonal Violence 3: Implications for Clinical Practice and Public Policy." *Behavioral Medicine,* 1997, *23,* 79–85.

Kim, L.I.C. "Psychiatric Care of Korean Americans." In A. C. Gaw (ed.), *Culture, Ethnicity, and Mental Health* (pp. 347–375). Washington, D.C.: American Psychiatric Association, 1993.

Kim, S. C. "Korean American Families." In E. Lee (ed.), *Working with Asian Americans: A Guide for Clinicians* (pp. 125–135). New York: Guilford Press, 1994.

Kington, R. S., and Smith, J. P. "Socioeconomic Status and Racial and Ethnic Differences in Functional Status Associated with Chronic Diseases." *American Journal of Public Health,* 1997, *87,* 805–810.

Kinzie, J. D. "Therapy with Southeast Asian Refugees." *Community Mental Health Journal,* 1988, *24*:2, 157–164.

Kinzie, J. D., and others. "Posttraumatic Stress Disorder Among Survivors of Cambodian Concentration Camps." *American Journal of Psychiatry,* 1984, *141*(5), 645–650.

Kinzie, J. D., and others. "The Prevalence of Posttraumatic Stress Disorder and Its Clinical Significance Among Southeast Asian Refugees." *American Journal of Psychiatry,* 1990, *147*(7), 913–917.

Kirmayer, L. J. "Somatization and the Social Construction of Illness Experience." In S. McHugh and T. M. Vallis (eds.), *Illness Behavior: A Multidisciplinary Model* (pp. 111–134). New York: Plenum Press, 1985.

Kirmayer, L. J. "Confusion of the Senses: Implications of Ethnocultural Variations in Somatoform and Dissociative Disorders." In A. J.

Marsella and others (eds.), *Ethnocultural Aspects of Posttraumatic Stress Disorder: Issues, Research, and Clinical Applications* (pp. 131–164). Washington, D.C.: American Psychiatric Association, 1996.

Kirmayer, L. J., and Robbins, J. M. "Three Forms of Somatization in Primary Care: Prevalence, Co-Occurrence, and Sociodemographic Characteristics." *Journal of Nervous and Mental Disease*, 1991, *179*, 647–655.

Kirmayer, L. J., and Robbins, J. M. "Patients Who Somatize in Primary Care: A Longitudinal Study of Cognitive and Social Characteristics." *Psychological Medicine*, 1996, *26*, 937–951.

Kirmayer, L. J., Young, A., and Robbins, J. M. "Symptom Attribution in Cultural Perspective." *Canadian Journal of Psychiatry*, 1994, *39*, 584–585.

Klag, M. J., and others. "End-Stage Renal Disease in African-American and White Men." *Journal of the American Medical Association*, 1997, *277*, 1293–1298.

Klatsky, A. L., and Armstrong, M. A. "Cardiovascular Risk Factors Among Asian Americans Living in Northern California." *American Journal of Public Health*, 1991, *81*, 1423–1428.

Klein, J. "*Susto*—The Anthropological Study of Diseases of Adaptation." *Social Science and Medicine*, 1978, *12*, 23–28.

Kleinman, A. "Neurasthenia and Depression: A Study of Somatization and Culture in China." *Culture, Medicine and Psychiatry*, 1982, *6*(2), 117–190.

Kleinman, A. *Social Origins of Distress and Disease: Depression, Neurasthenia, and Pain in Modern China.* New Haven, Conn.: Yale University Press, 1986.

Kleinman, A. *Rethinking Psychiatry.* New York: Free Press, 1988.

Kleinman, A., Das, V., and Lock, M. (eds.). *Social Suffering.* Berkeley: University of California Press, 1997.

Kleinman, A., Eisenberg, L., and Good, B. "Culture, Illness, and Care: Clinical Lessons from Cross-Cultural Research." *Annals of Internal Medicine*, 1978, *88*(2), 251–258.

Kooiman, C., Van de Wetering, B., and Van der Mast, R. "Clinical and Demographic Characteristics of Emergency Department Patients in the Netherlands." *American Journal of Emergency Medicine*, 1989, *7*(6), 632–638.

Koonin, L., Smith, J., Ramick, M., and Strauss, L. *Abortion Surveillance—United States, 1995.* CDC Surveillance Series. July 3, 1998, *47*(SS-2), 31–39.

Koss, J. D. "Somatization and Somatic Complaint Syndromes Among Hispanics: Overview and Ethnopsychological Perspectives." *Transcultural Psychiatric Research Review*, 1990, *27*, 5–29.

Koss-Chioino, J. D. "Traditional and Folk Approaches Among Ethnic Minorities." In J. F. Aponte, R. Y. Rivers, and J. Wohl (eds.), *Psychological Interventions and Cultural Diversity* (pp. 145–163). Needham Heights, Mass.: Allyn & Bacon, 1995.

Kovar, M. G. "Mortality Among Minority Populations in the United States." *American Journal of Public Health,* 1992, *82,* 1168–1170.

Kunstadter, P. "Epidemiological Consequences of Migration and Rapid Cultural Change: Non-Refugee Hmong in Thailand and Refugees in California." Paper presented at the Australian Center for International and Tropical Health and Nutrition, University of Brisbane, July 16–19, 1997.

Kuo, W. H. "Prevalence of Depression Among Asian-Americans." *Journal of Nervous and Mental Disease,* 1984, *172,* 449–457.

Lambrew, J., and others. "The Effects of Having a Regular Doctor on Access to Primary Care." *Medical Care,* 1996, *34*(2), 138–151.

Lapham, S. J. *The Foreign-Born Population in the United States, 1990.* Washington, D.C.: U.S. Bureau of the Census, Ethnic and Hispanic Branch, 1990.

Lasseter, J., Pyles, J., and Galijasevic, S. "Emergency Medicine in Bosnia and Herzegovina." *Annals of Emergency Medicine,* 1997, *30*(4), 527–530.

Lavizzo-Mourey, R., and MacKenzie, E. "Cultural Competence—An Essential Hybrid for Delivering High Quality Care in the 1990s and Beyond." *Transactions of the American Clinical and Climatological Association,* 1995, *107,* 226–237.

Laws, A., and Patsalides, B. "Medical and Psychological Examination of Women Seeking Asylum: Documentation of Human Rights Abuses." *Journal of the American Medical Women's Association,* 1997, *52*(4), 185–187.

Lazarus, R. S., and Folkman, S. *Stress, Appraisal, and Coping.* New York: Springer, 1984.

Lecca, P., Quervalu, I., Nunes, J., and Gonzales, H. *Cultural Competency in Health, Social, and Human Services: Directions for the Twenty-First Century.* New York: Garland, 1998.

LeClere, F., Jensen, L., and Biddlecom, A. "Health Care Utilization, Family Context, and Adaptation Among Immigrants to the United States." *Journal of Health and Social Behavior,* 1994, *35,* 370–384.

Lee, E. "A Social Systems Approach to Assessment and Treatment for Chinese American Families." In M. McGoldrick, J. K. Pearce, and J. Giordano (eds.), *Ethnicity and Family Therapy* (pp. 527–551). New York: Guilford Press, 1982.

Lee, E. *Working with Asian Americans: A Guide for Clinicians.* New York: Guilford Press, 1997.

Lee, E., and Lu, F. "Assessment and Treatment of Asian American Survivors of Mass Violence." *Journal of Traumatic Stress,* 1989, *2*(1), 93–120.

Lee, E., and Lu, F. "Family Therapy with Southeast Asian Families." In M. P. Mirkin (ed.), *The Social and Political Context of Family Therapy* (pp. 331–354). Needham Heights, Mass.: Allyn & Bacon, 1990.

Lee, M. M. "Diet, Physical Activity and Body Size in Chinese." *Asia Pacific Journal of Clinical Nutrition,* 1994, *3,* 145–148.

Lee, M. M., and others. "Comparison of Dietary Habits, Physical Activity and Body Size Among Chinese in North America and China." *International Journal of Epidemiology,* 1994, *23,* 984–990.

Lee, R. D., and Nieman, D. C. "Counseling Theory and Technique." In *Nutritional Assessment.* Dubuque, Iowa: W. C. Brown, 1993.

Lee, S. "Neurasthenia and Chinese Psychiatry in the 1990s." *Journal of Psychosomatic Research,* 1994, *38,* 487–491.

Lee, S., and Wong, K. C. "Rethinking Neurasthenia: The Illness Concepts of Shenjing Shuairuo Among Chinese Undergraduates in Hong Kong." *Culture, Medicine and Psychiatry,* 1995, *19*(1), 91–111.

Leong, F., Wagner, N., and Tata, S. "Racial and Ethnic Variations in Help-Seeking Attitudes." In J. G. Ponterotto, J. M. Casas, L. A. Suzuki, and C. M. Alexander (eds.), *Handbook of Multicultural Counseling* (pp. 415–438). Thousand Oaks, Calif.: Sage, 1995.

Levy, C. "Prop. 187 Can Spread TB, Says Health Official." *Oakland* (California) *Tribune,* Nov. 29, 1994.

Liao, Y., and others. "Mortality from Coronary Heart Disease and Cardiovascular Disease Among Adult U.S. Hispanics: Findings from the National Health Interview Survey (1986 to 1994)." *Journal of the American College of Cardiology,* 1997, *30*(5), 1200–1205.

Lightfoot-Klein, H. *Prisoners of Ritual.* New York: Harrington Park Press, 1989.

Like, R., Steiner, P., and Rubel, A. "Recommended Core Curriculum Guidelines on Culturally Sensitive and Competent Health Care." *Family Medicine,* 1996, *27,* 291–297.

Lin, K. M. *"Hwa-byung:* A Korean Culture-Bound Syndrome?" *American Journal of Psychiatry,* 1983, *140*(1), 105–107.

Lin, K. M., Carter, W., and Kleinman, A. "An Exploration of Somatization Among Asian Refugees and Immigrants in Primary Care." *American Journal of Public Health,* 1985, *75,* 1080–1084.

Lin, K. M., Ihle, L., and Tazuma, L. "An Exploration of Somatization Among Asian Refugees in a Primary Care Clinic." *American Journal of Medicine,* 1985, *78,* 41–44.

Lin, K. M., Inui, T. S., Kleinman, A. M., and Womack, W. M. "Sociocultural Determinants of the Help-Seeking Behavior of Mental Illness." *Journal of Nervous and Mental Disease,* 1982, *170*(2), 78–85.

Lin, T. Y. "The Shaping of Chinese Psychiatry in the Context of Politics and Public Health." In T. Y. Lin and L. Eisenberg (eds.), *Mental Health Planning for One Billion People* (pp. 13–24). Vancouver: University of British Columbia Press, 1985.

Lin, T. Y. "Neurasthenia Revisited: Its Place in Modern Psychiatry." *Psychiatric Annuals,* 1992, *22*(4), 173–187.

Lindsay, R. "The Burden of Osteoporosis: Cost." *American Journal of Medicine,* 1995, *98*(Suppl. 2a), 9s–11s.

Lipowski, Z. J. "Somatization: The Concept and Its Clinical Application." *American Journal of Psychiatry,* 1988, *145,* 1358–1368.

Londero, M. T., and Damond, M. E. "Recent Immigrant Hispanics and HIV/AIDS Preventive Education: Program and Impact Evaluation That Works." Paper presented at the International Conference on AIDS in Yokohama, Japan. Abstract in the conference syllabus, 1996, *11,* 191 (abstract no. MO-D-1799).

Longworth, D. L., and Weller, P. F. "Hyperinfection Syndrome with Strongyloidiasis." *Current Clinical Topics in Infectious Diseases,* 1986, *7,* 1–26.

Loo, C., Tong, B., and True, R. "A Bitter Bean: Mental Health Status and Attitudes in Chinatown." *Journal of Community Psychology,* 1989, *17,* 283–296.

Looker, A. C., and others. "Calcium Intakes of Mexican Americans, Cubans, Puerto Ricans, Non-Hispanic Whites, and Non-Hispanic Blacks in the United States." *Journal of the American Dietetic Association,* 1993, *93,* 1274–1279.

Looker, A. C., and others. "Prevalence of Low Femoral Bone Density in Older U.S. Women from NHANES III." *Journal of Bone and Mineral Research,* 1995, *10,* 796–802.

Loue, S., and Oppenheim, S. "Immigration and HIV Infection: A Pilot Study." *AIDS Education and Prevention,* 1994, *6,* 74–80.

Luluquisen, E. M., Groessl, K. M., and Puttkammer, N. H. *The Health and Well-Being of Asian and Pacific Islander American Women.* Oakland, Calif.: Asians and Pacific Islanders for Reproductive Health, 1995.

Machizawa, S. "Neurasthenia in Japan." *Psychiatric Annuals,* 1992, *22*(4), 190–191.

MacKinnon, K. "Rape, Genocide, and Women's Human Rights." *Harvard Women's Law Journal,* 1994, *17*(5).

Maduro, R. "Curanderismo and Latino Views on Disease and Curing." *Western Journal of Medicine,* 1983, *139,* 868–874.

Magana, A., and Clark, N. "Examining a Paradox: Does Religiosity Contribute to Positive Birth Outcomes in Mexican American Populations?" *Health Education Quarterly*, 1995, *22*(1), 96–109.

Mahabir, D., and Gulliford, M. C. "Use of Medicinal Plants for Diabetes in Trinidad and Tobago." *Pan American Journal of Public Health*, 1997, *1*(3), 174–179.

Malgady, R., Rogler, G., and Constantino, G. "Ethnocultural and Linguistic Bias in Mental Health Evaluation of Hispanics." *American Psychologist*, 1987, *42*(3), 228–234.

Manfiletto, E. "Profit in Diversity." *Managed HealthCare*, July 1995, pp. 6–46.

Mann, J., Melnick, G., Bamezai, A., and Zwanziger, J. "Managing the Safety Net: Hospital Provision of Uncompensated Care in Response to Managed Care." In *Advances in Health Economics and Health Research* (Vol. 15, pp. 49–77). Greenwich, Conn.: JAI Press, 1995.

Marin, G. "Defining Culturally Appropriate Community Interventions: Hispanics as a Case Study." *Journal of Community Psychology*, 1993, *21*, 149–161.

Marin, G., Perez-Stable, F., and Marin, B. "Cigarette Smoking Among San Francisco Hispanics: The Role of Acculturation and Gender." *American Journal of Public Health*, 1989, *79*, 196–198.

Marin, L. "Identifying Immigrant Battered Women." In D. L. Jang, L. Marin, and G. Pendleton (eds.), *Domestic Violence in Immigrant and Refugee Communities: Asserting the Rights of Battered Women* (pp. 5–15). San Francisco: Family Violence Prevention Fund, 1997.

Markides, K., Levin, J., and Ray, L. "Determinants of Physician Utilization Among Mexican-Americans: A Three-Generations Study." *Medical Care*, 1985, *23*(3), 236–246.

Marotolli, R. A., Berkman, L. F., and Cooney, L. M. "Decline in Physical Function Following Hip Fracture." *Journal of the American Geriatric Society*, 1992, *40*, 861–866.

Marsella, A. J. "Depressive Experience and Disorder Across Cultures." In H. Triandis and J. Draguns (eds.), *Handbook of Cross-Cultural Psychology* (Vol. 6, pp. 237–290). Needham Heights, Mass.: Allyn & Bacon, 1979.

Marsella, A. J., Friedman, M. J., Gerrity, E. T., and Scurfield, R. M. (eds.). *Ethnocultural Aspects of Post-Traumatic Stress Disorder Issues, Research, and Clinical Applications*. Washington, D.C.: American Psychological Association, 1996.

Martin, L. M., Calle, E. E., Wingo, P. A., and Heath, C. W. "Comparison of Mammography and Pap Test Use from the 1987 and 1992 National Health Interview Surveys: Are We Closing the Gaps?" *American Journal of Preventive Medicine*, 1996, *12*, 82–90.

Martinez, N. "Diabetes and Minority Populations." *Nursing Clinics of North America*, 1993, *28*(1), 87–95.

Marx, J. L., and others. "Effects of California Proposition 187 on Ophthalmology Clinic Utilization at Inner-City Urban Hospitals." *Ophthalmology*, 1996, *10*, 847–851.

Massachusetts Department of Public Health. *The Office of Refugee and Immigrant Health: A Program Description*. Boston: Massachusetts Department of Public Health, 1995.

Mathiasen, S. S., and Lutzer, S. *The Survivors: Violations of Human Rights in Tibet—Healing in the Tibetan Exile Community*. Esbjereg, Denmark: Sudjysk Universistetscenter of Forfatterne, 1992.

Matsumoto, D., and others. "Cultural Differences in Attitudes, Values, and Beliefs About Osteoporosis in First and Second Generation Japanese-American Women." *Women and Health*, 1995, *23*(4), 39–56.

Matsuoka, J. "Differential Acculturation Among Vietnamese Refugees," *Social Work*, 1990, *35*(4), 341–345.

Matsuoka, J., Breaux, C., and Ryujin, D. "National Utilization of Mental Health Services by Asian Americans/Pacific Islanders." *Journal of Community Psychology*, 1997, *25*(2), 141–145.

Maxmen, J. S., and Ward, N. G. *Essential Psychopathology and Its Treatment*. (Rev. ed.) New York: Norton, 1995.

Maxwell, A. E., Bastani, R., and Warda, U. S. "Breast Cancer Screening and Related Attitudes Among Filipino-American Women." *Cancer Epidemiology, Biomarkers and Prevention*, 1997, *6*, 719–726.

Maxwell, A. E., Bastani, R., and Warda, U. S. "Mammography Utilization and Related Attitudes Among Korean-American Women." *Women and Health*, 1998, *27*(3), 89–107.

Mayeno, L., and Hirota, S. M. "Access to Health Care." In N.W.S. Zane, D. T. Takeuchi, and K.N.J. Young (eds.), *Confronting Critical Health Issues of Asian and Pacific Islander Americans* (pp. 347–375). Thousand Oaks, Calif.: Sage, 1994.

McAfee, R. "Physician's Role in the Fight Against Domestic Violence." *North Carolina Medical Journal*, 1994, *55*, 398–399.

McBride, A. "Mental Health Effects of Women's Multiple Roles." *American Psychologist*, 1990, *45*(3), 381–384.

McCaig, L., and Stussman, B. "National Hospital Ambulatory Medical Care Survey: 1996." Emergency Department Summary. *Advance Data*, Dec. 17, 1997, pp. 1–20.

McCall, M. A., and Sorbie, J. "Educating Physicians About Women's Health. Survey of Canadian Family Medicine Residency Programs." *Canadian Family Physician,* 1994, *40,* 900–905.

McCranie, E. W., Hyer, L. A., Boudewyns, P. A., and Woods, M. G. "Negative Parenting Behavior, Combat Exposure, and PTSD Symptom Severity, Test of a Person-Event Interaction Model." *Journal of Nervous and Mental Disease,* 1992, *180*(7), 431–438.

McLeer, S. V., and Anwar, R. "The Role of the Emergency Physician in the Prevention of Domestic Violence." *Annals of Emergency Medicine,* 1987, *16*(10).

McNally, R. J., and Saigh, P. A. "On the Distinction Between Traumatic Simple Phobia and Posttraumatic Stress Disorder." In J.R.T. Davidson and E. B. Foa (eds.), *Posttraumatic Stress Disorder: DSM IV and Beyond* (pp. 207–212). Washington, D.C.: American Psychiatric Press, 1993.

McPhee, S. J., and others. "Pathways to Early Cancer Detection for Vietnamese Women: Such Khoe La Vang! (Health Is Gold!)." *Health Education Quarterly,* 1996, *23*(suppl.), S60–S75.

McPhee, S. J., and others. "Barriers to Breast and Cervical Cancer Screening Among Vietnamese-American Women." *American Journal of Preventive Medicine,* 1997, *13,* 205–213.

Meleis, A. I., Lipson, J. G., and Paul, S. M. "Ethnicity and Health Among Five Middle Eastern Immigrant Groups." *Nursing Research,* 1992, *41*(2), 98–103.

Mghir, R., Freed, W., Raskin, A., and Katon, W. "Depression and Posttraumatic Stress Disorder Among a Community Based Sample of Adolescent and Young Adult Afghan Refugees." *Journal of Nervous and Mental Disease,* 1995, *183*(1), 24–30.

Michael, S., and others. "Meeting Immigrant Health Challenges: An Integrated Model in New York City." *Innovation,* 1993, *6*(1) 55–56.

Miller, J. B. "The Development of Women's Sense of Self." In J. V. Jordan and others (eds.), *Women's Growth in Connection* (pp. 11–26). New York: Guilford Press, 1991.

Millon-Underwood, S. "Educating for Sensitivity to Cultural Diversity." *Nurse Educator,* 1992, *17*(3), 7.

Minuchin, S. *Families and Family Therapy.* Cambridge, Mass.: Harvard University Press, 1974.

Mitchell, B. D., and others. "Diabetes and Coronary Heart Disease Risk in Mexican Americans." *Annals of Epidemiology,* 1992, *2,* 101–106.

Mo, G. M. "Peculiar Features of Mental Disorders in Guangdong Area." *Journal of Hong Kong College of Psychiatry,* 1992, *2,* 58–59.

Mollica, R. F., Caspi-Yavin, R. Y., and Bollini, P. "The Harvard Trauma Questionnaire: Validating a Cross Cultural Instrument for Measuring Torture Trauma, and Post-Traumatic Stress Disorder in Indochinese Refugees." *Journal of Nervous and Mental Disease,* 1992, *180,* 111–116.

Mollica, R. F., and others. "Indochinese Versions of the Hopkins Screening Instrument for Psychiatric Care of Refugees." *American Journal of Psychiatry,* 1987, *122*(4), 497–500.

Moore, L. J., and Boehnlein, J. K. "Posttraumatic Stress Disorder, Depression, and Somatic Symptoms in U. S. Mien Patients." *Journal of Nervous and Mental Disease,* 1991, *179*(12), 728–733.

Morakinyo, O. "A Psychophysiological Theory of a Psychiatric Illness (the *Brain Fag* Syndrome) Associated with Study Among Africans." *Journal of Nervous and Mental Disorders,* 1980, *168*(2), 84–89.

Morrison, J. "Childhood Sexual Histories of Women with Somatization Disorder." *American Journal of Psychiatry,* 1989, *146,* 239–241.

Morrow, L. "Immigrants, Like Those Who Came Before Them, the Newest Americans Bring a Spirit and an Energy That Preserve the Nation's Uniqueness." *Time Magazine,* July 8, 1985, p. 25.

Moscicki, E. K., Locke B. Z., Rae, D. S., and Boyd, J. H. "Depressive Symptoms Among Mexican Americans: The Hispanic Health and Nutrition Examination Survey." *American Journal of Epidemiology,* 1989, *130,* 348–360.

Moss, N., Baumeister, L., and Biewener, J. "Perspectives of Latina Immigrant Women on Proposition 187." *Journal of the American Women's Medical Association,* 1996, *51*(4), 161–165.

Moussa, H. *Storm and Sanctuary: The Journey of Ethiopian and Eritrean Women Refugees.* Dundes, Ontario, Canada: Artemis Enterprises, 1993.

Muecke, M. A. "In Search of Healers—Southeast Asian Refugees in the American Health Care System." *Western Journal of Medicine,* 1983, *139,* 835–840.

Mull, J. D., and Mull, D. S. "A Visit with a Curandero." *Western Journal of Medicine,* 1983, *139,* 730–736.

Munoz, R., and Ying. Y. *The Prevention of Depression: Research and Practice.* Baltimore: Johns Hopkins University Press, 1993.

Murase, K., Egawa, J., and Tashima, N. "Alternative Mental Health Service Models in Asian/Pacific Communities." In T. Owan (ed.), *Southeast Asian Mental Health: Treatment, Prevention, Services, Training, and Research* (pp. 229–259). Washington, D.C.: U.S. Department of Health and Human Services, 1985.

Murillo-Rohde, I. "Health Care for the Hispanic Patient." *Critical Care Update,* May 1980, pp. 29–36.

Nakyonyi, M. M. "HIV/AIDS Education Participation by the African Community." *Canadian Journal of Public Health,* 1993, *84*(Suppl. 1), S19–23.

Narayan, U. "'Male-Order' Brides: Immigrant Women, Domestic Violence and Immigration Law." *Hypatia,* 1997, *10*(1), 104–119.

National Asian Women's Health Organization. *Executive Summary: A National Tobacco-Use Survey Among Asian Americans.* San Francisco: National Asian Women's Health Organization, 1998.

National Association of County Health Officials. *NACHO Multicultural Health Project Recommendations and Case Study Reports.* Washington, D.C.: National Association of County Health Officials, 1992.

National Association of Public Hospitals. *Preserving America's Safety Net Health Systems: A White Paper of NAPH.* Washington, D.C.: National Association of Public Hospitals, 1997a.

National Association of Public Hospitals. *Understanding the Welfare and Illegal Immigration Reform Acts of 1996.* Washington, D.C.: National Association of Public Hospitals and Health Systems, 1997b.

National Center for Health Statistics. *Health, United States: 1996–7.* Hyattsville, Md.: U.S. Department of Health and Human Services, 1997.

National Coalition of Hispanic Health and Human Services Organizations. *Delivering Preventive Health Care to Hispanics: A Manual for Providers.* Washington, D.C.: National Coalition of Hispanic Health and Human Services Organizations, 1990.

National Coalition of Hispanic Health and Human Services Organizations. "Meeting the Health Promotion Needs of Hispanic Communities." *American Journal of Health Promotion,* 1995, *9*(4), 300–311.

National High Blood Pressure Education Program. *The Sixth Report of the Joint National Committee on Prevention, Detection, Evaluation and Treatment of High Blood Pressure.* NIH No 98–4080. Bethesda, Md.: U.S. Department of Health and Human Services, 1997.

National Institutes of Health. *Heart Memo: Taking It to the Streets: Community-Based Interventions.* Bethesda, Md.: National Heart, Lung, and Blood Institute, 1997.

National Osteoporosis Foundation. Web Site. [http://www.nof.org]. 1998.

National Public Health and Hospital Institute. *Interpretation and Translation Services in Health Care: A Survey of U.S. Public and Private Teaching Hospitals.* Washington, D.C.: National Public Health and Hospital Institute, Mar. 1995a.

National Public Health and Hospital Institute. *Urban Social Health.* Washington, D.C.: National Public Health and Hospital Institute, 1995b.

National Research Council. *Recommended Dietary Allowances.* Washington, D.C.: National Academy Press, 1989.

Nelson, K. R., Bui, H., and Samet, J. H. "Screening in Special Populations: A "Case Study" of Recent Vietnamese Immigrants." *American Journal of Medicine,* 1997, *102,* 435–440.

New York City Department of City Planning. *The Newest New Yorkers 1990–1994.* New York: New York City Department of City Planning, 1996.

Ngor, H. S., with Warner, R. *A Cambodian Odyssey.* New York: Macmillan, 1987.

Nguyen, M. D. "Culture Shock—A Review of Vietnamese Culture and Its Concepts of Health and Disease." *Western Journal of Medicine,* 1985, *142,* 409–412.

Noble, K. B. "Attacks Against Asian-Americans Are Rising." *New York Times,* Dec. 13, 1995.

Norton, S. A., Kenney, G. M., and Ellwood, M. R. "Medicaid Coverage of Maternity Care for Aliens in California." *Family Planning Perspectives,* 1996, *28*(3), 108–12.

O'Donohue, W., and Elliot, A. "The Current Status of Post-Traumatic Stress Disorder as a Diagnostic Category: Problems and Proposals." *Journal of Traumatic Stress,* 1992, *5*(3), 421–439.

O'Hare, W. P. "America's Minorities—The Demographics of Diversity." *Population Bulletin,* 1992, *47*(4), 1–47.

Olson, L., and others. "Increasing Emergency Physician Recognition of Domestic Violence." *Annals of Emergency Medicine,* 1996, *27*(6), 741–746.

Olujic, M. "The Croatian War Experience." In C. Nordstrom and A. Robben (eds.), *Fieldwork Under Fire: Contemporary Studies of Violence and Survival.* Berkeley: University of California Press, 1995.

Oquendo, M. "Differential Diagnosis of Ataque de Nervios." *American Journal of Orthopsychiatry,* 1994, *65*(1), 60–65.

Orloff, L. E., and Kelly, N. "A Look at the Violence Against Women Act and Gender-Related Political Asylum." *Violence Against Women,* 1995, *1*(4), 380–400.

Osteoporosis and Related Bone Diseases National Resource Center. Web Site. [http://www.osteo.org]. 1998.

Pak, A. W., Dion, K. L., and Dion, K. K. "Correlates of Self-Confidence with English Among Chinese Students in Toronto." *Canadian Journal of Behavioural Science,* 1985, *17*(4), 369–378.

Pane, G. A., Farner, M. C., and Salness, K. A. "Health Care Access Problems of Medically Indigent Walk-in Patients." *Annals of Emergency Medicine,* 1991, *20*(7), 730–733.

Pappas, G., and others. "The Increasing Disparity in Mortality Between Socioeconomic Groups in the U.S." *New England Journal of Medicine,* 1993, *329*(2), 103–109.

Parrillo, V. N. "The Immigrant Family: Securing the American Dream." *Journal of Comparative Family Studies,* 1991, 22(2), 131–145.

Parson, E. R. "Ethnicity and Traumatic Stress: The Intersecting Point in Psychotherapy." In E. R. Parson (ed.), *Trauma and Its Wake.* Vol. 1: *The Study and Treatment of Post-Traumatic Stress Disorder* (pp. 314–377). New York: Brunner/Mazel, 1985.

Pavich, E. G. "A Chicana Perspective on Mexican Culture and Sexuality." *Journal of Social Work and Human Sexuality,* 1986, *4,* 47–65.

Pawliuk, N., and others. "Acculturation Style and Psychological Functioning in Children of Immigrants." *American Journal of Orthopsychiatry,* 1996, *66*(1), 111–121.

Payne, R. L., and Jones, J. G. "Measurement and Methodological Issues in Social Support." In S. N. Kasl (ed.), *Stress and Health: Issues in Research Methodology* (pp. 167–205). New York: Wiley, 1987.

Pereira, W. *Inhuman Rights: The Western System and Global Human Rights Abuse.* Goa, India: Other India Press, 1997.

Perez-Stable, E. J., Otero-Sabogal, R., Sabogal, F., and Napoles-Springer, A. "Pathways to Early Cancer Detection for Latinas: En Accion Contra el Cancer." *Health Education Quarterly,* 1996, *23*(Suppl.), S41–S59.

Perez-Stable, E. J., VanOss Marin, B., and Marin, G. "A Comprehensive Smoking Cessation Program for the San Francisco Bay Area Latino Community: Programo Latino Para Dejar de Fumar." *American Journal of Health Promotion,* 1993, 7(6), 430–442, 475.

Perkins, C. I., Morris, C. R., and Wright, W. E. *Cancer Incidence and Mortality in California by Race/Ethnicity, 1988–1993.* Sacramento: California Department of Health Services, Cancer Surveillance Section, Mar. 1996.

Perkins, C. I., Morris, C. R., Wright, W. E., and Young, J. L. *Cancer Incidence and Mortality in California by Detailed Race/Ethnicity, 1988–1992.* Sacramento: California Department of Health Services, Cancer Surveillance Section, Apr. 1995.

*Personal Responsibility and Work Opportunity Reconciliation Act.* Public Law 104–193, 1996.

Peters, K., and others. "Births and Deaths: United States, July 1995–June 1996." *Monthly Vital Statistics Report,* 1997, *45*(10, suppl. 2).

Pickwell, S. "Positive PPD and Chemoprophylaxis for Tuberculosis Infection." *American Family Physician,* 1995, *51*(8), 1929–1934.

Pimental, B. "Culture Clash Ends in Death of Five-Week-Old: Laotian Infant Had Been in Foster Care After Abuse Charge." *San Francisco Chronicle,* Feb. 12, 1994.

Pitman, R. K. "Biological Findings in Posttraumatic Stress Disorder: Implications for DSM IV Classification." In J.R.T. Davidson and E. B. Foa (eds.), *Posttraumatic Stress Disorder: DSM IV and Beyond* (pp. 173–189). Washington, D.C.: American Psychiatric Press, 1993.

Poirier, L. "The Importance of Screening for Domestic Violence in All Women." *Nurse Practitioner,* 1997, *22*(5), 105–108.

Polednak, A. "Cardiovascular Diseases." In *Racial and Ethnic Differences in Disease.* New York: Oxford University Press, 1989.

Pongpaew, P., and others. "Parasitic Infection and Socio-Demographic Characteristics of Urban Construction Site Workers." *Southeast Asian Journal of Tropical Medicine and Public Health,* 1993, *24,* 573–576.

Portes, A., and Rumbaut, R. G. *Immigrant America.* Berkeley: University of California Press, 1990.

Poss, J. E., and Rengel, R. "A Tuberculosis Screening and Treatment Program for Migrant Farmworker Families." *Journal of Health Care for the Poor and Underserved,* 1997, *8*(2), 133–140.

Preciado, J., and Henry, M. "Linguistic Barriers to Health Education and Services." In J. G. Garcia and M. C. Zea (eds.), *Psychological Interventions and Research with Latino Populations* (pp. 235–254). Needham Heights, Mass.: Allyn & Bacon, 1997.

Pressman, A., and Adams, A. *Clinical Assessment of Nutrition Status: A Working Manual.* Baltimore: Williams and Wilkins, 1990.

Prochaska, J., DiClemente, C., and Norcross, J. "In Search of How People Change: Applications to Addictive Behaviors." *American Psychologist,* 1992, *47*(9), 1102–1114.

Quillian, J. P. "Screening for Spousal or Partner Abuse in a Community Health Setting." *Journal of the American Academy of Nurse Practitioners,* 1996, *8*(4), 155–160.

Radloff, L. S. "The CES-D Scale: A Self-Report Depression Scale for Research in the General Population." *Applied Psychological Measurement,* 1977, *1,* 385–401.

Raisz, L. G. "The Osteoporosis Revolution." *Annals of Internal Medicine,* 1997, *126,* 458–462.

Ramakrishna, J., and Weiss, M. G. "Health, Illness and Migration: East Indians in the United States." *Western Journal of Medicine,* 1992, *157*(3), 265–270.

Ranck, J. "The Politics of Memory and Justice in Post-Genocide Rwanda." Unpublished doctoral dissertation, University of California at Berkeley, 1998.

Rask, K., Williams, M., Parker, R., and McNagny, S. "Obstacles Predicting Lack of a Regular Provider and Delays in Seeking Care for Patients at an Urban Public Hospital." *Journal of the American Medical Association,* 1994, *271*(24), 1931–1933.

Recker, R., and others. "Bone Gain in Young Adult Women." *Journal of the American Medical Association,* 1992, *268,* 2403–2408.

Reeves, K. "Hispanic Utilization of an Ethnic Mental Health Clinic." *Journal of Psychosocial Nursing,* 1986, *24,* 23–26.

Reinert, B. "The Healthcare Beliefs and Values of Mexican-Americans." *Home Healthcare Nurse,* 1986, *4*(5), 23, 26–27, 30–31.

Reinli, K., and Block, G. "Phytoestrogen Content of Foods—A Compendium of Literature Values." *Nutrition and Cancer,* 1996, *26*(2), 123–148.

*Report of the Secretary's Task Force on Black and Minority Health, 1985.* Washington, D.C.: U.S. Government Printing Office, 1985.

Richards, J. "Emergency Medicine in Vietnam." *Annals of Emergency Medicine,* 1997, *29*(4), 543–548.

Richman, J. "State Loses Out on Court Ruling." *Oakland Tribune,* Aug. 13, 1998.

Riddick, S. "A Community Approach to Training Medical Interpreters." Paper presented at American Public Health Association Annual Meeting, New York, Oct. 1990.

Riddick, S. "Language Barriers in Hospital Care: Strategies for Change." Paper presented at Language Rights Conference of Asian–Pacific American Legal Center of Southern California, Los Angeles, Apr. 1991.

Rivera-Arzola, M., and Ramos-Grenier, J. "Anger, *Ataques de Nervios,* and *La Mujer Puertorriquena:* Sociocultural Considerations and Treatment Implications." In J. G. Garcia and M. C. Zea (eds.), *Psychological Interventions and Research with Latino Populations* (pp. 125–141). Needham Heights, Mass.: Allyn & Bacon, 1997.

Robins, L. N., Helzer, J. E., Croughan, J. L., and Ratcliff, K. S. "National Institute of Mental Health Diagnostic Interview Schedule: Its History, Characteristics and Validity." *Archives of General Psychiatry,* 1981, *38,* 381–389.

Robins, L. N., Wing, J., Wittchen, H. U., and Helzer, J. E. "The Composite International Diagnostic Interview: An Epidemiologic Instrument Suitable for Use in Conjunction with Different Diagnostic Systems and in Different Cultures." *Archives of General Psychiatry,* 1988, *45,* 1069–1077.

Rogler, L. H., Malgady, R. G., Constantino, G., and Blumenthal, R. "What Do Culturally Sensitive Mental Health Services Mean? The Case of Hispanics." *American Psychologist,* 1987, *42,* 565–570.

Romero-Gwynn, E. "Obesity Increased Among Acculturated Mexican Americans." Paper presented at Minority Health Issues for an Emerging Majority, the Fourth National Forum on Cardiovascular Health, Pulmonary Disorders, and Blood Resources, June 26–27, 1992.

Rosaldo, R. *Culture and Truth: The Remaking of Social Analysis.* Boston: Beacon Press, 1989.

Rosenberg, M., Stark, E., and Zahn, M. "Interpersonal Violence: Homicide and Spouse Abuse. In J. M. Last (ed.), *Public Health and Preventive Medicine.* (12th ed.) Norwalk, Conn.: Appleton-Century-Crofts, 1986.

Rosenstock, I., Strecher, V., and Becker, M. "Social Learning Theory and the 'Health' Belief Model." *Health Education Quarterly,* 1988, *15*(2), 175–183.

Ross, P. D. "Osteoporosis: Frequency, Consequences, and Risk Factors." *Archives of Internal Medicine,* 1996, *156,* 1399–1411.

Rossiter, J. C. "Attitudes of Vietnamese Women to Baby Feeding Practices Before and After Immigration to Sydney, Australia." *Midwifery,* 1992, *8*(3), 103–12.

Rousseau, C., Drapeau, A., and Corin, E. "School Performance and Emotional Problems in Refugee Children." *American Journal of Orthopsychiatry,* 1996, *66*(2), 239–251.

Rozee, P., and Van Boemel, G. "The Psychological Effects of War Trauma and Abuse on Older Cambodian Refugee Women." *Women and Therapy,* 1990, *8*(4), 23–46.

Ruiz, P. "Access to Health Care for Uninsured Hispanics: Policy Recommendations." *Hospital and Community Psychiatry,* 1993, *44*(10), 958–962.

Rumbaut, R., and Weeks, J. R. "Unraveling a Public Health Enigma: Why Do Immigrants Experience Superior Health Outcomes?" Research in the *Sociology of Health Care,* 1989.

Salgado de Snyder, V. N. "Factors Associated with Acculturative Stress and Depressive Symptomatology Among Married Mexican Immigrant Women." *Psychology of Women Quarterly,* 1987, *11*(4), 475–488.

Salladay, R. "New Fears over 187's Vise Grip." *Oakland Tribune,* Nov. 16, 1994.

*San Francisco Examiner.* Dec. 16, 1997, pp. A–1, A–8.

Sandler, S. G., and Fang, C. "Preventing Transfusion-Transmitted Infections: Issues Related to Migrating Populations and Increasing World Travel." *Haematologia,* 1991, *24,* 197–210.

Sanjur, D. "Ethnicity and Food Habits." In *Social and Cultural Perspectives in Nutrition*. Englewood Cliffs, N.J.: Prentice Hall, 1982.

Sanjur, D. *Hispanic Food Ways: Nutrition and Health*. Needham Heights, Mass.: Allyn & Bacon, 1995.

Sarason, I. G., Pierce, G. R., and Sarason, B. R. "General and Specific Perceptions of Social Support." In R. Avison and I. H. Gotlib (eds.), *Stress and Mental Health: Contemporary Issues and Prospects for the Future* (pp. 151–177). New York: Plenum Press, 1994.

Saunders, S. "Applicant's Experience of the Process of Seeking Therapy." *Psychotherapy*, 1993, *30*(4), 554–564.

Schauffler, H., and others. *The State of Health Insurance in California*. Los Angeles: Health Insurance Policy Program, Center for Health Policy Research, University of California, 1998.

Schoenbaum, M., and Waidmann, T. "Race, Socioeconomic Status, and Health: Accounting for Race Differences in Health." *Journal of Gerontology*, 1997, *52B*, 61–73.

Schornstein, S. L. *Domestic Violence: A Primer for Health Care Professionals*. Thousand Oaks, Calif.: Sage, 1997.

Schultz, S. L. "How Southeast-Asian Refugees in California Adapt to Unfamiliar Health Care Practices." *Health Social Work*, 1982, *7*, 148–156.

Schwartz, A., Eilenberg, J., and Thompson Fullilove, M. "Gloria's Despair: Struggling Against the Odds." *American Journal of Psychiatry*, 1996, *153*(10), 1334–1338.

Scribner, R., and Dwyer, J. "Acculturation and Low Birthweight Among Latinos in the Hispanic HHANES." *American Journal of Public Health*, 1989, *79*, 1263–1267.

Segura, D. "Chicanas in White-Collar Jobs: 'You Have to Prove Yourself More.'" *Sociological Perspectives*, 1992, *35*(1), 163–182.

Shaw, E. "Female Circumcision: What Kind of Maternity Care Do Circumcised Women Need and Can United States Caregivers Provide It?" *American Journal of Nursing*, 1985, *85*(6), 684–687.

Shaw, G., Velie, E., and Wasserman, C. "Risk for Neural Tube Defect–Affected Pregnancies Among Women of Mexican Descent and White Women in California." *American Journal of Public Health*, 1997, *87*(9), 1467–1471.

Shepherd, J. "Post-Traumatic Stress Disorder in Vietnamese Women." In E. Cole, O. M. Espin, and E. Rothblum (eds.), *Refugee Women and Their Mental Health: Shattered Societies, Shattered Lives* (pp. 281–296). Binghamton, N.Y.: Haworth Press, 1992a.

Shepherd, J. "Post-Traumatic Stress Disorder in Vietnamese Women." *Women and Therapy*, 1992b, *13*(1,2), 281–296.

Shepherd, J., and Faust, S. "Refugee Healthcare and the Problem of Suffering." *Bioethics Forum,* 1993, *9*(3), 3–7.

Sheran, M., and others. "Undocumented Immigrants with HIV Infection in New York City: A Program Report." Paper presented at the International Conference on AIDS. Abstract in the conference syllabus, 1994, *10,* 241 (abstract no. PCO327).

Shils, M. E., and Young, V. R. (eds.). *Modern Nutrition in Health and Disease.* (7th ed.) Philadelphia: Lea and Febiger, 1998.

Shimada, J., Jackson, J. C., Goldstein, E., and Buchwald, D. "Strong Medicine: Cambodian Views of Medicine and Medical Compliance." *Journal of General Internal Medicine,* 1995, *10*(7), 369–374.

Sieng, S., and Thompson, J. "Traces of Khmer Women's Imaginary: Finding Our Way in the West." *Women and Therapy,* 1992, *13*(1–2), 129–139.

Silverman, J., Torres, A., and Forrest, J. D. "Barriers to Contraceptive Services." *Family Planning Perspectives,* 1987, *19*(3), 94–102.

Simon, G. E., and VonKorff, M. "Somatization and Psychiatric Disorder in the NIMH Epidemiological Catchment Area Study." *American Journal of Psychiatry,* 1991, *148,* 1494–1500.

Simoni, J., and others. "Women's Self-Disclosure of HIV Infection: Rates, Reasons, and Reactions." *Journal of Consulting and Clinical Psychology,* 1995, *63*(3), 474–478.

Skaer, T. L., Robison, L. M., Sclar, D. A., and Harding, G. H. "Financial Incentive and the Use of Mammography Among Hispanic Migrants to the United States." *Health Care for Women International,* 1996, *17,* 281–291.

Slutsker, L., and others. "Malaria in East African Refugees Resettling to the United States: Development of Strategies to Reduce the Risk of Imported Malaria." *Journal of Infectious Disease,* 1995, *171,* 489–493.

Sluzki, C. "Migration and Family Conflict." *Family Process,* 1979, *18*(4), 379–390.

Sluzki, C. "Disruption and Reconstruction of Networks Following Migration/Relocation." *Family Systems Medicine,* 1992, *10*(4), 359–363.

Smith, K., and McGraw, S. "Smoking Behavior of Puerto Rican Women: Evidence from Caretakers of Adolescents in Two Urban Areas." *Hispanic Journal of Behavioral Sciences,* 1993, *15*(1), 140–149.

Smith-Fawzi, M. C., and others. "The Validity of Posttraumatic Stress Disorder Among Vietnamese Refugees." *Journal of Traumatic Stress,* 1997, *10*(1), 101–108.

Snow, L. "Folk Medical Beliefs and Their Implications for Care of Patients." *Annals of Internal Medicine,* 1972, *81,* 82–96.

Snowden, L. R. "Ethnic Minority Populations and Mental Health Outcomes." In D. M. Steinwachs, L. M. Flynn, G. S. Norquist, and E. A. Skinner (eds.), *Using Client Outcomes Information to Improve Mental Health and Substance Abuse Treatment* (pp. 79–87). New Directions for Mental Health Services, no. 71. San Francisco: Jossey-Bass, 1996.

Snowden, L. R., and Hu, T. "Ethnic Differences in Mental Health Service Use Among the Severely Mentally Ill." *Journal of Community Psychology,* 1997, *25*(3), 235–247.

Solis, J., Marks, G., Garcia, M., and Shelton, D. "Acculturation, Access to Care, and Use of Preventive Services by Hispanics: Findings from HHANES, 1982–1984." *American Journal of Public Health,* 1990, *80*(Suppl.), 11–19.

Song-Kim, Y. I. "Battered Korean Women in Urban United States." In S. M. Furuto and others (eds.), *Social Work Practice with Asian Americans* (pp. 213–226). Thousand Oaks, Calif.: Sage, 1992.

Soskolne, V., and Shtarkshall, R. A. "Essentials of Cross-Cultural Cooperation in Developing Preventive Programs in Multi-Cultural Settings." Paper presented at the International Conference on AIDS. Abstract in the conference syllabus, 1994, *10,* 424 (abstract no. PDO306).

Spetz, J., and others. *The Effect of Proposition 187 on the Use of Prenatal Care by Foreign-Born Mothers in California.* San Francisco: Public Policy Institute of California, 1997.

Spielvogel, A., Dickstein, L., and Robinson, G. "A Psychiatric Residency Curriculum About Gender and Women's Issues." *Academic Psychiatry,* 1995, *19,* 187–201.

Spizzichino, L., and others. "Immigrants and HIV Infection: The Role of Counselling." Paper presented at the International Conference on AIDS in Yokohama, Japan. Abstract in the conference syllabus, 1996, *11,* 413 (abstract no. TU-D-2903).

Stark, E., Flitcraft, A., and Frazier, W. "Medicine and Patriarchal Violence." *International Journal of Health Services,* 1979, *9,* 461–493.

Starrett, R., and others. "The Role of Environmental Awareness and Support Networks in Hispanic Elderly Persons' Use of Formal Social Services." *Journal of Community Psychology,* 1990, *11,* 218–225.

Stein, T. "A Curriculum for Learning in Psychiatric Residencies About Homosexuality, Gay Men and Lesbians." *Academic Psychiatry,* 1994, 18, 59–70.

Stellman, S. D. "Proportional Mortality Rates Among Korean Immigrants to New York City, 1986–1990." *Yonsei Medical Journal,* 1996, *37,* 31–37.

Stiglmayer, A. (ed.) *Mass Rape: The War Against Women in Bosnia-Herzegovina.* Lincoln: University of Nebraska Press, 1994.

Straus, M., and Gelles, R. "Violence in American Families: How Much Is There and Why Does It Occur?" In E. W. Nunnally, C. S. Chilman, and F. M. Cox (eds.), *Troubled Relationships. Families in Trouble Series* (pp. 141–162). Thousand Oaks, Calif.: Sage, 1988.

Straus, S. E. "The Chronic Mononucleosis Syndrome." *Journal of Infectious Disease,* 1988, *157,* 405–412.

Suarez, L. "Pap Smear and Mammogram Screening in Mexican-American Women: The Effects of Acculturation." *American Journal of Public Health,* 1994, *84,* 742–746.

Suarez, L., Roche, R. I., Nichols, D., and Simpson, D. M. "Knowledge, Behavior, and Fears Concerning Breast and Cervical Cancer Among Older Low-Income Mexican-American Women." *American Journal of Preventive Medicine,* 1997, *13,* 137–142.

Sue, S., Fujino, D., Hu, L., and Takeuchi, D. "Community Mental Health Services for Ethnic Minority Groups: A Test of the Cultural Responsiveness Hypothesis." *Journal of Consulting and Clinical Psychology,* 1991, *59*(4), 533–540.

Sue, S., and Sue, D. *Counseling the Culturally Different: Theory and Practice.* (2nd ed.) New York: Wiley, 1990.

Sue, S., and Zane, N. "The Role of Culture and Cultural Techniques in Psychotherapy: A Critique and Reformulation." *American Psychologist,* 1987, *42*(1), 37–45.

Sue, S., Zane, N., and Young, K. "Research with Culturally Diverse Populations." In A. Bergin and S. Garfield (eds.), *Handbook of Psychotherapy and Behavior Change* (pp. 783–817). New York: Wiley, 1994.

Surrey, J. L. "The Self in Relation: A Theory of Women's Development." In J. V. Jordan and others (eds.), *Women's Growth in Connection* (pp. 51–66). New York: Guilford Press, 1991.

Susskind, Y. "Demanding Justice: Rape and Reconciliation in Rwanda." *MADRE,* 1997–1998, *13*(2), 6–8.

Szapocznik, J., and others. "Bicultural Effectiveness Training: A Treatment Intervention for Enhancing Intercultural Adjustment in Cuban American Families." *Hispanic Journal of Behavioral Sciences,* 1984, *6*(4), 317–344.

Szapocznik, J., and others. "Family Effectiveness Training: An Intervention to Prevent Drug Abuse and Problem Behaviors in Hispanic Adolescents." *Hispanic Journal of Behavioral Sciences,* 1989, *11*(1), 4–27.

Szasz, T., and Hollender, M. "A Contribution to the Philosophy of Medicine: Basic Models of the Doctor-Patient Relationship." *Archives of Internal Medicine,* 1956, *24,* 585–592.

Takagi, T. "Women of Color and Violence Against Women." In C. Moliner (ed.), *Violence Against Women Supplement* (pp. 51–56). St. Paul,

Minn.: National Network of Women's Funds and Foundations/Corporate Philanthropy, 1991.

Takeuchi, D., Wang, Y. X., and Chun, C.-A. *Stress-Health Relationships in Chinese Americans: Testing Acculturative Differences.* Poster session presented at the Eighth Annual Convention of the American Psychological Society, Aug. 1996.

Terry, R. D. *Introductory Community Nutrition.* Dubuque, Iowa: William C. Brown, 1993.

Thiagarajan, S. *Barnga: A Simulation Game of Cultural Clashes.* Yarmouth, Me.: Intercultural Press, 1990.

Thomas, T. N. "Acculturative Stress in the Adjustment of Immigrant Families." *Journal of Social Distress and the Homeless,* 1995, *4*(2), 131–142.

Thompson, J. "A Curriculum for Learning About American Indians and Alaska Natives in Psychiatry Residency Training." *Academic Psychiatry,* 1996, *20,* 5–14.

Tien, L. "Southeast Asian American Refugee Women." In L. Comas-Diaz and B. Greene (eds.), *Women of Color: Integrating Ethnic and Gender Identities in Psychotherapy* (pp. 479–503). New York: Guilford Press, 1994.

Tobias, J. H., Cook, D. G., Chambers, T. J., and Dalzell, N. "A Comparison of Bone Mineral Density Between Caucasian, Asian, and Afro-Caribbean Women." *Clinical Science,* 1994, *87,* 587–591.

Torres-Matrullo, C. "Acculturation and Psychopathology Among Puerto Rican Women in Mainland United States." *American Journal of Orthopsychiatry,* 1976, *46*(4), 710–719.

Tosomeen, A. H., Marquez, M. A., Panser, L. A., and Kottke, T. E. "Developing Preventive Health Programs for Recent Immigrants." *Minnesota Medicine,* 1996, *79,* 46–48.

Toubia, N. "Female Circumcision as a Public Health Issue." *New England Journal of Medicine, 331* (11), 712–716.

Tracy, L. "An Integrative Model of Traumatic Stress." Unpublished paper. Berkeley: School of Social Welfare, University of California, 1997.

Tracy, L. "Tradition and Change Among Tibetan Youth and Families Living in Exile." Paper presented at the Annual Conference of the Western Psychological Association. Albuquerque, N.M., Apr. 16, 1998.

Tran, T. V. "Psychological Traumas and Depression in a Sample of Vietnamese People in the United States." *Health and Social Work,* 1995, *18*(3), 184–194.

Trevino, F. M., and Moss, A. *Health Insurance Coverage and Physician Visits Among Hispanics and Non-Hispanics.* Hyattsville, Md.: National Center for Health Statistics, 1983.

Triandis, H. C., and others. "Individualism and Collectivism: Cross-Cultural Perspectives on Self-Intergroup Relationships." *Journal of Personality and Social Psychology,* 1988, *54*(2), 323–338.

True, R. H. "Psychotherapeutic Issues with Asian American Women." *Sex Roles,* 1990, *22*(7), 477–486.

True, R. H., and Guillermo, T. "Asian/Pacific Islander American Women." In M. Bayne-Smith (ed.), *Race, Gender, and Health* (pp. 94–120). Thousand Oaks, Calif.: Sage, 1996.

Truman, B. I., Wing, J. S., and Keenan, N. L. "Asians and Pacific Islanders." In U.S. Department of Health and Human Services, *Chronic Disease in Minority Populations.* Atlanta, Ga.: Centers for Disease Control and Prevention, 1994.

Truong, D. H., and others. "Tuberculosis Among Tibetan Immigrants from India and Nepal in Minnesota, 1992–1995." *Journal of the American Medical Association,* 1997, *277,* 735–738.

Tseng, W. S., and Hsu, J. *Culture and Family: Problems and Therapy.* New York: Haworth Press, 1991.

Tucker, M. E. "Separating Somatization from Depression: Acculturation Key in Hispanic Women." *Clinical Psychiatry News,* 1997, *25,* 17.

Tung, M.P.M. "Symbolic Meanings of the Body in Chinese Culture and 'Somatization.'" *Culture, Medicine, and Psychiatry,* 1994, *18,* 483–492.

Tyrance, P., Himmelstein, D., and Woolhandler, S. "U.S. Emergency Department Costs: No Emergency." *American Journal of Public Health,* 1997, *86*(11), 1527–1531.

Uba, L. "Meeting the Mental Health Needs of Asian Americans: Mainstream or Segregated Services." *Professional Psychology,* 1982, *13,* 215–222.

Uba, L. *Asian Americans: Personality Patterns, Identity, and Mental Health.* New York: Guilford Press, 1994.

U.S. Bureau of the Census. *Statistical Abstract of the United States, 1990 Census.* (113th ed.) Washington, D.C.: U.S. Government Printing Office, 1993.

U.S. Bureau of the Census. *The Earnings Ladder: Who's at the Bottom? Who's at the Top?* Washington, D.C.: Department of Commerce, 1994.

U.S. Bureau of the Census. *The Nation's Asian and Pacific Islander Population—1994.* Washington, D.C.: Department of Commerce, 1995.

U.S. Bureau of Population, Refugees, and Migration. *U.S. Policy Initiatives Related to Refugee Women.* Washington, D.C.: U.S. Government Printing Office, 1997.

U.S. Conference of Mayors. *Status Report on Hunger and Homelessness in America's Cities: 1996*. Washington, D.C.: U.S. Government Printing Office, 1996.

U.S. Conference of Mayors and U.S. Conference of Local Health Officers. *Language and Culture in Health Care/Coping with Linguistic and Cultural Differences: Challenges to Local Health Departments*. Washington, D.C.: U.S. Conference of Mayors and U.S. Conference of Local Health Officers, 1993.

U.S. Congress. House of Representatives. *Access to Emergency Medical Services Act of 1997*. 105th Cong., H.R. 815, 1997a.

U.S. Congress. House of Representatives. 105th Cong., H.R. 931 IH (companion S.B. 392), 1997b. "To provide an exception to the restriction on eligibility for public benefits for certain legal aliens."

U.S. Congress. House of Representatives. *Patients' Bill of Rights*. 105th Cong., H.R. 3605, 1998.

U.S. Congress. Office of Technology Assessment. *Does Health Insurance Make a Difference?* Washington, D.C.: U.S. Government Printing Office, 1992.

U.S. Congress. Office of Technology Assessment. *Hip Fracture Outcomes in People Age 50 and Over—Background Paper*. Washington, D.C.: U.S. Government Printing Office, 1994.

U.S. Department of Agriculture. American Nutrition Information Service. *Composition of Foods: Raw, Processed, Prepared*. USDA Agriculture Handbook no. 8. Washington, D.C.: U.S. Government Printing Office, 1976–1987.

U.S. Department of Agriculture. *The Food Guide Pyramid*. Home and Garden Bulletin, no. 252. Hyattsville, Md.: U.S. Department of Agriculture, 1992.

U.S. Department of Health and Human Services. *Healthy People 2000: National Health Promotion and Disease Prevention Objectives*. Washington, D.C.: U.S. Government Printing Office, 1990.

U.S. Department of Health and Human Services. "Diabetes and Chronic Disabling Conditions." *Healthy People Progress Review*. Washington, D.C.: U.S. Government Printing Office, 1996.

U.S. Department of Health and Human Services. Public Health Service. *Healthy People Progress Review: Hispanic Americans*. Washington, D.C.: U.S. Government Printing Office, 1997.

U.S. Department of Justice. *Violence Against Women: Estimates from the Redesigned Survey*. National Crime Victimization Survey. Washington, D.C.: Office of Justice Programs, 1995.

U.S. Department of Justice. Immigration and Naturalization Service. *Statistical Yearbook of the Immigration and Naturalization Service, 1996*. Washington, D.C.: U.S. Government Printing Office, 1996.

U.S. Preventive Services Task Force. *Guide to Clinical Preventive Services.* (2nd ed.) Alexandria, Va.: International Medical Publishing, 1996.

U.S. Surgeon General. *Surgeon General's Report on Nutrition and Health.* Washington, D.C.: U.S. Government Printing Office, 1988.

Valensi, P., and others. "Silent Myocardial Ischemia and Left Ventricular Hypertrophy in Diabetic Patients." *Diabetes and Metabolism,* 1997, *23*(5), 409–616.

Van Arsdale, P. W. "Secondary Migration and the Toll of Voluntary Agencies in the Resettlement Process." In W. H. Holtzman and T. H. Bornemann (eds.), *Mental Health of Immigrants and Refugees* (pp. 66–77). Austin: Hogg Foundation for Mental Health, University of Texas, 1990.

van der Veer, G. *Counselling and Therapy with Refugees: Psychological Problems of Victims of War, Torture and Repression.* New York: Wiley, 1992.

Vargas-Willis, G., and Cervantes, R. "Consideration of Psychosocial Stress in the Treatment of the Latina Immigrant." *Hispanic Journal of Behavioral Sciences,* 1987, *9*(3), 315–329.

Vega, W. A., and Rumbaut, R. G. "Ethnic Minorities and Mental Health." *Annual Review of Sociology,* 1991, *17*, 351–383.

Vega, W. A., and others. "Perinatal Drug Use Among Immigrant and Native-Born Latinas." *Substance Use and Misuse,* 1997, *32*(1), 43–62.

Ventura, S., Martin, J., Curtin, S., and Mathews, T. "Report of Final Natality Statistics, 1995." *Monthly Vital Statistics Report,* 1997, *45*(11), 1–84.

Villarruel, A. M., and Ortiz de Montellano, B. "Culture and Pain: A Mesoamerican Perspective." *Advances in Nursing Science,* 1992, *15*(1), 21–32.

Wagner, J., and others. "Dietary Soy Protein and Estrogen Replacement Therapy Improve Cardiovascular Risk Factors and Decrease Aortic Cholesteryl Ester Content in Ovariectomized Cynomolgus Monkeys." *Metabolism: Clinical and Experimental,* 1997, *46*(6), 698–705.

Walker, A., and Parmar, P. *Warrior Marks: Female Genital Mutilation and the Sexual Blinding of Women.* Orlando, Fla.: Harcourt Brace, 1993.

Walker-Moffat, W. *The Other Side of the Asian American Success Story.* San Francisco: Jossey-Bass, 1995.

Wallen, J. "Providing Culturally Appropriate Mental Health Services for Minorities." *Journal of Mental Health Administration,* 1992, *19*(3), 288–295.

Ware, N., and Kleinman, A. "Culture and Somatic Experience: The Social Course of Illness in Neurasthenia and Chronic Fatigue Syndrome." *Psychosomatic Medicine,* 1992a, *54*(5), 546–560.

Ware, N., and Kleinman, A. "Depression in Neurasthenia and Chronic Fatigue Syndrome." *Psychiatric Annals,* 1992b, *22*(4), 202–208.

*Washington Post,* July 6, 1997, p. A3.

*Washington Post,* Apr. 10, 1998.

Webster, R. A., McDonald, R., Lewin, T. J., and Carr, V. J. "Effects of a Natural Disaster on Immigrant and Host Population." *Journal of Nervous and Mental Disease,* 1995, *183*(6), 390–397.

Weidman, H. H. *"Falling-Out:* A Diagnostic and Treatment Problem Viewed from a Transcultural Perspective." *Social Science and Medicine,* 1979, *13B,* 95–112.

Weis, S. E., and others. "The Effect of Directly Observed Therapy on the Rates of Drug Resistance and Relapse in Tuberculosis." *New England Journal of Medicine,* 1994, *330,* 1179–1184.

Weitzman, B. C., and Berry, C. A. "Health Status and Health Care Utilization Among New York City Home Health Attendants: An Illustration of the Needs of the Working Poor, Immigrant Women." *Women's Health,* 1992, *19*(2/3), 87–105.

Wells, K. B., and others. "Which Mexican-Americans Underutilize Health Services?" *American Journal of Psychiatry,* 1987, *144*(7), 918–922.

Westermeyer, J. "Migration and Psychopathology." In C. L. Williams and J. Westermeyer (eds.), *Refugee Mental Health in Resettlement Countries* (pp. 39–56). Cambridge, Mass.: Hemisphere Publishing Corporation, 1986.

Westermeyer, J. *Cultural Factors in Psychiatric Assessment of Refugees and Others.* Minneapolis: Refugee Mental Health Technical Assistance Center, University of Minnesota, 1987.

Westermeyer, J. "DSM-III Psychiatric Disorders Among Hmong Refugees in the United States." *American Journal of Psychiatry,* 1988, *145,* 197–202.

Westermeyer, J. J. "Cross-Cultural Psychiatric Assessment." In A. C. Gaw (ed.), *Culture, Ethnicity and Mental Illness* (pp. 125–144). Washington, D.C.: American Psychiatric Press, 1993.

Wild, S., and others. "Mortality from CHD and Stroke for Ethnic Groups in California, 1985 to 1990." *Annals of Epidemiology,* 1995, *5*(6), 432–439.

Willet, W. *Nutritional Epidemiology.* New York: Oxford University Press, 1990.

Williams, T. *Chinese Medicine.* Rockport, Mass.: Element, 1995.

Wilson, J. P., Harel, A., and Kahana, B. (eds.). *Human Adaptation to Extreme Stress.* New York: Plenum Press, 1988.

Wilson, M. E. *A World Guide to Infections: Diseases, Distribution, Diagnosis.* New York: Oxford University Press, 1991.

Wilson-Ford, V. "Health Protective Behaviors of Rural Black Elderly Women." *Health and Social Work,* 1991, *17*(1), 28–36.

Wismer, B. A., and others. "Mammography and Clinical Breast Examination Among Korean American Women in Two California Counties." *Preventive Medicine*, 1998a, *27*, 144–151.

Wismer, B. A., and others. "Rates and Independent Correlates of Pap Smear Testing Among Korean American Women." *American Journal of Public Health*, 1998b, *88*.

Witmer, A., and others. "Community Health Workers: Integral Members of the Health Care Work Force." *American Journal of Public Health*, 1995, *85*(8), 1055–1058.

Wolfe, M. S. "Tropical Diseases in Immigrants and Internationally Adopted Children." *Medical Clinics of North America*, 1992, *6*, 1463–1480.

Wolff, C. T., Friedman, S. B., Hofer, M. A., and Mason, J. W. "Relationships Between Psychological Defenses and Mean Urinary 17–Hydroxycorticosteroid Excretion Rates: Part 1. A Predictive Study of Parents of Children with Leukemia." *Psychosomatic Medicine*, 1964, *26*, 576–591.

Woloshin, S., and others. "Language Barriers in Medicine in the United States." *Journal of American Medical Association*, 1995, *273*(9), 724–728.

Women's Health Initiative. "Backgrounder." [http://www.nhlbi.nih.gov/nhlbi/whi1/factsht.htm]. 1997.

Wong, H. "Asian and Pacific Americans." In L. R. Snowden (ed.), *Reaching the Underserved: Mental Health Needs of Neglected Populations*. Thousand Oaks, Calif: Sage, 1985.

Woodwell, D. "National Ambulatory Medical Care Survey: 1995 Summary." *Advance Data*, 1997, *286*, 1–25.

World Cancer Research Fund. *Food, Nutrition and the Prevention of Cancer: A Global Perspective*. Washington, D.C.: American Institute for Cancer Research, 1997.

World Health Organization. Division of Mental Health. *International Classification of Diseases*. (9th ed.) Geneva, Switzerland: World Health Organization, 1978.

World Health Organization. *International Classification of Diseases*. (10th ed.) *Classification of Mental and Behavioral Disorders, Clinical Descriptions, and Diagnostic Guidelines*. Geneva, Switzerland: World Health Organization, 1996.

Xu, Y. X., and Zhon, Y. B. "Some Recommendations with Regard to the Diagnostic Criteria for Several Types of Neurosis." *Chinese Journal of Neurology and Psychiatry*, 1983, *16*, 236–238.

Yan, H. Q. "The Necessity of Retaining the Diagnostic Concept of Neurasthenia." *Culture, Medicine and Psychiatry*, 1989, *13*, 139–145.

Yao, E. L. "Adjustment Needs of Asian Immigrant Children in the Schools." *Elementary School Guidance and Counseling*, 1985, *19*, 222–227.

Yim, S. B. "Korean Battered Wives: A Sociological and Psychological Analysis of Conjugal Violence in Korean Immigrant Families." In H. H. Sunoo (ed.), *Korean Women in a Struggle for Humanization* (pp. 213–226). Memphis, Tenn.: Association of Korean Christian Scholars in North America, 1978.

Ying, Y. "Depressive Symptomatology Among Chinese-Americans as Measured by the CES-D." *Journal of Clinical Psychology*, 1988, *44*, 739–746.

Ying, Y. "Explanatory Models of Major Depression and Implications for Help-Seeking Among Immigrant Chinese-American Women." *Culture, Medicine and Psychiatry*, 1990, *14*, 393–408.

Ying, Y. "Chinese American Adults' Relationship with Their Parents." *International Journal of Social Psychiatry*, 1994, *40*(1), 35–45.

Ying, Y. "Cultural Orientation and Psychological Well-Being in Chinese-Americans." *American Journal of Community Psychology*, 1995, *23*(6), 893–911.

Ying, Y. "Intergenerational Relationship in Immigrant Families—Chinese Parent Scale." Unpublished manuscript, 1998.

Ying, Y. "Strengthening Intergenerational/Intercultural Ties in Migrant Families: A New Intervention for Parents." *Journal of Community Psychology*. Forthcoming.

Ying, Y., Akutsu, P., Zhang, X., and Huang, L. "Psychological Dysfunction in Southeast Asian Refugees Mediated by Sense of Coherence." *American Journal of Community Psychology*, 1997, *25*(6), 839–859.

Ying, Y., and Chao, C. "Intergenerational Relationship in Iu Mien American Families." *Amerasia Journal*, 1996, *22*(3), 47–64.

Ying, Y., and Hu, L. "Public Outpatient Mental Health Services: Use and Outcome Among Asian Americans." *American Journal of Orthopsychiatry*, 1994, *64*(3), 448–455.

Ying, Y., and Miller, L. S. "Help-Seeking Behavior and Attitude of Chinese Americans Regarding Psychological Problems." *American Journal of Community Psychology*, 1992, *20*(4), 549–556.

Ying, Y., and Zhang, X. "Mental Health in Rural and Urban Chinese Families: The Role of Intergenerational Personality Discrepancy and Family Solidarity." *Journal of Comparative Family Studies*, 1995, *26*(2), 233–246.

Young, C. "Emergency! Says Who? Analysis of the Legal Issues Concerning Managed Care and Emergency Medical Services." *Journal of Contemporary Health Law and Policy*, 1997, *13*, 553–579.

Youssef, G. E., and others. "Chronic Enterovirus Infection in Patients with Postviral Fatigue Syndrome." *Lancet*, 1988, *1*, 146–150.

Yu, L. C., and Harburg, E. "Acculturation and Stress Among Chinese Americans in a University Town." *International Journal of Group Tensions*, 1980, *10*, 1–4, 99–119.

Zaldivar, A., and Smolowitz, M. "Perceptions of the Importance Placed on Religion and Folk Medicine by Non-Mexican-American Hispanic Adults with Diabetes." *Diabetes Educator*, 1994, *20*(4), 303–306.

Zambrana, R. "Ethnic Differences in the Substance Use Patterns of Low-Income Pregnant Women." *Family and Community Health*, 1991, *13*, 1–11.

Zambrana, R., and others. "The Relationship Between Psychosocial Status of Immigrant Latino Mothers and Use of Emergency Pediatric Services." *Health and Social Work*, 1994, *19*(2), 93–102.

Zepeda, M. "Selected Maternal-Infant Care Practices of Spanish-Speaking Women." *JOGN*, Nov.–Dec. 1982, pp. 371–374.

Zheng, Y. P., and Lin, K. M. "Comparison of the Chinese Depression Inventory and the Chinese Version of the Beck Depression Inventory." *Acta Psychiatrica Scandinavia*, 1991, *84*, 531–536.

Zheng, Y. P., and others. "Neurasthenia in Chinese Students and Visiting Scholars in the United States." *Psychiatric Annals*, 1992, *22*(4), 194–198.

Zheng, Y. P., and others. "An Epidemiological Study of Neurasthenia in Chinese-Americans in Los Angeles." *Comprehensive Psychiatry*, 1997, *38*(5), 249–259.

Ziegler, R. G., and others. "Migration Patterns and Breast Cancer Risk in Asian-American Women." *Journal of the National Cancer Institute*, 1993, *85*(22), 1819–1827.

Zimmerman, R., and Clover, R. "Adult Immunizations—A Practical Approach for Clinicians: Part I and Part II." *American Family Physician*, 1995, *51*(4–5), 859–867, 1139–1148.

Ziv, T. A., and Lo, B. "Denial of Care to Illegal Immigrants: Proposition 187 in California." *New England Journal of Medicine*, 1995, *332*(16), 1095–1098.

Zola, I. "Problems of Communication, Diagnosis and Patient Care: The Interplay of Patient, Physician and Clinic Organization." *Journal of Medical Education*, 1963, *38*, 829–838.

Zola, I. "Culture and Symptoms—An Analysis of Patients' Presenting Complaints." *American Sociological Review*, 1966, *31*, 615–630.

Zuniga, M. "'Dichos' as Metaphorical Tools for Resistant Latino Clients." *Psychotherapy*, 1991, *28*(3), 480–483.

# Name Index

## A

Abbey, S. E., 243
Abbott, J., 179
Abraham, M., 179
Abrams, B., 128
Accreditation Council of Graduate Medical Education, 322
Acierno, R., 179, 186, 188
Ackerman, L. K., 90, 95
Acosta, F., 60
Adams, A., 116, 118
Adams, C., 117
Aday, L., 44
Adler, P., 286
Adrien, A., 109
Advisory Committee on Immunization Practices (ACIP), 96
Africa Watch Women's Rights Project, 192
Agger, I., 183
Ahern, M., 49
Ahluwallia, K., 185–186
Aitchison, R., 191
Akutsu, P. D., 54, 57
Albers, L., 49
Aldwin, C., 285
Almstrom, B., 109
American College of Emergency Physicians, 186
American Diabetes Association, 161
American Medical Association, 184, 186
American Medical Women's Association, 147
American Psychiatric Association, 211, 220, 222–223, 233, 234, 242, 249

American Thoracic Society, 103
Amering, M., 207–208
Andersen, R., 44, 138
Anderson, J., 158
Anderson, N.L.R., 131
Andreski, P., 224
Andrulis, D. P., 52, 68, 330
Angel, R., 235
Anwar, R., 186
Applewhite, S. L., 29, 31
Armstrong, M. A., 152
Aronow, W. S., 140
Aronson, L., 272
Arullendran, P., 112
Asch, S., 74, 75
Association of State and Territorial Health Officials, 35, 42, 262
Atrash, K., 128
Austin, J. E., 116
Avery, R. K., 97

## B

Bachman, R., 179
Badger, L. W., 239
Bailey, R. L., 112
Baker, D., 48
Bakris, G., 151
Balady, G. L., 147
Bamford, K., 60
Barker, J., 321
Barsky, A. J., 241, 273
Bastani, R., 169
Bateman, W. B., 155, 321
Baughan, D. M., 271
Baumeister, L., 76
Bazron, B. J., 19, 20
Beard, G. M., 242, 247

Becerra, J., 128
Becerra, R. M., 29
Becker, M., 120
Ben-Porath, E., 105
Ben-Porath, Y. S., 8, 9, 283
Berger, L., 23
Berk, M., 49
Berkman, L. F., 170
Berlin, E. A., 324, 326
Berry, C. A., 11
Berry, J. W., 9, 24, 287
Biddlecom, A., 44–45
Biewener, J., 76
Bindman, A., 51, 70
Binkin, N. J., 103
Bird, J. A., 302
Blazer, P., 224
Block, G., 116, 118
Bochner, S., 208
Boehnlein, J. K., 207
Bogen, E., 5
Boudewyns, P. A., 226
Boyd, M., 9
Boyd-Franklin, N., 21
Bradshaw, C. K., 57
Bramwell, K. J., 48, 49
Breaux, C., 54
Breslau, N., 224
Bridges, K. W., 239
Brillon, L., 283, 284, 287
Brook, R., 48
Brown, J. S., 134
Browne, A., 184
Brownmiller, S., 190
Bui, H., 103, 104
Buldwald, D., 30
Burdman, P., 74
Bureau of Primary Health Care (BPHC), 47
Burgess, P., 225
Burk, M., 126, 130, 133
Burt, V. L., 151, 152
Butler, C. D., 171

C

Calle, E. E., 164
Campbell, D. W., 180

Campbell, J. C., 180
Campbell, T. L., 178
Campis, L. K., 291
Camus-Jacques, G., 191
Canda, E. R., 23
Canino, I. A., 239
Canino, J., 57
Cannistra, L. B., 147
Cantwell, M. F., 98
Carlson, E. B., 207, 224
Carpenter, C.C.J., 108
Carr, J. E., 251
Carr, V. J., 220, 225
Carter, W., 57, 236, 240
Cascardi, M., 183
Castillo, R., 236, 238–239
Castro de Alvarez, V., 16
Catalano, R., 74, 76
Cauthen, G. M., 98
Center for Family and Community Health, 295, 296
Centers for Disease Control (CDC), 51–52, 90, 92, 93, 96, 98, 103, 106, 110, 112, 139–140, 142, 143–144, 145, 199
Cervantes, R., 57, 60, 62, 224, 225
Chambers, T. J., 172
Chan, C., 63
Chan, L., 246
Chan, T. C., 48, 49
Chao, C., 282, 284, 285
Chavez, L. R., 48–49, 50, 125, 166, 167, 168
Chechile, D., 190, 194
Chemtov, D., 105, 109
Chen, A. M., 295, 299
Chen, M. S., 144
Cheung, F. M., 57, 239, 247
Cheung, P., 246
Chin, A. L., 247
Chin, K., 181
Chin, R., 247
Chittick, J. B., 109
Chohan, S., 109
Chrischilles, E. A., 171
Chun, C. A., 239, 240–241, 247
Chun, K. M., 54, 56

Chung, R. C., 60, 180, 246
Clancy, C., 49
Clark, N., 128
Clark, R. F., 48, 49
Clarkson, T., 146
Clinton, B., 312, 341
Clover, R., 96
Cohen, J., 49
Coll, C. G., 30
Columbia, L., 240
Comas-Diaz, L., 21, 58, 60, 63
Compton, K. M., 190, 194
Congressional Conference, 201
Connor, E. M., 109
Consensus Development Confer-
    ence, 170
Constantino, G., 60
Cook, D. G., 172
Cooney, L. M., 170
Corey, C., 44
Cornelius, W., 48–49, 50, 125
Cornell, C. P., 178
Corr, J. E., 207
Cosgrove, J., 22
Council on Scientific Affairs, 127, 128
Creamer, M., 225
Crespo, C. J., 152
Crites, L. L., 183, 184
Cross, L., 50
Cross, T. L., 19, 20
Croughan, J. L., 224
Cunningham, P., 49
Curtin, S., 125

**D**

Dahl, S., 224
Dalzell, N., 172
Damond, M. E., 109
Dana, R., 20
Dasen, P. R., 24
Dasgupta, S. D., 183
D'Avanzo, C. D., 180
Davidson, J.R.T., 224
Davis, B. D., 164
Davis, C. E., 146
Davis, C. S., 171
Davis, G. C., 224

DeGruy, F., 240
Del Monte, M. L., 150
DeLay, P., 83
Delmas, P. D., 174
DelVecchio, A., 208
Dempster, D. W., 172
Dennis, K. W., 19, 20
DeQuatro, V., 154
Derk, S., 186
Desjarlais, 191
Dickinson, P., 240
DiClemente, C., 55
Doherty, W. J., 178
Dorkenoo, E., 201
Drachman, D., 282, 283, 284
Draguns, J. G., 246
Duncan, L., 144
Dunham, N., 188
Duran, D., 237
Dutton, M., 186
Dwyer, J., 11

**E**

Eastman, K., 56
Echeverry, J., 55, 57, 58, 60, 61
Eisenberg, D. M., 154
Eisenberg, L., 15
Eisenbruch, M., 224, 230
Elliot, A., 223
Ellwood, M. R., 131
Enas, E., 143, 145
Enomoto, K., 239, 240–241
Erikson, E. H., 288
Escobar, J. I., 205, 234, 235, 236, 238–
    239
Eskenazi, B., 11
Espin, O., 62
Evans, L., 60

**F**

Fang, C., 111
Faust, S., 82, 83, 85, 86, 87, 231, 271
Fenton, C. R., 74, 76
Fenton, J. J., 75
Fernandez, M., 178
Ferran, E., 19
Fieldhouse, P., 114

Finkler, K., 238
Flaskerud, J., 57
Flowers-Bowie, 341
Folkman, S., 225
Forbes, K., 49
Fourcroy, J., 197
Fowkes, E. G., 324, 326
Foy, D. W., 183
Francis, M., 261
Freed, W., 207
Freeman, H., 44
Freudenberg, N., 16
Friedson, E., 15
Frisancho, A. R., 118
Froman, R., 109
Fruchter, R. G., 13–14, 166
Frye, B. A., 180
Fujino, D., 55, 62
Fujomoto, W., 157
Fulton, J., 46
Furbee, P., 186
Furnham, A., 208

G

Galijasevic, S., 46
Gany, F., 30, 34, 167
Gany, F. M., 19
Garcia Coll, C. T., 283, 284, 287
Garcia, J. G., 57
Garcia, M., 44, 45
Garcia, N., 113, 115, 120
Garcia-Preto, N., 21
Gardner, G., 137
Garfinkel, P. E., 243
Garza-Trevino, E., 13, 321
Gaviria, M., 129, 132
Gaw, A., 217, 249, 252, 253, 254
Gelberg, L., 74
Gelles, R. J., 178
George, L. K., 224
Geringer, E., 241, 273
Giatras, I., 151
Gil, R. M., 15
Gillum, R., 138
Ginsberg, C., 40, 41–42, 265
Ginzburg, E., 127, 134
Gjerdingen, D., 86

Goff, D. C., 142, 147
Goldberg, D. P., 239
Goldberg, K., 147
Goldstein, E., 30, 218
Goletti, D., 98
Gonzales, H., 24
Good, B., 15, 208
Gooding, S. S., 49, 50
Gordon, S., 29, 158
Gould, J., 11
Grant, G., 283
Gray, E., 22
Gray, R. J., 147
Green, B., 217
Green, L. W., 296
Greenberger, E., 285
Greene, B., 60
Greenlund, K. J., 138
Griffith, J. L., 241
Griffith, M. E., 241
Grinberg, L., 219
Grinberg, R., 219
Groessl, K. M., 180
Guarnaccia, P. J., 235
Guendelman, S., 11, 44, 128
Guerney, B. G., Jr., 288
Guerney, L., 288, 289
Guillermo, T., 114, 180
Gulliford, M. C., 156, 159
Gupta, R., 185
Gurin, P., 178
Gutierrez, L. M., 63

H

Ha, N.-T., 302
Hahn, R. A., 12, 13
Haines, D. W., 9
Hames, C. G., 138
Harding, G. H., 304
Hardt, E., 21, 27
Harel, A., 223
Hargreaves, W., 74, 76
Harkness, S., 287
Harris, R., 162
Harrison, A. O., 283, 284
Hart, B. J., 184
Harwood, A., 15

Havas, S., 154
Haywood, Y., 186
Hazuda, H. P., 152
He, J., 151
Health Care Advisory Board, 49
Heaney, R., 172
Heath, C. W., 164
Heise, L., 180
Helzer, J. E., 224
Henderson, S. M., 134
Hendry, K., 52
Herbst, P. R., 230
Herman, J. L., 223
Hernandez-Guzman, L., 285
Hiatt, R. A., 166, 169, 302
Higginbotham, J. C., 31
Himmelstein, D., 51
Hirota, S. M., 180, 304
Ho, M. K., 22, 23, 25
Hocevar, D., 285
Hodes, R. M., 104, 109, 111
Hogeland, C., 17
Hogue, C., 128
Hollender, M., 15
Hong, W., 246
Hoover, C. R., 233
Horn-Ross, P. L., 163
Hornstein, L., 107
Horowitz, M. J., 223, 226
Houskamp, B. M., 183
Howard, K., 55
Hoyert, D., 142, 145
Hsu, J., 22, 182
Hu, L., 54, 55
Hu, T., 55
Huang, S., 113
Hubbell, F. A., 44, 45, 166, 167, 168
Hudes, M., 11
Hughes, D., 224
Hui, K. K., 154
Hulme, P. A., 237
Hyer, L. A., 226
Hyman, A., 184

**I**

Iglehart, A. P., 29
Ihle, L., 57

Institute of Medicine, 44
Inui, T. S., 57
Isaacs, M. R., 19, 20
Ishisaka, H., 58
Ivey, S. L., 3, 44, 66, 70, 82, 137, 178, 335

**J**

Jacalyn, L., 16
Jackson, J. C., 30
Jamerson, K., 154
James, S., 128
Janoff-Bulman, R., 226
Jayakar, K., 57
Jenkins, C., 28, 30
Jensen, L., 44–45
Jerrell, J., 55
Johnson Foundation, Robert Wood, 324, 326
Johnson, T., 21, 27
Jones, J. F., 243
Jones, O., 48–49, 50, 125
Jones, P., 49
Jones, S., 49
Jones, W., 199
Juarbe, T., 44
Jun, S., 294

**K**

Kagan, A., 113, 137, 138, 143
Kagawa-Singer, M., 180
Kahana, B., 223
Kaiser Family Foundation, 67, 337
Kamya, H. A., 23
Kang, S. H., 166, 294
Kanis, J. A., 170
Kanuha, V., 179, 180, 183
Kaptchuk, T. J., 159
Karno, M., 206
Katon, W., 207, 234, 236, 238, 239
Katschnig, H., 207–208
Katz, S. S., 112
Keane, V. P., 104
Keegan, L., 126, 130, 133
Keenan, N. L., 163
Kelly, A. W., 301–302
Kelly, N., 182

Kelsey, J. L., 162, 164
Kenney, G. M., 131
Kessler, R. C., 205–206, 207, 224, 240
Key, L., 201
Khalil, H. G., 75
Khazoyan, C. M., 131
Kilpatrick, D., 179, 186, 188
Kim, S. C., 57
Kim, U., 9, 287
Kington, R. S., 153
Kinzie, J. D., 220, 226
Kirmayer, L. J., 207, 208, 235, 236, 237, 238, 239, 240
Klag, M. J., 153
Klatsky, A. L., 152
Klein, J., 255
Kleinman, A., 15, 21, 24, 25, 27, 28, 57, 84, 207, 208, 235, 236, 237–238, 239, 240, 243, 244, 245, 246, 247
Ko, R., 121
Kooiman, C., 46
Koss, J. D., 237
Koss-Chioino, J. D., 59
Kottke, T. E., 301
Kovar, M. G., 144
Kramer, E. J., 3, 19, 70, 155, 170, 322, 336
Kreuter, M. W., 296
Krishel, S. J., 48, 49
Kung, H., 142, 145
Kunstadter, P., 115
Kwon-Ahn, Y. H., 282, 283, 284

**L**

Lambrew, J., 51
Lasseter, J., 46
Lau, J., 151
Lavizzo-Mourey, R., 20
Laws, A., 193
Lazarus, R. S., 225
Leake, B., 74
Lecca, P., 24
LeClere, F., 44–45
Lee, E., 25, 57, 224
Lee, M. M., 113, 115

Lee, S., 242
Leetch, L., 188
Leininger, L., 162
Leong, F., 57
Levey, A. S., 151
Levin, J., 48
Levy, C., 73
Lew, R., 294
Lewin, T. J., 220, 225
Liao, Y., 140
Lieberman, D., 150
Lightfoot-Klein, H., 199
Like, R., 322
Lin, K. M., 57, 60, 236, 240, 247, 253
Lin, T. Y., 242, 243–244
Lindsay, R., 171, 172
Lipowski, Z. J., 236, 238
Lipson, J. G., 7
Liu, F., 138
Lo, B., 73, 184
Londero, M. T., 109
Longworth, D. L., 107, 111
Loo, C., 58
Looker, A. C., 170, 171, 173
Lor, V., 86
Loria, C. M., 152
Loue, S., 105, 109
Lu, F., 25, 224
Luluquisen, E. M., 180
Lutzer, S., 224
Lyman, R. D., 291

**M**

Mabey, D.C.W., 112
Machizawa, S., 244
MacKenzie, E., 20
Maduro, R., 15
Magana, A., 128
Magnuson, K., 30
Mahabir, D., 156, 159
Malgady, R. G., 60
Manfiletto, E., 268
Marin, G., 11, 59, 143, 145, 161
Marin, L., 180, 181
Markides, K., 48

Marks, G., 44, 45
Marotolli, R. A., 170
Marquez, M. A., 302
Marsella, A. J., 207
Martin, J., 125
Martin, L. M., 164
Marx, J. L., 75
Massachusetts Department of Public Health, 263
Mathews, T., 125
Mathiasen, S. S., 224
Matsuoka, J., 21, 22
Mattar, S., 205
Maxmen, J. S., 206, 207, 213, 214, 215, 218
Maxwell, A. E., 169
Mayeno, L., 180
McAfee, R., 188
McCaig, L., 46, 48
McCall, M. A., 16
McCoy, H. V., 49
McCranie, E. W., 226
McDonald, R., 220, 225
McEnvoy, L., 224
McGraw, S., 144
McLeer, S. V., 186
McNagny, S., 48, 51, 70
McNally, R. J., 223
McPhee, S. J., 168, 301
Meleis, A. I., 7
Meyer, E. C., 283, 284, 287
Mghir, R., 207
Michael, S., 15
Milan Study on Atherosclerosis and Diabetes, 146
Millon-Underwood, S., 323
Min, K., 295
Minde, T., 9, 287
Minuchin, S., 22
Mishra, S. I., 166, 167, 168
Mitchell, B. D., 138
Mitchell, B. , 186
Mizoguchi, N., 72
Mo, G. M., 251
Mok, D., 9, 287
Mollica, R. F., 271, 273

Moore, L. J., 207
Morakinyo, O., 255
Morita, S., 244
Morris, C. R., 163, 164
Morrison, J., 236
Moskowitz, J. M., 295
Moss, A., 44
Moss, N., 75, 76
Muecke, M. A., 238
Mulinare, J., 13
Mull, D. S., 29, 31
Mull, J. D., 29, 31
Munoz, R., 290
Murillo-Rohde, I., 126
Murray, E. T., 163
Mutapcic, A., 224

**N**

Nakyonyi, M. M., 109
Napoles-Springer, A., 303
Narayan, U., 182
National Asian Women's Health Organization, 144
National Association of County Health Officials, 42, 262
National Association of Public Hospitals and Health Systems (NAPH), 47–48, 67, 68
National Center for Health Statistics, 140, 144
National Coalition of Hispanic Health and Human Services Organizations, 35, 36, 42, 155, 237
National High Blood Pressure Education Program, 150–151, 152, 153, 154
National Institute of Mental Health (NIMH), 54, 246
National Institutes of Health (NIH), 145
National Osteoporosis Foundation, 173
National Public Health and Hospital Institute (NPHHI), 52, 265, 266
National Registry of Myocardial Infarctions, 147

National Research Council, 118
Nelson, K. R., 103, 104
New York City Department of City Planning, 6
Ng, A. T., 249
Ngor, H. S., 191
Nguyen, M. D., 15
Nguyen, Q., 58
Nguyen, T., 55
Nichols, D., 167
Norcross, J., 55
Norton, S. A., 131
Novotny, T. E., 295
Nunes, J., 24

**O**

O'Donohue, W., 223
O'Hare, W. P., 61
Okazaki, S., 62
Okimoto, J., 58
O'Leary, K. D., 183
Olson, L., 180
Onorato, I. M., 98
Oppenheim, S., 105, 109
Oquendo, M., 56
Organista, K., 57
Orloff, L. E., 182
Ortiz de Montellano, B., 129
Osteoporosis and Related Bond Diseases National Resource Center, 173
Otero-Sabogal, R., 302, 303
Ovando, C., 285

**P**

Padilla, A. M., 224, 225
Pan, M., 121
Panser, L. A., 301
Pappas, G., 142
Parker, R., 48, 51, 70
Parmar, P., 199
Parrillo, V. N., 282
Pasic, J., 154
Patsalides, B., 193
Pattison, P., 225
Paul, S. M., 7

Paulino, A., 282, 283, 284
Pawliuk, N., 22
Pereira, W., 181
Perez, N., 128
Perez-Stable, F., 11, 143, 145, 161, 303
Perkins, C. I., 163, 164
Peters, K., 137
Peterson, E., 224
Peyrot, M., 49
Phaobtang, T., 23
Pickwell, S., 92
Pimental, B., 23
Pitman, R. K., 223
Poirier, L., 180
Polednak, A., 137, 138, 142, 143, 144
Pongpaew, P., 107
Poortinga, Y. H., 24
Portes, A., 9
Poss, J. E., 127
Prentice-Dunn, S., 291
Pressman, A., 116, 118
Prochaska, J., 55
Puttkammer, N. H., 180
Pyles, J., 46

**Q**

Quervalu, I., 24
Quillian, J. P., 180

**R**

Radloff, L. S., 291
Raisz, L. G., 170, 173, 174
Ramakrishna, J., 6
Ranck, J., 190
Rask, K., 48, 51, 70
Raskin, A., 207
Ratcliff, K. S., 224
Rau, E., 270
Ray, L., 48
Ray, L. A., 31
Recker, R., 172
Reeves, K., 57
Reinert, B., 29
Reinli, K., 146
Rengel, R., 127

Resnick, H., 179, 186, 188
Richards, J., 46
Richman, J., 71
Riddick, S., 35, 257, 266, 267
Robbins, J. M., 238, 239, 240
Robins, L. N., 224
Robison, L. M., 304
Roche, R. I., 167
Rogler, G., 60
Romero-Gwynn, E., 114, 115
Rosen, C., 109
Rosen, G., 238, 239
Rosen, H., 105
Rosen, K., 17
Rosenstock, I., 120
Ross, P. D., 170, 171, 172
Rosser-Hogan, R., 207, 224
Rossiter, J. C., 134
Rozee, P., 222, 271
Rubel, A., 321
Ruiz, P., 13, 61, 322
Rumbaut, R. G., 9, 206
Ryujin, D., 54

**S**

Sabogal, F., 302
Saigh, P. A., 223
Salgado de Snyder, V. N., 224, 225
Salladay, R., 74
Saltzman, L. E., 179
Samet, J. H., 103, 104
*San Francisco Examiner,* 68
Sanchez-Sosa, J. J., 285
Sandler, S. G., 111
Sanjur, D., 113, 114, 120
Saunders, S., 55
Schauffler, H., 309
Schei, B., 224
Schensul, S. L., 129, 132
Schillinger, D., 184
Schluter, R., 270
Schmitt, S., 112
Schornstein, S. L., 178, 182
Schultz, S. L., 15
Schur, C., 49
Schwalbe, J., 44

Sclar, D. A., 304
Scribner, R., 11
Segall, M. H., 24
Shaw, G., 128
Shaw, 202
Shelton, D., 44, 45
Shepherd, J., 227, 230, 231, 271, 281
Sheran, M., 109
Sherwin, R., 154
Shils, M. E., 118
Shimada, J., 30
Shtarkshall, R. A., 109
Siegler, E. L., 150, 170
Sieng, S., 63
Sikora, R., 186
Silver, D., 16
Simmons, M., 144
Simon, E., 235, 236–237
Simoni, J., 58
Simpson, D. M., 167
Singer, M. K., 246
Skaer, T. L., 304
Skilbeck, W., 60
Slutsker, L., 106
Sluzki, C., 9, 22, 83, 282
Smith, D. B., 49
Smith, J. P., 153
Smith, K., 144
Smith-Fawzi, M. C., 224
Smolowitz, M., 158
Snider, D. E., Jr., 98
Snow, L., 15
Snowden, L. R., 25, 55, 57
Solis, J., 44, 45
Song-Kim, Y. I., 181
Sorbie, J., 16
Soskolne, V., 109
Spetz, J., 74–75
Spielvogel, A., 321
Spizzichino, L., 109
Srinivasan, S., 178
Starrett, R., 58
Stein, T., 322
Steiner, P., 321
Stellman, S. D., 143
Stern, G., 129, 132

Stevens, C., 48
Stiglmayer, A., 190
Straus, M., 178
Straus, S. E., 243
Strecher, V., 120
Stussman, B., 46, 48
Suarez, L., 167
Sue, S., 54, 55, 56, 61, 62, 63, 239, 240–241
Super, C., 287
Susskind, Y., 190
Szapocnik, J., 285
Szasz, T., 15

**T**

Tager, I. B., 295
Takagi, T., 182
Takeuchi, D., 55, 247
Tan, E. K., 251
Tata, S., 57
Taylor, F., 121
Tazuma, L., 57
Terry, R. D., 116
Teutsch, S., 13
Thiagarajan, S., 287
Thiel-deBocanegra, H., 30, 34, 167
Thompson, J., 63, 322
Tien, L., 60
Tobias, J. H., 172
Tong, B., 58
Tosomeen, A. H., 301
Toubia, N., 196, 197, 198, 199
Tracy, L., 22, 205, 212, 220, 226
Tracy, L. C., 3, 19
Trevino, F. M., 31, 44
Triandis, H. C., 284
True, R. H., 58, 63, 180
Truman, B. I., 163
Truong, D. H., 103
Tseng, W. S., 22
Tucker, M. E., 237
Tung, M.P.M., 237
Tyrance, P., 51

**U**

Uba, L., 55, 57, 58, 60, 61

U.S. Bureau of Population, Refugees, and Migration, 180
U.S. Bureau of the Census, 5, 12, 14, 179, 307, 338, 340
U.S. Conference of Local Health Officers, 42, 262
U.S. Conference of Mayors, 42, 68, 262
U.S. Congress, 50, 66, 171
U.S. Department of Agriculture (USDA), 117, 118
U.S. Department of Health and Human Services (DHHS), 114, 119, 155, 156, 162–163, 319
U.S. Department of Justice, 179
U.S. Preventive Services Task Force, 90, 162
U.S. Surgeon General, 113, 114

**V**

Valdez, R. B., 166, 167, 168
Valensi, P., 146
Van Arsdale, P. W., 9, 10
Van Bohmel, G., 222, 271
Van de Wetering, B., 46
Van der Mast, R., 46
VanOss Marin, B., 11, 143, 145, 161
Vargas-Willis, G., 57, 60, 62
Vega, W. A., 131, 206
Velie, E., 128
Venegas-Samuels, K., 13, 322
Ventura, S., 125
Villaruel, A. M., 129
Vitaliano, P., 207
VonKorff, M., 235, 236–237

**W**

Wagner, J., 146
Wagner, N., 57
Waitzkin, H., 236, 238–239
Walker, 199
Wallace, R. B., 171
Wallen, J., 59
Wang, C., 246
Wang, G., 56
Wang, Y. X., 247

Ward, N. G., 206, 207, 213, 214, 215, 218
Warda, U. S., 169
Ware, N., 243, 246
Warner, R., 191
Warren, B., 113, 115, 120
Warrier, S., 183
*Washington Post,* 5, 6, 12, 66
Wasserman, C., 128
Webster, R. A., 220, 225
*Webster's College Dictionary,* 19
Wegner, E., 49
Weidman, H. H., 255
Weis, S. E., 104
Weiss, M. G., 6
Weitzman, B. C., 11
Weller, P. F., 107, 111
Wells, K. B., 61
Westermeyer, J., 9, 57, 212
Whelton, P. K., 151
White, D., 151
Whittle, H. C., 112
Wieser, P., 126, 130, 133
Wild, S., 138
Wilets, M., 49
Willet, W., 113, 116
Williams, J., 186
Williams, M., 48, 51, 70
Williams, T., 31
Wilson, J. P., 223
Wilson, M. E., 97, 105, 110, 111
Wilson, P., 73
Wing, J., 224
Wing, J. S., 163
Wingo, P. A., 164
Wismer, B. A., 162, 168, 295, 296
Witmer, A., 37
Wittchen, H. U., 224
Wolfe, M. S., 97
Woloshin, S., 41
Womack, W. M., 57
Women's Health Initiative, 174
Wong, H., 61

Wong, K. C., 242
Woods, M. G., 226
Woodwell, 46
Wool, C. A., 241, 273
Woolhandler, S., 51
World Cancer Research Fund, 114
World Health Organization (WHO), 170, 196, 243, 249
Wright, W. E., 163, 164

**X**

Xu, Y. X., 245, 246

**Y**

Yamamoto, J., 60
Yan, H. Q., 246
Yao, E. L., 282, 285
Yew-Schwartz, P., 242
Yim, S. B., 181
Ying, Y., 24, 25, 54, 56, 206, 282, 284, 285, 290, 291, 336
Yoder, L., 49
Young, A., 238, 239
Young, J. L., 164
Young, K., 54, 62
Young, V. R., 118
Youssef, G. E., 243

**Z**

Zaldivar, A., 158
Zambrana, R., 49, 131
Zane, N., 54, 61, 63
Zea, M. C., 57
Zepeda, M., 133
Zheng, D. C., 246
Zheng, Y. P., 208, 243, 246, 247
Zhon, Y. B., 245, 246
Ziegler, R. G., 11
Zimmerman, R., 96
Ziv, T. A., 73
Zola, I., 15
Zuniga, M., 62

# Subject Index

## A

Abdominal exam, 102

Abortion: Asian use of, 122; Caucasian use of, 122; due to fetal defect, 129; Latina use of, 122; methods of obtaining, 124–125; rates of, among minority women, 124; therapeutic, 124–125

Abuse. *See* Child abuse; Domestic violence; Race

Access to health care: barriers to, 14–18, 25, 44–45, 51, 129–130, 308–309; barriers to, in domestic violence, 180, 182, 185–186; barriers to, in mental health, 56–59, 60–61; health counselors and, 298; for limited-English-proficient clients, 35–43, 259–270; preservation of, 51–53; for reproductive care, 121, 125; of traditional practitioners, 31; utilization and, 44–45, 51–53; welfare and immigration reform and, 66–77, 340–341. *See also* Health services utilization; Health-seeking behaviors; Mental health services utilization

Accreditation Council of Graduate Medical Education, 322

Acculturation: assessment of, 32; bottle feeding and, 133, 134; breast and cervical cancer screening and, 167, 168; cardiovascular disease and, 137–138, 142–143; diabetes and, 157; diet, health, disease and, 113–115, 137–138, 157; hypertension and, 152–153; intergenerational conflict and, 22–23, 282–285, 287; mental health outcomes and, 207; migration and, 8–9; neurasthenia *versus* depression and, 247; somatization and, 237; stress and, 208–209; utilization and, 44–45

Acupuncture, 30, 31, 231

Acute care, costs of, 50–51

Adenopathy, 102

Adoptees, international, 135

Adoption practices, 134–135

Adult Medical Services at Hotel Oakland (AMSHO), 312

Advocacy: in mental health treatment, 218–219; to promote access to care, 318

Affective disorders. *See* Anxiety and anxiety disorders; Depression

Afghanistan, Hepatitis B incidence in, 88

Africa: culture-bound syndromes in, 255–256; female genital mutilation in, 194; Hepatitis B incidence in, 88; infectious diseases in, 99–100; malaria incidence in, 106

African Americans: adoption among, 135; California population of, 73; cardiovascular disease in, 138, 139, 140, 141, 142; diabetes in, 156; falling-out syndrome in, 255–256; FQHC utilization of, 47; health beliefs of, 27, 29; health status of, 319; hypertension in, 142, 151, 153; infant mortality of, 128; mental health service utilization of, 55; myocardial infarction in, 147; time orientation of, 24

Age, hypertension and, 151

Agency for Health Care Policy and Research, 338–339

Ahluwallia, Kirinjit, domestic violence case, 185–186

Aid to Families with Dependent Children, 68

AIDS (acquired immunodeficiency syndrome): in pregnancy, 127–128; stigma of, as barrier to access, 16

Alameda County, California, 306; Asian Health Services in, 305–321; Asian Pacific Islanders in, 307–311; ethnic distribution in, 306–307; Korean Breast and Cervical Cancer Screening Project, Health Is Strength project in, 295–301; primary care funding in, 315

Alameda Health Consortium, 312

Alcohol use: domestic violence and, 179; limiting, in hypertension, 154

Alpha fetoprotein, 105, 128

Alta Bates Medical Center, 314

Amazon basin, hepatitis D in, 105

Ambulatory visit rates, 45–46

American College of Obstetrics and Gynecology, 202

American Medical Association, 73, 201–202

American Medical Women's Association, 201–202

American Nurses Association, 201–202

American Public Health Association, 73

American Thoracic Society/Centers for Disease Control consensus statement on tuberculosis prophylaxis, 103

Amniocentesis, 128–129

Amoebic dysentery, 107

Amoebic liver abscess, 106, 107

*Amok,* 252

Amulets, 30

Anemia: hypochromic, microcytic type *versus* thalassemia, 91; screening protocols for, 86, 91; treatment of, 91

Anger: culture and suppression of, 253–254; Korean *hwa-byung* syndrome and, 253–254

Angiotension-converting enzyme inhibitors, 151

Anglo-Americans, time orientation of, 24

Anthropometaric measurements, 118

Antidepressants, 215–217, 247

Anti-immigrant backlash, 18, 72–73

Antiretorviral therapy, 108, 128

*Antojos,* 126–127

Anxiety and anxiety disorders, 205–219; assessment of, 212, 214–215; case study of, 211–212; comorbidity with, 206–207; cultural issues in, 207–208; culture-bound syndromes and, 253; domestic violence and, 188; DSM-IV categories of, 210–212; epidemiology of, 205–207; female genital mutilation and, 198; prevalence of, in women *versus* men, 205; psychosocial context of, 208–209; risk factors for, 207; somatic expression of, 238–239; somatization and, 206–208, 213, 214, 233, 236–237, 238–239, 240; symptoms of, 210–211; treatment of, 214–215, 215–219

Arizona, prevalence of undocumented immigrants in, 10

*Ascaris,* 106, 107

Asia: diet in, 113–114; infectious diseases in, 100; neurasthenia in context of, 243–245

Asian Health Services (AHS), 305–321; advocacy of, 318; capital development project of, 320;

Asian Health Services (AHS), (*continued*)

categorical programs of, 316–317; Community Care Fund, 310; community role of, 311–313; funding of, 314–317, 318–319, 320; Korean Breast and Cervical Cancer Screening Project, Health Is Strength project of, 295–301; overview of, 305–306; service delivery of, 313–314; user population of, 306–311

Asian Immigrant Women Advocates, 309

Asian immigrants/Asian Americans: abortion among, 122; breast and cervical cancer screening programs for, 295–304; in California, 73, 307–311; coping strategies of, 58; depression in, 206; diabetes in, 156–157; FQHC utilization of, 47; hypertension in, 152; intergenerational conflict among, 282–294; ischemic heart disease in, 139–140; male sterilization among, 122–123; mental health service strategies for, 59; mental health service utilization of, 58; osteoporosis in, 171–172; physical inactivity in, 145; somatization in, 236, 239, 240; thrombolytic agents and, 147; time orientation of, 24

Asian Pacific Islander American Health Forum, 318

Asian Pacific Islanders (APIs): breast cancer in, 163–164; in California, 307–311; cardiovascular disease mortality rates of, 140, 141, 142; cervical cancer in, 163–164; health problems of, 311; hypertension in, 152; mental health service utilization of, 54–64; tobacco use of, 144; women's shelters for, 179–180

Asplenia, 96

Assessment: of acculturation, 32; of anxiety, 212, 214–215; of cardiovascular disease risk factors, 143; of coronary heart disease symptoms, 146–147; cultural, 32–33; of cultural competence, 330–335; of depression, 212, 213–214; dietary, 113, 115–119; of ethnicity, 32; of health status, 10–11; in initial visit, 83–86; of intergenerational conflict, 291–292; of language, client's, 32; of language, provider's, 36–37; of loss, 33; of migration and premigration history, 32–33, 82–85, 86–87; of newcomers, 82–96; of posttraumatic stress disorder, 227–228, 273–275; screening protocols for, 86, 87, 88, 90–93; in second and third visits, 86–90; of suicidality, 213–214, 273; of support systems, 33; of trauma, 33, 227–228, 273–275; of work and financial history, 33, 84. *See also* Gynecological examination; History taking; Laboratory tests; Physical examination; Screening protocols

Association of Asian Pacific Community Organizations, 318

Asylum seekers: defined, 8; gender persecution and, 182

*Ataque de nervios,* 254

AT&T Language Line, 265, 269

Attitudes, culturally competent, 327

Atypical antidepressants, 216

Atypical culture-bound reactive syndromes, 249

Avoidance symptoms, 222–223, 225–226

Azithromycin, 112

**B**

Bacillus of Calmette-Guérin (BCG) vaccine, 84

Balance theories of health, 27–28

Bangladesh immigrants, proportion of men *versus* women, 5

Barnga simulation game, 287, 288

"Battered aliens" category, 69

BCG vaccine, 92, 96

Behavioral ethnicity, 20–21

Behavioral Risk Factor Surveillance System, 51, 145

Behavioral Risk Factor Surveys (BRFS), 164

Belief systems: about health and treatment, 24–31, 33–34, 337; about mental health problems and treatment, 25, 56, 64; about somatization, 25–26, 233, 237–238, 240–241; exploration of, in initial assessment, 84

Beth Israel Hospital, 331

Betrayal, sense of, female genital mutilation and, 198

Bible, 198

Bilingual and bicultural providers: in Asian Health Services, 305, 306; in community health centers, 259–262; funding for, 260; in health care organizations, 339–340; for health services, 36–38, 42–43; in hospitals, 265; in Medicaid managed care organizations, 268–270; for mental health services, 60, 64; in public health departments, 263, 264. *See also* Interpreters

Bilingual health education materials, 41, 43, 263, 264–265, 269

Biomedical science, 339

Bipolar disorder, 252

Birth defects, 128–129

Birth outcomes: after passage of California's Proposition 187, 74–75; Latina, African American, and Caucasian compared, 128

Birth spacing, 122–123

Birth weights, 128

Bisphophonates, 174

*Black* classification, 13–14

Blacks: breast and cervical cancer in, 163; diabetes prevention objectives for, 156; emergency department utilization of, 48; osteoporosis in, 171

Blood donation, 111

Blood drawing: anxiety about, 86; Chinese beliefs about, 34

Body measurements, 118

Body metaphors, 238

Body work, 29, 31; for posttraumatic stress disorder, 231, 276, 280

Bone mineral density testing, 172–173

Border control, 70

Borreliosis, 101

Bosnia: gatekeepers in, 46; Hepatitis B incidence in, 88; posttraumatic stress disorder and, 225; rape in, 190

Bottle feeding, 133–134

Brain fag, 255

Breast cancer, 162–169; educational materials on, 296–297, 302–303; hormone replacement therapy and, 146; incidence and mortality rates of, 163–164; incidence of, among black women in New York, 13–14; incidence of, in U.S. *versus* Asian countries, 11; screening behaviors of immigrant women for, 167–169, 296; screening estimates for, 164–166; screening for, 162–163; screening programs for, 295–304

Breastfeeding, 133–134

Brucellosis, 101

Buddhism, Morita therapy and, 244

Buddhist priests, 30

Buproprion, 216

Bureau of Primary Health Care (BPHC), 47, 313

Bush medicines, 158–159

**C**

Cabbage, 126
*Caida de la mollera,* 29, 133
Calcitonin, 174
Calcium, 132, 173
California: breast and cervical cancer in, 163; breast and cervical cancer screening in, 164, 166, 167, 169; female genital mutilation legislation in, 200; FQHC utilization in, by race, 47; Korean breast and cervical cancer screening demonstration in, 295–301; prenatal coverage in, denial of, 53, 74–75; prevalence of immigrants in, 6, 7; prevalence of undocumented immigrants in, 10. *See also* Alameda County; San Francisco
California Health Facilities Mortgage Insurance Program (Cal-Mortgage), 320
California Medical Association, 73
California Nurses Association, 73
California's Birth public Use files, 74–75
California's Proposition 187, 17, 67, 71, 72–77; arguments for and against, 73; impact of, 73–77; medical professionals' opposition to, 73–74; passage and context of, 72–73; provisions of, 72
Cambodian refugees/Cambodian Americans: breast and cervical cancer screening program for, 301–302; concentration camp survivor, 220; cultural bereavement of, 224; health and mental health problems of, 271, 272; health and mental health risks of, 271; posttraumatic stress disorder in, 225, 226, 228, 230, 271–273; posttraumatic stress disorder support group for, 271–281; traditional health practices of, 29–30, 230
Canada, health care services in, 16

Canadian immigrants, percentage of undocumented, 10
Cape Verdean immigrants, HIV-2 in, 109
Capital campaign, Asian Health Services, 320
Cardiac exam, 102
Cardiovascular disease (CVD), 137–149; assessment of symptoms of, 146–147; genetic *versus* environmental factors in, 138–143; mortality rates and prevalence of, 137, 138–143; prevention of, 145, 148–149; risk factors for, in immigrant women, 143–145
Caribbean Islands: culture-bound syndromes in, 254, 255–256; diabetes in, 156; diabetes traditional treatments in, 158–159; health-seeking behaviors in, 30
Case management, in mental health services, 218–219
Case presentations, 327
Caucasians: abortion among, 122; breast and cervical cancer in, 163; California population of, 73; cardiovascular disease mortality rates of, 140, 141, 142; emergency department utilization of, 48; FQHC utilization of, 47; male sterilization among, 122–123; osteoporosis in, 171; somatization in, 239
Census issues, 339
Center for Epidemiological Studies-Depression Scale (CES-D), 207, 246, 291
Center for Family and Community Health (CFCH), 295, 300
Central America, infectious diseases in, 99, 111
Central American immigrants: posttraumatic stress disorder in, 225; prenatal care of, 125
Cerebrovascular disease, 137; mortality rates of, by race, 141, 142

Cervical cancer, 162–169; educational materials on, 296–297; incidence and mortality rates of, 163–164; incidence of, in black women in New York, 13–14; screening behaviors of immigrant women, 167–169, 295; screening estimates, 164–166; screening for, 162–163; screening programs for, 295–304

Chagas' disease, 111

Chancroid, 110, 112

Chest exam, 102

*Chi qong,* 280

Child abuse: cultural differences and, 22–23; female genital mutilation and, 195; somatization and, 236. *See also* Female genital mutilation

Child development education, 288

Childbirth, 125, 126, 131–132; home *versus* institutional, 125, 131; infibulation and, 197–198, 203

Childbirth preparation classes, 125–126

Children: acculturation of, and intergenerational conflict, 22–23, 282–285; establishing structure for, 289; parents' unavailability to, 283; parents' understanding of, 287–288; pressures on, 284–285; rewarding, 289; role reversal of, 283; rules and limits for, 289; special time for, 289, 293. *See also* Intergenerational conflict

Children's Health Initiative Program (CHIP), 310, 340

Children's Hospital of Oakland, 314

China: depression in, 245; diet in, 115; *koro* epidemics in, 251; neurasthenia in, 244–246; as origin of immigrants in New York, 6. *See also* Chinese immigrants

Chinese American Psychiatric Epidemiological Study, 246, 247

*Chinese Classification of Mental Disorders* (CCMD-2), 245

Chinese immigrants/Chinese Americans, 246–247; birth experience of, 132; breast cancer in, 164; cardiovascular disease in, 141; contraception among, 122, 123; culture-bound syndromes in, 250–252; depression in, 247; diabetes pilot program for, 159–160; diabetes traditional treatment of, 157–158, 159, 160, 161; dietary acculturation of, 115; health beliefs and practices of, 27, 28, 29, 31, 34, 56, 126, 132–133, 157–158; intergenerational conflict among, 282–283, 285–292; neurasthenia in, 208, 237–238, 246–247; in New York, 6; percentage of women, 5; postpartum experience of, 132–133; prenatal care of, 125, 126; prenatal education classes for, 126; resettlement distribution of, 6, 7; somatization in, 237; traditional practitioners used by, 31

*Chinese-English Terminology of Traditional Chinese Medicine,* 244

Chistosomiasis, 106

Chlamydial infection, 110, 112

Chloroquine, 106

Cholangiocarcinoma echinococcosis, 106

Cholelithiasis, 127

Cholesterol, treatment for high, 119

Chronic diseases, 135–174

Chronic fatigue syndrome (CFS), 243

Churches, Korean, breast and cervical cancer information dissemination in, 297–298, 300–301

Civil rights violations, as domestic violence, 178

Class A conditions, 90

Class B conditions, 90

Clinical breast examination (CBE), 162

Clinton administration: health care reform, 51, 311; welfare and immigration reform, 76–77, 342

Cognitive behavioral approaches: for anxiety and depression, 217–218; for posttraumatic stress disorder, 229, 273; for somatization, 241

Cognitive processing model, 225–226

Coining, 29, 86, 272

Collectivism: domestic violence services and, 182–184; female genital mutilation and, 195; intergenerational conflict and, 284

Colombian immigrants, resettlement distribution of, 7

*Comadres*, 132

Communication, cross-cultural. *See* Cross-cultural communication

*Community Health Advisors: Health Promotion and Disease Prevention* (CDC), 51–52

*Community Health Advisors: Models, Research, and Practice* (CDC), 51–52

Community Health Center program, 314

Community health centers, 46, 47; Asian Health Services case study of, 305–321; linguistic strategies in, 259–262; welfare and immigration reform and, 70

Community health workers, 37, 42, 130

Community House Calls program, 337

Community Interpretation Services (CIS), 267–268

Community networking, 300–301, 311–313, 318

Community outreach programs, for breast and cervical cancer screening, 295–304

Compensation, for bilingual skills, 38

Composite International Diagnostic Interview (CIDI), 224

Concentration camps, refugee stressor of, 9, 222, 225

Condoms: Chinese American view of, 122; Latino use of, 123

Confidentiality: and family interpreters, 40–41; and mental health service utilization, 58

Contraception: barriers to use of, 123–124; forms of, used by different immigrant groups, 121–123; support for choice in, 123

Conversion disorder, 256

Coping strategies: for mental illness, 56–59, 64; somatization as, 237–238; for stress and anxiety, 215; for traumatic stress, 225–226

Coronary heart disease (CHD), 137; assessment of symptoms of, 146–147; estrogen and hormone replacement and, 145–146; genetic *versus* environmental factors in, 138–143; prevention of, 145, 148–149; risk factors for, in immigrant women, 143–145. *See also* Cardiovascular disease

Coronary revascularization procedures, 147

Corporate fundraising, 320

Costs: of acute care for nonqualifying immigrants, 50–51; as barrier to access, 61; of domestic violence, 188; of hip fractures, 171; of hiring interpreters, 39

Countries of origin: Hepatitis B incidence by, 88; of immigrants, 4–7; of undocumented immigrants, 10

Crafts, 276–279

Credibility: achieved, 63; ascribed, 63; of psychotherapists, 63

Croatian women, rape of, 190

Crocheting and knitting, 276–279

Cross-cultural communication, clinician-patient, 31–33, 34. *See also* Bilingual and bicultural providers; Cultural competence; Language and linguistics

Cross-cultural encounter simulation, 286

Cuba, Hepatitis B incidence in, 88

Cuban immigrants: calcium intake of, 173; diabetes in, 155; hypertension control in, 152; percentage of women, 5; prenatal care of, 125; resettlement distribution of, 7; tobacco use of, 143–144

Cultural assessment, 32–33

Cultural barriers, 15–16. *See also* Access to health care

Cultural bereavement, 224

Cultural competence, 19–34; in Asian Health Services, 311; assessment of, 330–335; behavioral *versus* ideological ethnicity and, 20–21; cross-cultural communication and, 31–33; cultural issues and, 21–24; culturally diverse learning organization and, 334; defined, 19–20, 330–331; formalized internal action for, 333; health belief systems and, 24–31, 33–34, 338; for immigrant parents, 287, 292–293; inaction stage of, 332; initiatives for, 333; in mental health services, 59–60, 64; stages of, in organizations, 332–334; symbolic stage of, 332; training in, 42, 269–270, 322–329, 330, 338

Cultural competence curriculum, 322–329; attitudes component of, 327; educational objectives of, 324–327; knowledge component of, 324–325; learner evaluation for, 328–329; learning experiences for, 327–329; skills component of, 326, 328–329; teaching approaches for, 322–323

Cultural competence self-assessment, 330–333; implications of, 334–335; objectives of, 331–332, 334–335; protocol for, 331–334

Cultural diversity in health care, 331–332. *See also* Bilingual and bicultural providers; Cultural competence

Cultural proverbs, 62

Cultural relativism, 204

Culturally diverse learning organization, 334

Culture: and contraceptive use, 123–124; defined, 19; food and, 113; health-related beliefs and, 24–31, 33–34; issues of, that affect health care, 15–16, 21–24; somatization and, 25–26, 233, 237–238

Culture-bound syndromes, 249–256; African, 255–256; anxiety and depression and, 208; Chinese *(koro),* 250–252; defined, 249; explanatory belief models and, 25–26, 29; impact of, 249–250; Korean *(hwa-byung),* 253–254; Latin and South American, 254–255; Malay *(amok),* 252; in males, 249–250, 251, 252

Cupping, 29, 86, 272

*Curanderos,* 30–31

Curriculum: for cultural competence, 322–329; of Strengthening of Intergenerational/Intercultural Ties in Immigrant Chinese American Families (SITICAF), 285–290

**D**

Data collection: on health status, limitations, 12–14; on utilization, limitations of, 45–46

Debt management, 320

Decision making, health, cultural differences in, 15–16, 25, 29, 30

Delaware, female genital mutilation legislation in, 200

Delusional disorder, 251

Demonstration and pilot projects, 316

Dengue fever, 101

Depo-Provera injection, 122

Deportation, fear of: as barrier to health care access, 17, 73–74, 131;

Deportation, fear of (*continued*): as barrier to mental health service utilization, 58; as barrier to seeking domestic violence care, 180, 182

Depression, 205–219; case study of, 209–210; chronic fatigue syndrome and, 243; comorbidity with, 206–207; cultural issues in, 207–208; culture-bound syndromes and, 252, 253, 254; domestic violence and, 180, 183, 188; DSM-IV categories of, 209–210; epidemiology of, 205–207; female genital mutilation and, 198; neurasthenia and, 208, 244, 245, 246–247; prevalence of, in women *versus* men, 205; psychosocial context of, 208–209; rape and, 192; risk factors for, 207; somatic expression of, 238–239; somatization and, 206–208, 213, 214, 233, 236–237, 238–239, 240; symptoms of, 209; treatment of, 212, 213–215–219

Desensitization exercises, 276

Detainment of new immigrants, conditions warranting, 90

Diabetes, gestational, 127

Diabetes mellitus, 155–161; cardiovascular disease and, 144–145; comorbid with hypertension, 151, 153; Healthy People 2000 objectives for, 155, 156; incidence of, 155–157, 311; patient education for, 160–161; pilot study of, in Chinese immigrants, 159–160; traditional treatments for, 157–159, 160, 161; treatment for, 119; tuberculosis risk and, 92

Diabetic retinopathy, 156

Diagnosis, explaining, to patient, 87–88

*Diagnostic and Statistical Manual of Mental Disorders* (DSM-II), 242

*Diagnostic and Statistical Manual of Mental Disorders* (DSM-III), 220, 224–225, 242, 246

*Diagnostic and Statistical Manual of Mental Disorders* (DSM-III-R), 246

*Diagnostic and Statistical Manual of Mental Disorders* (DSM-IV), 208, 209–211, 233, 234, 239, 249, 253, 255

Diagnostic Interview Schedule (DIS), 207, 224

Diaphragm (contraceptive), Latina view of, 122

Diarrheal diseases, 108

*Dichos*, 62

Diet. *See* Nutrition and diet

Digestive disorders, culture-bound, 29, 253–254

Diphtheria, tetanus, pertussis (DTP) immunization, schedule of, 94

Directly observed therapy (DOT): advantages of, 112; for tuberculosis, 103–104

Disadvantaged Minority Health Act, 1990, 318

Discharge instructions, 89–90

Discrimination, in-group *versus* outgroup distinction and, 284

Disease: diet and, 113–115; illness *versus*, 27; immigrant variation in, 114. *See also* Chronic diseases; Illness; Infectious diseases

Disproportionate share (DSH) funds, 67

Dissociative syndromes, 254, 255–256

Distribution patterns, 6, 7

Djibouti, 191–192

Documented immigrants, defined, 7

Domestic violence, 178–189; case example of, 185–186; cultural differences in meanings of, 22–23, 180–181; culturally sensitive approaches to, 183–189; defined, 178–179; federal legislation and, 69; gender roles and, 180–181, 182; legal barriers to seeking care for, 182; mandatory reporting of, 184–185; medical clues of, 188; obstacles to obtaining care for,

180, 182, 185–186; prevalence of, 179–180; role of tradition in, 181–182; screening issues in, 186–188; somatic complaints of, 188; Western model of services for, 182–184

Dominican Republic immigrants: in New York, 6; resettlement distribution of, 7

Dong Quai, 133

Dysthymia, 209, 253. *See also* Depression

**E**

East Bay Asian Consortium, 312

East Indian immigrants. *See* Indian immigrants

Eastern Europe: anxiety in, case study, 211–212; Hepatitis B incidence in, 88; infectious diseases in, 100

Eastern European immigrants, cardiovascular disease risk factors of, 144

Eating disorders, from domestic violence, 188

Education, provider. *See* Cultural competence curriculum; Cultural competence self-assessment; Training

Educational levels, of immigrant women, 14

Educational materials: bilingual and translated, 41, 43, 263, 264–265, 269, 306; on breast and cervical cancer, 297, 300, 301–303

Eggs, raw, 31

El Salvador immigrants: percentage of undocumented, 10; percentage of women, 6; resettlement locations of, 7

Electronic database on immigrant health, 337

Emergency care: acute care *versus*, 70; legislation regarding, 50, 67, 69

Emergency departments (EDs): non-emergency care in, 49–50, 70; as

safety-net providers, 46, 48–50, 67–68; utilization of, 48–50, 68

Emergency medical transfer laws, 50

Emergency Medical Treatment and Active Labor Act (EMTALA), 67, 69

*Empacho*, 29

Empowerment: in dietary therapy, 119; in oral history method, 230; of women in psychotherapy, 62–63, 64, 218–219

*En Accion Contra el Cancer*, 302

Endocarditis, 111

English as a Second Language (ESL) interactive education, in post-traumatic stress disorder support group, 276, 277, 279

English language ability, of women *versus* men immigrants, 14. *See also* Language and linguistics; Limited-English-proficient clients

*Entamoeba histolytica*, 107

*Enterobius*, 107

Epidemiological Catchment Area (ECA) studies, 205, 206, 235, 236

Epstein-Barr virus, 243

Eritrean prostitutes, 190

Eritrean refugee women, rape of, 191–192

Estrogen: coronary heart disease and, 145–146; for osteoporosis, 174

Ethiopia, tuberculosis program in, 104

Ethiopian immigrants: health practices of, 111; hepatitis incidence in, 104–105

Ethiopian refugee women, rape of, 191–192

Ethnic matching, in psychotherapy relationship, 61–62

Ethnic neurosis, 249

Ethnic psychosis, 249

Ethnicity: assessment of, 32; behavioral *versus* ideological, 20–21; classification of, 12–13

EthnoMed, 337

European Americans, mental health service utilization of, 54, 55
Evidence-based medicine, 339
Evil eye, 29
Evil spirits, 254
EWIs (entry without inspection), 8
Exercise, for osteoporosis, 173–174. *See also* Physical activity
Exotic psychotic syndromes, 249
Expanded access to primary care (EAPC), 315
Explanatory belief models, 25–31, 33–34, 338
Expressive therapies, 218
Extended families, domestic violence and, 178, 181. *See also* Families
Extremities, examination of, 102
Eye exam, 102

**F**
Fairy tales, 287, 293
*Fajeros,* 133
Falciparum malaria, 106
Falling-out syndrome, 255–256
Families: in Asian cultures, 283, 284; cultural issues of, that affect health care, 22–23; culture-bound syndromes and, 249–250; intergenerational conflict in, 22–23, 282–293; as interpreters, 40–41, 265; involving, in depression and anxiety treatment, 218; involving, in posttraumatic stress disorder treatment, 229–230; involving, in treatment planning, 89, 229–230; in Latino culture, 57–58, 284. *See also* Domestic violence
Familism, 58
Family formation, 122–123
Family planning programs, 123
Family reunification, 9
Famine, refugee stressor of, 9
Far East Asia, infectious diseases in, 100
Fat consumption: cardiovascular disease and, 138; high, 114; hypertension and, 154

Febrile illness, acute: causes of, 101, 106, 108; pregnancy and, 110
Federal Breast and Cervical Cancer Control Program, 297
Federal Office of Refugee Resettlement, 273
Federal Prohibition of Female Genital Mutilation Act of 1995, 199
Federally qualified health centers (FQHCs), 46–47; financial problems of, 53; funding of, 53, 316; utilization of, 47; welfare and immigration reform and, 67–68, 70
Female circumcision, 196. *See also* Female genital mutilation
Female genital mutilation, 194–204; age of, 197; assessment of, 86; defined, 196; effects of, 196–197; health consequences of, 197–198; health policy and guidelines for, 201–204; historical and contemporary justifications for, 198–199; legislative responses to, 69, 199–201; overview of, 196–197; prevalence of, in United States, 199; psychological consequences of, 198; purposes of, 194, 198–199; rape and, 192; reporting of, 202–203; social and cultural imperatives associated with, 194–195, 198–199; underground market for, 203
Feminist psychotherapy, 62–63
Filial piety, 283, 284
Filial therapy, 287–289
Filipino immigrants/Filipino Americans: breast and cervical cancer screening in, 164–165, 169; breast cancer in, 164; breastfeeding diet of, 134; cardiovascular disease in, 141; health beliefs of, 28, 29; hypertension in, 114, 142; mental health service utilization of, 54; percentage of undocumented, 10; percentage of women, 5; prenatal care of, 125

Financial barriers, to accessing health care, 16–17, 44

Financial history, 33

Florida: breast and cervical cancer screening rates in, 165, 166; falling-out syndrome in, 255–256; prevalence of immigrants in, 6, 7; prevalence of undocumented immigrants in, 10

Fluoride, 174

Folk illnesses. *See* Culture-bound syndromes

Folk medicine. *See* Traditional and folk medicine

Fontanel, fallen, 29

Food: cultural meanings of, 113; for postpartum care, 132–133; as traditional medicine, 126, 158

Food analysis, 117–118

Food consumption tables, 117–118

Food cravings, 126–127

Food diary, 116–117

Food frequency questionnaires, 116

Food groups, 118

*Food Guide Pyramid* (USDA), 118

Food stamp program, 68–69, 341

Fortune tellers, 30

Fourth International Women's Conference (Beijing), 189

Friends, as interpreters, 40–41, 265

Funding: of Asian Health Services, 314–317, 318–319, 320; for bilingual and interpretation services, 43; for bilingual services in community health centers, 260; for categorical programs, 315–316; criteria and data sets for, 318–319; federal, 67–68, 69, 314–315, 340–341; for federally qualified health centers, 47; for indigent care, 3, 52–53, 315–317; for prenatal care, 130–131, 316; for primary care, 314–315

Fundraising, 320

**G**

Gangs, 285

Gastrointestinal culture-bound syndrome *(hwa-byung)*, 253–254

Gastrointestinal diseases, 108

Gatekeepers, in Bosnia, 46

Gender matching, in psychotherapy relationship, 61–62

Gender roles: addressing, in psychotherapy, 62–63; coping strategies and, 58; cultural differences in, that affect health care, 15–16, 21, 58, 180–181; culture-bound syndromes and, 250; domestic violence and, 180–181, 182; female genital mutilation and, 194–195; Westernization of, 21

Generalized anxiety disorder, 211. *See also* Anxiety and anxiety disorders

Genital herpes, 110

Genital retraction, 250–252

Genocide, rape as tool of, 190–191

George Washington University Medical Center screening protocol for domestic violence, 186–187

Ginger, 132

Glucose-6-phosphate dehydrogenase (G6PD) screen, 106

Gonorrhea, 110

Greater Atlantic health Service, 268

Grief resolution, 219

Guatemalan immigrants: percentage of undocumented, 10; resettlement locations of, 7

Guided imagery, 277, 279–280

Guyana immigrants, resettlement locations of, 7

Gynecological assessment, 85

Gynecological examinations: discomfort with, 32, 85; key elements of, 102; for sexually transmitted diseases, 110

**H**

*H. Influenzae B* immunization, recommended schedule for, 94

*Haemophilus influenzae* (HIB) vaccine, 96

Haiti, Hepatitis B incidence in, 88

Haitian immigrants: adoption among, 134; culture-bound syndrome in, 255–256; health beliefs of, 27; percentage of undocumented, 10; resettlement locations of, 7

Hansel and Gretel, 287

Hansen's disease, 110

Harborview Hospital (Seattle), 202–203

Harborview Medical Center, Community House Calls program, 337

Harvard Medical School, 331

Harvard Trauma Scale, 273, 274

Hawaiians, Native, 5; breast and cervical cancer screening in, 164–165; cardiovascular disease in, 141, 144–145; hypercholesterolemia in, 114; obesity in, 144–145; prenatal care of, 125

Hawaiians, Samoan, 49

Head and neck exam, 102

Healers. See Traditional practitioners

Health belief systems, 24–31, 33–34, 338; dietary therapies and, 120; exploration of, in initial assessment, 84; medication and, 217; prenatal care and, 126–127

Health care: cultural issues that affect, 21–24; culturally-based beliefs that affect, 24–31; federal funding for, 67–68; life cycle, 313–314; sources of, 46–50. See also Access to health care

Health care environment, competitive, 319

Health care system, barriers to accessing, 14–18, 16–17, 25, 44–45, 51. See also Access to health care

Health counselors, 298–299, 300–301

Health education pamphlets, bilingual, 41. See also Educational materials

Health Is Gold!, 302

Health services utilization, 44–53; factors in, 44–45; by sources of care, 46–50; studies on, limitations of, 45–46

Health status: before and after migration, 10–11; of Asian Pacific Islanders, 311, 319; California's Proposition 187 impact on, 76; data on, limitations of existing, 12–14; examination for, 10–11, 90; immigration policy on, 10; socioeconomic status and, 148

Health-seeking behaviors: cultural beliefs and, 24–31, 33–34; and mental health service utilization, 56–59; of perinatal and reproductive needs, 121. See also Access to health care; Utilization

Healthy migrant effect, 11. See also Acculturation

Healthy People 2000 (DHHS), 119, 155–157, 162–163

Healthy People 2000 objectives: for breast and cervical cancer screening, 162–163; for diabetes, 155–157

Heart disease. See Cardiovascular disease

Hennepin County Medical Center, 268, 269, 270

Hepatic metabolism, 216–217

Hepatitis A, 104, 105

Hepatitis B (HBV): incidence of, 88, 104–105, 310; pregnancy and, 110; recommended adult immunization schedule for, 95; recommended primary immunization schedule for, 94; screening protocols for, 86, 87, 88, 105; therapies for, 105; transmission of, 105

Hepatitis C (HCV), 104, 105–106

Hepatitis D (HDV), 104, 105

Hepatitis E, 104, 105

Herbal medicine: Asian, 28, 29, 30, 31, 34; assessment of use of, 84; comparative study of, 29; for dia-

betes, 158–159, 160, 161; for hypertension control, 154; for mental health problems, 57, 247; Mexican-American, 30–31; for postpartum period, 132–133
Herbalists, 36
Herzegovina, Hepatitis B incidence in, 88
High blood pressure. *See* Hypertension
Highland General Hospital, 314
Hip fractures, 171
Hiring: of professional interpreters, 38–39; of traditional practitioners, 36
*Hispanic* classification, 13
Hispanic Health and Nutrition Examination Survey (HHANES), 152, 156, 207
History taking: for dietary assessment, 116, 117; of immunizations, 84, 93; for infectious diseases, 101; in initial visit, 83–85; of medications, 84; of migration and premigration history, 32–33, 82–85, 86–87, 212; for osteoporosis assessment, 172; for traumatic stress, 227. *See also* Assessment
Hmong immigrants: coping responses of, to mental health problems, 57; dietary acculturation and disease in, 115; health decision-making of, 30
Homeless programs, 46–47
Hookworm, 107
Hopkins Short List Depression Inventory, 273
Hormonal contraception: Chinese American view of, 122; Latina use of, 122
Hormone replacement therapy (HRT): coronary heart disease and, 145–146; for osteoporosis, 174
Horn of Africa, rape in, 192
Hospital Interpretation Program, 267–268

Hospital visit rates, 45–46
Hospitals: language bank interpreters in, 37–38; linguistic strategies in, 37–38, 40, 265–268; volunteer interpreter programs in, 40. *See also* Public hospitals
Hot and cold theory, 27, 28; for postpartum care, 131–132; for prenatal care, 126–127
Hours of operation, for mental health service agencies, 61
Housing assistance restrictions, 68
HTLV-I, 109
*Hueseros*, 30
Human immunodeficiency virus (HIV) infection: Asian Health Services program for, 316; comorbid with syphilis, 110; comorbid with tuberculosis, 91–92, 93, 98; counseling about, 109; parasite infection and, 108; polio vaccine and, 96; pregnancy and, 110, 127–128; reluctance to reveal, 57–58; screening for, 108–109
Hunan Medical College, 245
Hutu genocidal campaign, 190
*Hwa-byung*, 253–254
Hyperarousal symptoms, 223, 225–226
Hypercholesterolemia, 114; as risk factor for cardiovascular disease, 138
Hypertension, 150–154; awareness and control of, 152–154; comorbidity with, 151, 153; consequences of, 151; defined, 150–151; diet and, 114; ethnicity and, 152–153; incidence of, 150–151, 152–153, 310; lifestyle modification for, 153–154; as risk factor for cardiovascular disease, 138; treatment for, 119, 151, 154
Hypochondriasis, 234

**I**

*Iberian* classification, 13
Ideological ethnicity, 21

Illegal Immigration Reform and Immigrant Responsibility Act (IIRIRA) of 1996, 66, 67, 69, 340; female genital mutilation and, 199–200, 201; PROCOL category and, 8

Illinois, prevalence of undocumented immigrants in, 10

Illness: cultural beliefs about, 24–31, 33–34, 338; disease *versus,* 27

Immersion learning, 323

Immigrant women, 3–4; barriers of, to access, 14–18, 44–45; culture-bound syndromes and, 249–250; hazardous occupations of, 11, 24; health risks of, 11; median age of, 5; mental health problems of, 11; origins of, 5–6; prevalence of, *versus* immigrant men, 5; recent, initial assessment of, 82–96. *See also* Newcomers

Immigrants: categories of, 7–8; defined, 5; diversity among, 6; migration patterns of, 4–5; origins of, 4–7; percentage of foreign born, 5; posttraumatic stress disorder risk of, *versus* refugees, 225; prevalence of, 5; refugees *versus,* 8–9; resettlement locations of, 6, 7

Immigration and Naturalization Service (INS): asylum provision of, for gender persecution, 182; documented immigrants and, 7; fear of, as barrier to accessing health care, 17, 58, 73–74; threat of reporting to, as domestic violence, 178–180; undocumented immigrants and, 8, 72

Immigration Reform and Control Act (IRCA) of 1986, employment of undocumented immigrants and, 10

Immigration/immigrant law and policy: as barrier to access, 17–18, 310; female genital mutilation and, 199–201; on health status

and screening, 10–11; immigrant policy *versus* immigration policy and, 70; 1996 and 1997 reforms of, 66–77, 340; 1920s to 1940s, 4; pending legislation on, 340–341; on prenatal care, 14, 53, 74–75; recommendations for, 341–342

Immune system, parasitic infection and, 108. *See also* Human immunodeficiency virus (HIV) infection

Immunizations: for adults, 93–96; assessment of history of, 84, 93; laboratory screening for, 86; recommended adult schedule for, 95; recommended primary schedule for, 93, 94; for tuberculosis, 92

Immunosuppressive medications: strongyloidiasis screening and, 107, 111; tuberculosis and, 111

In Action Against Cancer, 303

Income levels, of Asian Pacific Islanders in Alameda County, 308–309

India, infectious diseases in, 100

Indian immigrants (India): cardiovascular disease in, 141, 145; diversity among, 6; percentage of women, 5; resettlement locations of, 7

Individualism: domestic violence services and, 182–183; female genital mutilation and, 195; intergenerational conflict and, 284

Indo Chinese Psychiatry Clinic, Boston, 271, 273

Infant mortality, 128

Infectious diseases: blood transfusion and, 111; cross-cultural considerations in screening, 111–112; detection and treatment of, in newcomers, 97–112; geographic distribution of, 99–100; medical history and review of systems for, 101; in pregnancy, 110–111, 127–128; screening and treatment of, 97–112; special considerations in,

110–111; spread of, due to immigration reform, 73–74

Infertility, 134

Infibulation: defined, 196; ethical dilemmas of, 203; health consequences of, 197–198, 203. *See also* Female genital mutilation

Influenza, 101; immunization for, 95, 96

Informed consent, confusion about, 17–18

In-group *versus* out-group distinction, 284

Initial visit: for assessment of recent immigrant women, 82–86; examinations and laboratory assessments in, 86, 87, 88; history taking in, 83–85; for mental health services, 59–61, 64

Injectable polio vaccine (IPV), 96

In-laws, abuse by, 178

In-person surveys, limitations of, 12

Insulin resistance: as cardiovascular disease risk factor, 144–145; "thrifty" genotype and, 157

Insurance status: and access to mental health services, 61; of Asian Pacific Islanders in Alameda County, 309–310; impact of, on emergency department utilization, 49–50; impact of, on health services utilization, 44, 45

Interferon, 105

Intergenerational conflict: acculturation and, 22–23, 282–285; assessment of, 291–292; family educational program on, 285–293; mental health problems and, 283–284

Intergenerational Relationship in Immigrant Families-Chinese Parent Scale, 291

*International Classification of Disease* (ICD-9), 243

*International Classification of Disease* (ICD-10), 245, 249

International ladies Garment Workers Union, 309

Interpreters: in community health centers, 261, 313; for discharge instructions to recent immigrants, 89–90; for domestic violence screening, 186; for explaining lab results to recent immigrants, 86; funding of, 43; in health care organizations, 339–340; in hospitals, 37–38, 40, 265–268; language bank, 37–38; in Medicaid managed care organizations, 269–270; nonprofessional, 40–41; professional, 38–39; in public health departments, 263, 264; remote, 39–40; standards for, 39, 42–43; training of, 39, 42–43, 266, 267, 269–270. *See also* Bilingual and bicultural providers

Intrauterine device (IUD): Chinese American use of, 122; Latina use of, 122

Intrusive symptoms, 222, 225–226, 276

Involuntary migrants: defined, 8; migration and, 9

Iranian immigrant women, median age of, 5

Iraq, Hepatitis B incidence in, 88

Iron intake, 91

Ischemic heart disease: assessment of symptoms of, 146; mortality rates for, by race, 139–140, 141

Islamic cultures, gynecological exams and, 85

Isoniazid, 93

## J

Jamaican immigrants, percentage of women, 6

Japan, neurasthenia in, 243–244

Japanese immigrants/Japanese Americans: acculturation and diet of, 113–114; breast cancer in, 164; breast cancer screening in, 165;

Japanese immigrants/Japanese Americans (*continued*): cardiovascular disease in, 114, 138, 141, 142–143; diabetes in, 156–157; prenatal care of, 125
Joint Commission on Accreditation of Healthcare Organizations, 186
Joint National Committee on Prevention, Detection, Evaluation, and Treatment of High Blood Pressure (JNC VI), Sixth Report of the, 150–151, 153–154

**K**
Kaiser Family Foundation, Henry J., 337
*Kell,* 26
Knitting and crocheting, 276–279
Koran, 198
Korean Breast and Cervical Cancer Screening Project, Health Is Strength, 295–301; goals of, 295–296; program components of, 296–299; results of, 299–301
Korean churches, breast and cervical cancer information dissemination in, 297–298, 300–301
Korean "comfort women," 190
Korean Community Advisory Board (KCAB), 295, 299
Korean Health Survey, 1994, 295
Korean immigrants/Korean Americans: breast and cervical cancer screening behaviors of, 168–169, 296; breast and cervical cancer screening demonstration for, 295–301; breast cancer in, 164; cardiovascular disease in, 141, 143; culture-bound syndrome (*hwa-byung*) in, 253–254; health-seeking behaviors of, 57; percentage of women, 6
*Koro,* 250–252
Kru Khmer, 30

**L**
Labor support persons, 131–132

Laboratory tests, 86; for infectious disease, special considerations of, 111; for nutritional assessment, 118; protocols for, 86, 87, 88, 90–93
Lactation, 133–134, 217
Lactose intolerance, 173
Lamivudine, 105
Language and linguistics: assessment of, 32, 36–37; as barriers to access, 14–15; cross-cultural communication and, 31–33; hypertension treatment and, 150; issues of, 35–43; strategies for, in health care settings, 259–270, 310. *See also* Bilingual and bicultural providers; Interpreters; Limited-English proficient clients
Language bank interpreters, 37–38, 263
Language Cooperative Program, 313
Language-specific clinics, 269
Laotians: community outreach to, 312–313; posttraumatic stress disorder in, 226
Latin America, Hepatitis B incidence in, 88
Latin American countries, public health services in, 17
*Latin* classification, 13
Latina/Latino immigrants: adoption among, 135; affective disorders in, 206; barriers of, to access, 51; birth defect prevention of, 129; birth experience of, 131–132; breast and cervical cancer screening programs for, 303–304; breast cancer in, 163; breast cancer screening of, 163, 164, 166, 167–168; breastfeeding among, 133; California population of, 73; California's Proposition 187 impact on, 74–77; cardiovascular disease in, 138, 139, 140; cervical cancer in, 163; cervical cancer screening of, 163, 164, 166, 167–168; contraception among, 122, 123–125;

cultural barriers of, to access, 16, 57–58; culture-bound syndromes in, 254–255; diabetes education for, 161; diabetes in, 155–156; diabetes traditional treatments of, 158; diet of, 114–115; emergency department utilization of, 49; financial barriers of, to access, 44; FQHC utilization of, 47; health beliefs and practices of, 29, 126–127, 129, 133; health-seeking behaviors of, 29, 30; HIV infection in, 127–128; hypertension in, 152–153; infant mortality of, 128; intergenerational conflict among, 283, 285; mental health service strategies for, 59; mental health service utilization of, 54–64; mental illness beliefs of, 56; obesity of, 114–115; perceptions of, regarding California's Proposition 187, 76; postpartum experience of, 132; practitioner relationships and, 30; prenatal care of, 126–127, 131; somatization in, 237; substance use of, 131; time orientation of, 24

Latino Health Council, 263

LEARN (listen, explain, acknowledge, recommend, negotiate), 322–323, 325

Legal barriers: to accessing health care, 17–18; to seeking help for domestic violence, 182. *See also* Immigration law

Leptospirosis, 101

Lesbian relationships, domestic violence in, 180

Life cycle health care, 313–314

Lifestyle modification: for coronary heart disease prevention and control, 145; for hypertension control, 153–154; for neurasthenia, 247

Limited-English-proficient (LEP) clients, 35–43, 259–270; in Alameda County, California, 307;

bilingual and bicultural providers for, 36–37; community health center approaches to, 259–262; community health workers for, 37; hospital approaches to, 37–38, 40, 265–268; language bank interpreters for, 37–38; managed care approaches to, 268–270; nonprofessional interpreters for, 40–41; professional interpreters for, 38–39; public health department approaches to, 262–265; recommendations for, 42–43; remote consecutive interpretation for, 39–40; written translation materials for, 41

Linguistics. *See* Language and linguistics

Liver diseases, 104–106, 217. *See also* Hepatitis

Living situation, assessment of, 83–84

Local health departments, 262–265

Los Angeles: comparative study of folk medicines used in, 29; prenatal care utilization and birth outcomes in, after Proposition 187 passage, 75; somatization study in, 235

Los Angeles County Hospital, 53

Los Angeles County mental health system, utilization of, 54–55, 61–62

Loss: assessment of, 33; cultural bereavement and, 224; grief resolution for, 219; refugee stressor of, 9; resolution of, 228. *See also* Posttraumatic stress disorder; Trauma

Lymphogranuloma venereum, 110

**M**

Mailed surveys, limitations of, 12

Mail-order bride trade, 69

Major depression, 209–210; culture-bound syndromes and, 252, 253, 254; suicidality and, 213–214. *See also* Depression

*Mal ojo,* 29
*Mal puesto,* 29
Malaria, 101; incidence of, 106; in pregnant patients, 110; screening and treatment of, 106–107; transmission of, 106–107
Malaysian culture-bound syndrome *(amok),* 252
Male sterilization, 122–123
Mammogram facilities, 297
Mammograms, 162, 164–165, 166, 169, 296, 303–304
Managed care, 52–53, 311, 318; linguistic strategies in, 268–270; practice guidelines and, 338–339
Mandatory reporting: of domestic violence, 184–185; of female genital mutilation, 201
*Marianismo,* 58
Market model, 52
Marriage status: domestic violence and, 183; female genital mutilation and, 199
Massachusetts Department of Public Health (DPH), 263–265
Massachusetts, medical interpreter associations in, 39
Massage, 29, 31, 231, 280
Measles, mumps, rubella (MMR) immunization: recommended adult schedule for, 95; recommended primary schedule for, 94
Meat consumption, 115
Medicaid: disproportionate share payments from, 67; fear of using, 17; nonurgent emergency department utilization and, 49, 50; welfare and immigration reform and, 66, 67, 68, 70
Medicaid managed care, 52; approaches of, to limited-English-proficiency clients, 260, 268–270
Medi-Cal, 298, 309, 310, 317
Medical interpreter associations, 39
Medical records, race and ethnicity classifications in, 13

Medical schools: cultural competence training in, 322, 323, 327–328; diversity in, 339–340
Medicare: assistance in accessing, 298; welfare and immigration reform and, 66
Medicare managed care, 52
Medications: assessment of history of, 84; cultural views of, 217; ethnic differences in metabolism of, 216–217, 229; herbs used with, 161; immunocompromising or suppressive, 92; as osteoporosis risk factor, 172; for osteoporosis treatment, 174; prescribing, for recent immigrants, 89; for tuberculosis prophylaxis, 93. *See also* Psychopharmacology
Meditation, 31, 279–280
Mediums, 30
Meningococcal vaccine, 96
Menopause, 145–146, 172
Mental health problems: coping responses to, 56–59, 64; cultural beliefs about, 25, 56, 64, 240–241; from domestic violence, 180, 183, 188; from female genital mutilation, 198; of immigrant women, 11; intergenerational conflict and, 283–284; from rape, 192–193; recognition of, 56, 64; somatic presentation of, 238–239; stress and, 208–209. *See also* Anxiety and anxiety disorders; Culture-bound syndromes; Depression; Neurasthenia; Posttraumatic stress disorder; Somatization
Mental health service utilization, 54–64; awareness of service availability and, 58; in California, after Proposition 187 passage, 74; distrust and, 58–59; ethnic differences in, 54–56; for somatization, 239–240; stage model of, 55–64; studies of, 54–56; by type of service, 55; variables in, 55

Mental health services: accessibility and geographic location of, 60; case management in, 218–219; costs of, 61; engagement of, 61–63, 64; hours of operation of, 61; initial contact with, 59–61, 64; in multiservice centers, 61, 64. *See also* Psychotherapy

Mexican immigrants/Mexican Americans: anxiety disorders in, 206; breast and cervical cancer screening of, 167, 303–304; cardiovascular disease in, 140, 142; culturally sensitive psychotherapy for, 62; depression in, 206, 209–210; diabetes in, 144, 151, 155; diabetes traditional treatment of, 158; diet of, 114–115, 144, 173; emergency department utilization of, 48–49; folk illnesses of, 29; health beliefs and practices of, 27–28, 29, 158; hypertension in, 151, 152–153; mental health service utilization of, 55, 62; myocardial infarction in, 147; obesity in, 114–115, 144; osteoporosis in, 171; percentage of undocumented, 10; percentage of women, 5; posttraumatic stress disorder in, 225; practitioner relationships and, 30; prenatal care for, 125; *Salmonella* infection in, 111; somatization in, 235; substance use of, 131; time orientation of, 24; tobacco use of, 143, 144; traditional practitioners used by, 30–31

Midarm muscle circumference (MAMC) measurement, 118

Middle East: female genital mutilation in, 194; infectious diseases in, 100

Middle Eastern immigrants, diversity among, 6

Midwives, 30, 132

Mien immigrants: community outreach to, 311–312; coping responses of, to mental health problems, 57; posttraumatic stress disorder in, 226

Migrant health centers, 46, 47

Migration, 8–9; assessment of history of, 32–33, 82–85, 86–87, 212; health status before and after, 10–11; intergenerational conflict and, 23; mental health and, 207; stress and, 8–9, 208–209. *See also* Acculturation

Milk products, 173

Minneapolis Health Department, 268, 269

Minneapolis Metropolitan Health Plan (MHP), 268–270

Minnesota: breast and cervical cancer screening program in, 301–302; female genital mutilation legislation in, 200

Monkey King, 287, 293

Monoamine oxidase inhibitors (MAOIs), 215

Morita therapy, 244

Mourning, 219

Moxibustion, 86

Multiple Risk Factor Intervention Trial, 152–153

Multiservice centers, mental health service provision in, 61, 64

*Mycobacterium species*, 91

Myocardial infarction (MI), 147–148; mortality rates of, for Mexican American *versus* white women, 140, 142, 147

**N**

Narrative therapies, 218, 227, 228, 230, 241

National Ambulatory Medical Care Survey (NAMCS), 45–46

National Asian Women's Health Organization, 144

National Coalition of Hispanic Health and Human Services Organizations, 237

National Comorbidity Study (NCS), 205–206, 240
National Crime and Victimization Survey, 179
National data sets: race and ethnicity classifications in, 13; used for funding criteria, 318–319
National Death Index, 140
National Health Interview Survey (1990), 44–45, 140, 143–144
National Heart, Lung and Blood Institute, 174
National High Blood Pressure Education Program, 152
National Hospital Ambulatory Medical Care Survey (NHAMCS), 45–46
National Institute of Mental Health, 54, 246
National Medical Expenditure Survey, 49
National Osteoporosis Foundation, 173
National Public Health and Hospital Institute (NPHHI), 265, 266, 331
Native Americans, 5; ischemic heart disease and stroke in, 139
Nefazadone, 216
Nei Jing, 159
Neurasthenia, 242–248; in Asian context, 243–245; chronic fatigue syndrome and, 243; as coping mechanism, 237–238; depression and, 208, 244, 245, 246–247; etiology of, in Chinese context, 244–245; evaluation and treatment of, 247; as expression of distress, 244; history and etiology of, 242–243; research on, in Chinese populations, 246–247; symptoms of, 242, 243, 245
Neurologic exam, 102
New Jersey: prevalence of immigrants in, 6, 7; prevalence of undocumented immigrants in, 10

New York: prevalence of immigrants in, 6, 7; prevalence of undocumented immigrants in, 10
New York City: cervical cancer screening rates in, 166; immigrant health care network in, 336–337; prevalence of immigrants in, 6, 7
New York Task Force on Immigrant Health, 336–337
New York University School of Medicine, 336–337
Newcomers: assessment, screening, and immunization of, 82–96; dietary assessment and intervention for, 113–120; immunizations for, 93–96; infectious diseases of, 97–112; initial assessment of, 82–96; initial visit for, 82–86; prenatal care for, 121, 125–131; prescribing medications for, 89; providing discharge instructions to, 89–90; second and third visits for, 86–90; treatment planning for, 87, 89; visa-mandated medical examinations of, 90. See also Immigrant women; Immigrants
Newcomer's Guide to Health Care in Massachusetts, 264
Ni-Hon-San study, 138, 143
Nondihydropyridine calcium antagonists, 151
Nonimmigrant overstays, defined, 7–8
Nonprofessional interpreters, 40–41
North Dakota, female genital mutilation legislation in, 200
Nutrition and diet, 113–120; acculturation of, 113–115; for anemia, 91; assessment of, 115–119; cardiovascular disease and, 137, 138; for common diseases, 118–119; for diabetes, 161; discussion of, with recent immigrants, 89; disease and, 113–115; interventions in, 115, 119–120; during lacta-

tion, 134; for osteoporosis, 172–173; for prenatal care, 126–127; traditional Chinese, 31
Nutrition labels, 116–117

## O

Obesity: cardiovascular disease and, 138, 144–145; diabetes and, 156, 157; in Hispanic immigrants, 114–115; hypertension and, 153; measurement of, 118; as risk factor for chronic diseases, 157; treatment for, 119
Obsessive-compulsive disorder, 211, 253. *See also* Anxiety and anxiety disorders
Obstetrical history taking, 85
Occupations: assessment of, 33, 84; hazardous, of immigrant women, 11, 24; issues of that affect health care, 24
Office for Civil Rights, U.S. Department of Health and Human Services, 266, 267
Office of Refugee and Immigrant Health (ORIH), Massachusetts Department of Public Health, 263–265
Office of Women's Health, 3
Oophorectomy, 146
Opening Doors: Reducing Sociocultural Barriers to Health Care, 337
Ophthalmology clinic utilization, in California, after Proposition 187 passage, 75–76
Opisthorchiasis, 106
*Opisthorchis,* 107
Oral contraception, Chinese American view of, 122
Oral history method, 227, 230
Oral polio vaccine (OPV), 96
Organizational change, 338
Osteoporosis, 170–174; defining of, 170; ethnicity and risk for, 171–172; future study of, 174; preva-

lence of, 170–171; prevention and treatment of, 173–174; risk factors for, 172; screening for, 172–173
Osteoporosis and Related Bone Disease National Resource Center, 173
Outreach workers, 51–52

## P

*P. ovale* malaria, 106
Pain disorder, 234
Pakistani immigrants, proportion of women *versus* men, 5
Panic attacks, 210–211. *See also* Anxiety and anxiety disorders
Panic disorder, 211; culture-bound syndromes and, 253, 254. *See also* Anxiety and anxiety disorders
Papanicolaou (Pap) testing, 162, 165, 166, 167–168
Parasites, 107–108, 111, 311
Parental Locus of Control Scale, 291
Parenting: cultural differences in, 22, 287; filial therapy for, 288–289; intergenerational conflict and, 282–293; stress of, 289–290
*Parteras,* 30
Pathways to Cancer Screening for Four Ethnic Groups, 303
Patient input, in Asian Health Services, 312
Patient-physician relationship. *See* Practitioner-patient relationship
Pelvic inflammatory disease, 110
Personal Responsibility and Work Opportunity Reconciliation Act (PRWORA), 1996, 66, 67–69, 310
*Personalismo,* 30, 161
Phlebotomy, Chinese beliefs about, 34. *See* Blood drawing
Phobia, 211, 253. *See also* Anxiety and anxiety disorders
Physical activity/inactivity: cardiovascular disease and, 145;

Physical activity/inactivity (*continued*):
hypertension and, 154; osteoporosis and, 172, 173–174

Physical examinations: in initial visit, 85–86; key elements of, 102; for nutritional assessment, 116; for osteoporosis, 172–173; visa-mandated, 90

Phytoestrogens, 146

Pinching, 29

Pinworm, 107

*Plasmodium vivax* malaria, 106

Pneumococcal vaccination, 96

*Pneumocystis carinii* pneumonia (PCP), 109

Pneumonia, 101, 109

Pol Pot regime, 271, 272–273, 276

Polio immunization: for HIV-infected individuals, 96; recommended adult schedule for, 95; recommended primary schedule for, 94

Polish immigrants, percentage of undocumented, 10

Political asylum, 8; for gender persecution, 182; for politically related sexual violence, 193

Portal hypertension, 107

Postpartum care, 132–134

Posttraumatic stress disorder (PTSD), 220–231; assessment of, 227–228, 273–275; comorbidity with, 221; cultural issues of, 224; culture-bound syndromes and, 255; domestic violence and, 180, 183, 188; DSM-IV diagnosis of, 222–223; epidemiology of, 224–225; rape and, 192; risk of, 220–222; somatization and, 236; support group model for, 231, 271–281; symptom categories of, 222–223; treatment of, 227–231, 271–281

Practice guidelines, 338–339

Practitioner-patient relationship: cross-cultural communication and, 31–33, 34; cultural differences in, 30. *See also* Providers; Psychotherapists; Traditional practitioners

Praziquantel, 107

Pregnancy: assessment for, 85; complications of, 128; folk traditions about, 126–127, 129; infectious diseases and, 110–111, 127–128; prenatal care and, 125–131; psychopharmacology and, 217; substance use during, 131

Premigration history assessment, 32–33, 82–83

Prenatal care, 121, 125–131; adherence to, 129–131; birth defects and, 128–129; California's Proposition 187 and, 53, 74–75; in different cultures, 125; folk traditions of, 126–127, 129; funding of, 130–131, 316; immigration law and, 14, 342; infectious disease prevention and, 110–111, 127–128; initiation of, 125; nutrition education for, 127

Present State Examination (PSE), 246

Preterm labor, 128

Preventive care: barriers to, 129–130; for cardiovascular disease, 145, 148–149; for hypertension, 151; lack of access to, 51; for osteoporosis, 173–174; prenatal, 129–130

Primaquine, 106

Primary care: in Asian Health Services, 313–315; somatization in, 239–241

Primary care clinics, utilization of in California, after Proposition 187 passage, 75–76

Professional interpreters, 38–39

Program evaluation, 337–338. *See also* Cultural competence self-assessment

*Promotoras,* 301
Proposition 187. *See* California's Proposition 187
Prostitution, 192
Providence Ambulatory Health Care Foundation, 260–262
Providers: bilingual and bicultural, 36–38, 42–43, 60, 64; cultural competence self-assessment for, 330–335; culturally competent, 59–60, 64. *See also* Bilingual and bicultural providers; Practitioner-patient relationship; Psychotherapy relationship; Traditional practitioners
PRUCOL (permanently residing in the United States, under color of law), 8
Psychoeducation: for anxiety and depression, 215, 217; for posttraumatic stress disorder, 229
Psychogenic blindness, 222, 271, 278
Psychopharmacology: for anxiety and depression, 215–217; for posttraumatic stress disorder symptoms, 229
Psychotherapists: credibility of, 63; ethnically matched, 62–63; gender-matched, 62–63
Psychotherapy: for anxiety and depression, 215, 218; client education about, 60; culturally sensitive, 62; engagement in, 61–63; for *koro* syndrome, 252; for posttraumatic stress disorder, 229, 230, 271–281; for somatization, 241. *See also* Mental health services
PTSD Assessment and Treatment Program for Immigrants and Refugees, 271–281
PTSD Symptom Checklist, 224–225
Public assistance: California's Proposition 187 and, 72–77; welfare and immigration reform and, 66–71

Public health departments, linguistic strategies in, 262–265
Public health needs assessments, in Massachusetts, 263–264
Public Health Service Act, 46, 314
Public hospitals: financial problems of, 52–53; as safety net providers, 46, 47–48, 67, 70; utilization of, 48. *See also* Hospitals
Public housing programs, 47
Public sector funding, 52
Puerto Ricans: *ataque de nervios* in, 254; calcium intake of, 173; diabetes in, 155, 156; health beliefs of, 27, 56; health-seeking behaviors of, 58; hypertension control in, 152; as immigrants, 5; practitioner relationships of, 30; somatization in, 235; time orientation of, 24; tobacco use of, 143–144
Purified protein derivative (PPD) test, 91–92, 93, 103, 127
Push and pull migration factors, 8–9

**Q**
Qi gong, 31
Quality assurance, for interpreter services, 43

**R**
Race, classification of, 13–14
Radio cancer information, 302
Rape, 190–193; of Cambodian women, 271; cultural responses to, 192; documentation of, 193; posttraumatic stress disorder and, 227, 271; psychosocial and physical health for survivors of, 192–193; refugee experience of, 9, 191–192; as tool of genocide, 190–191
Recruitment, of bilingual/bicultural staff, 36, 42
Redding, California, 337
Reeducation camps, refugee stressor of, 9

Refugee Act of 1980, *refugees* defined in, 8

Refugee camps, 82–83; diarrheal disease in, 108

Refugee Clinic. *See* San Francisco General Hospital (SFGH) Refugee Clinic

Refugee Health Advisory Committee, 263

Refugees: culturally relevant treatment of, 227–228; defined, 8; immigrants *versus*, 8–9; initial assessment of, 82–96; mental health problems of, 206; posttraumatic stress disorder in, 224–225; rape of, 9, 191–192; screening protocols for, 86, 87, 88; somatization in, 235–236; traumatic stress of, 9, 11, 220–231. *See also* Cambodian refugees

Relapsing fever, 101

Relaxation exercises, 276, 277, 279–280

Religion and spirituality, 23; contraception and, 124; cultural competence and, 23; female genital mutilation and, 198; infant mortality and, 128; for traumatic stress, 230

Remote consecutive interpretation, 39–40

Renal disease, hypertension and, 153

*Report of the Secretary's Task Force on Black and Minority Health* (DHHS), 319

Reproductive health care, 121–135. *See also* Breast cancer; Cervical cancer; Pregnancy; Prenatal care

Research, Action, and Information Network for Bodily Integrity of Women (RAINBO), 199

Research, community-sensitive, 299–300

Resettlement locations: of immigrants, 6, 7; of undocumented immigrants, 10

Residence, duration of, and health services utilization, 44–45

Residency, medical, 322, 323, 327–328

Resolution of trauma, 228

Resource allocation, 340

*Respecto,* 30

Rheumatic fever, 111

Rheumatic heart disease, 139

Rhode Island, female genital mutilation legislation in, 200

Ritualistic prayers, 31

Robert Wood Johnson Foundation, 337

Roma women, cardiovascular disease risk factors of, 144

Roman Catholicism, contraception and, 124

Rubella vaccine, 95

Russia, Hepatitis B incidence in, 88

Russian immigrants: health beliefs of, 28, 29; percentage of women, 5. *See also* Soviet Union (former) immigrants

**S**

*S. pneumoniae,* recommended adult immunization schedule for, 95

Safety net providers, 45, 46; financial problems of, 52–53; welfare and immigration reform and, 67–68, 69

*Salmonella,* 96, 108, 111

Samoans: cardiovascular disease in, 141, 144–145; emergency department utilization of, 49; obesity in, 144–145

San Francisco: Asian Pacific Islander population in, 307–308; breast and cervical cancer screening programs in, 302–303; emergency department utilization in, 68; mental health service utilization in, after Proposition 187, 74; provider familiarity with female genital mutilation in, 202

San Francisco General Hospital (SFGH) Family Health Center, 277

San Francisco General Hospital (SFGH) Refugee Clinic: formation of, 271–272; medication provision at, 89; screening protocols of, 86, 87, 88, 90–93, 105

San Francisco General Hospital (SFGH) Refugee Clinic, Posttraumatic stress disorder support group, 231, 271–281; assessment and referral to, 273–275; average stay in, 275; craft activities in, 276–279; funding of, 276, 277; induction into, 275–277; interactive ESL in, 276, 277, 279; outcomes of, 280–281; social contact in, 277–279; stress reduction/guided imagery exercises in, 276, 277, 279–280; structured activities of, 275–277

Scarification, ritual, 86

Schistosomiasis, 107

Schizophrenia, 251, 252

Screening examinations: cross-cultural considerations in, 111–112; for health status determination, 10–11, 90; review of overseas, 85. *See also* Assessment; Gynecological examinations; Laboratory tests; Physical examinations; Screening protocols

Screening protocols and screening: for anemia, 86, 91; for birth defects, 128–129; for breast cancer, 162–169, 295–304; for cervical cancer, 162–169, 295–304; for domestic violence, 186–188; for hepatitis B, 86, 87, 88, 105; for HIV, 108–109, 127–128; for infectious diseases, 97–112; for infectious diseases in pregnant patients, 110–111, 127–128; for malaria, 106; for osteoporosis, 172–173; for parasites, 107–108;

for sexually transmitted diseases, 110; for tuberculosis, 91–92, 98, 103–104, 127

Seasonal farmworkers, 70

Seattle: EthnoMed electronic database in, 337; hospital linguistic strategies in, 266–268

Secondhand smoke, assessment of, 84

Selective estrogen receptor modulators, 174

Selective serotonin reuptake inhibitors (SSRIs), 216

Self-Esteem Inventory, 291

Senegalese somatization syndrome, 25–26

Sephardic Jews, malaria incidence in, 106

Serbian "ethnic cleansing," 190

Sexual disorders, 251

Sexual history taking, 85

Sexual violence. *See* Domestic violence; Rape

Sexually transmitted disease (STD): in pregnancy, 127–128; screening and treatment for, 110, 127–128

Sexually transmitted diseases (STDs), hepatitis B as, 104, 105

Shamans, 36, 57, 230, 337

Shame: about domestic violence, 183, 185; about female genital mutilation, 195; about gender issues, 62–63; about mental health problems, 57; about rape, 192; about seeking mental health service, 60

Shasta Community Health Center, 337

*Shenjingshuairou,* 245

*Shi jin jitsu,* 280

*Shinkeisuijaku,* 243–244

Shock, Mexican-American syndrome of, 29

*Simpatica,* 58

Skin exam, 102

Sleep disturbance, 275, 276

*Sobadores,* 30

Social Security Act, Title XIX, 69

Socioeconomic status (SES): of Asian Pacific Islanders in Alameda County, 308–309; health status and, 148; hypertension and, 152–153; somatization and, 235; and utilization, 44

Sodium intake, 154

Sodium metabolism, 142

Somali immigrants and refugees: female genital mutilation in, 202–203; malaria incidence in, 106; rape of, 192

Somatic Symptom Index (SSI), 234–235

Somatic therapeutic approaches, for posttraumatic stress disorder, 231

Somatization and somatization disorders, 233–241; anxiety and, 206–208, 213, 214, 233, 236–237, 238–239, 240; belief systems and, 25–26, 240–241; as coping strategy, 237–238; culture and, 25–26, 233, 237–238, 240–241; culture-bound syndromes and, 253; defined, 233; depression and, 206–208, 213, 214, 233, 236–237, 238–239, 240; diagnosis of, presentation of, 87, 89; from domestic violence, 188; DSM-IV diagnosis of, 233, 234–235; mental health services utilization and, 239–240; as presentation of mental disorders, 238–239, 240; prevalence of, 235–236; in primary care, 239–240; psychological distress and, 236–237; from rape, 192; sociogenic, 236; traumatic stress and, 227, 233, 235–236, 274–275; treatment of, 240–241

Somatization disorder (SD), 234–235

Somatoform disorder, 255

Sorcerers, 30

South America: culture-bound syndromes in, 254–255; infectious diseases in, 99, 111

South American immigrants, prenatal care of, 125

Southall Black Sisterhood, 185

Southeast Asia: Hepatitis B incidence in, 88; infectious diseases in, 100

Southeast Asian immigrants: in Alameda County, California, 308; breast cancer in, 164; cultural bereavement of, 224; depression in, 238; liver diseases in, 106; mental health service utilization of, 54; neurasthenia in, 246; posttraumatic stress disorder in, 226; refugee, mental health problems of, 206, 207, 224, 271; tobacco use of, 311. See also Cambodian refugees

"Southern medicine" (Vietnamese), 28

Soviet Union (former), Hepatitis B incidence in, 88

Soviet Union (former) immigrants: MMR vaccine for, 95; in New York, 6; resettlement locations of, 7

Soy products, 146

Stage model of utilization, 55–64; agency contact stage in, 59–61, 64; coping response stage in, 56–59, 64; problem recognition stage in, 56, 64; service engagement stage of, 61–63, 64

Standards, for medical interpreters, 42–43

State of California Breast Cancer Early Detection Program, 297

State of Health Insurance in California, The (Schauffler), 309

State public health agencies, 262–265

States: female genital mutilation legislation in, 200; immigrant distribution in, 6, 7; immigration reform in, 342; primary care funding by, 315; undocumented immigrant distribution in, 10

Stigma of illness: as barrier to access, 16, 25; and mental health service utilization, 57, 61; neurasthenia and, 247, 248; of tuberculosis, 104

Stool O&P exam, 107, 108, 111

Strengthening of Intergenerational/ Intercultural Ties in Immigrant Chinese American Families (SITICAF): curriculum of, 285–290; outcomes of, 291–294

Stress: anxiety and depression and, 215; cognitive process model of, 225–226; coping with intergenerational, 290–294; of immigrants and refugees, 9, 208–209, 215, 271; reactions to severe, 220–222, 223; somatization and, 239. *See also* Posttraumatic stress disorder; Trauma

Stress reduction exercises, 276, 277, 279–280

Stroke mortality rates, 139

Strongyloidiasis, 107, 111

Structural barriers, to accessing health care, 44

Substance use: assessment of, 84; domestic violence and, 188; during pregnancy, 131

*Suc Khoe La Vang!*, 302

Suicidality: assessment of, 213–214, 273; from domestic violence, 188

*Suk-yeong*, 250–252

Summit Hospital, 314

Supplemental security income (SSI), welfare and immigration reform and, 66, 340, 341

Support groups for traumatized refugee women, 231, 271–281. *See also* San Francisco General Hospital Refugee Clinic

Support systems: assessment of, 33; use of, for mental health problems, 57

Supportive therapy, for anxiety and depression, 215, 218

Surveys, limitations of, 12

Sustained-release hormonal contraception, 122

*Susto*, 29, 254–255

Symptom description, cultural differences in, 146–147

Syphilis, 110

**T**

*Taenia solium*, 107

*Tang-neo bing*, 159

Tapeworms, 107

Teaching approaches, for cultural competence, 323–324

Telephone surveys, limitations of, 12

Telephone systems, bilingual, 268–269

Television cancer education, 303

Temporary Assistance to Needy Families (TANF), 68

Tennessee, female genital mutilation legislation in, 200

Testimony method, 228, 230

Tetanus immunoglobulin (TIG) injection, 93, 95

Tetanus-diphtheria immunization, adult, 93, 94, 95

Texas: breast and cervical cancer screening in, 167; FQHC utilization in, by race, 47; prevalence of immigrants in, 6, 7; prevalence of undocumented immigrants in, 10

Thailand: diet in, 115; parasitic infection in, 107

Thalassemia, 91, 310

Thiabendazole, 111

Third National Health and Nutrition Examination Survey (NHANES III), 151, 152

Thrombolytic agents, 147

Tibetan immigrants, tuberculosis incidence in, 103

Time orientation: cultural differences in, 24; preventive care utilization and, 130

Title XIX, Social Security Act, 69

Tobacco use: among Southeast Asians, 311; assessment of, 84, 143; cessation of, for hypertension control, 154; and osteoporosis,

172; as risk factor for cardiovascular disease, 138, 143–144

Tongan women, obesity and cardiovascular disease in, 144–145

Torture, refugee stressor of, 9

Toxoplasmosis, 112

*Toy* somatization syndrome, 25–26

Trachoma, 112

Traditional and folk medicine: for birth defect prevention, 129; comparative study of, 29; consideration of, in infectious disease screening, 111–112; for diabetes, 157–159, 160; health belief systems and, 27–30, 337; for postpartum care, 132–133; for pregnancy, 126–127; stigmata of, found in physical examination, 86; for traumatic stress, 228, 230

Traditional Chinese Medicine: for diabetes, 159, 160, 161; neurasthenia in, 244–245, 247. *See also* Herbal medicine; Traditional and folk medicine

Traditional Chinese pharmacies, 31, 160

Traditional practitioners: accessibility of, 31; Cambodian, 30; Chinese, 31; community center relationship with, 336; health-seeking behaviors and, 30; hiring, for limited-English-proficiency clients, 36, 42; Mexican American, 30–31; use of, 30–31; use of, for mental health problems, 57, 59

Training: of bilingual/bicultural staff, 42, 263, 264; in cultural competence, 42, 269–270, 322–329, 330, 338; of interpreters, 39, 42–43, 266, 267, 269–270. *See also* Cultural competence curriculum

Trauma: assessment of, 33, 227–228, 273–275; experienced by refugees, 9, 11, 12, 220–222, 271, 272–273; levels and duration of,

226; resolution of, 228; responses to, 220–222, 225–226. *See also* Domestic violence; Posttraumatic stress disorder; Rape; Stress

Trauma treatment centers, 227–228, 231

Treatment planning, for recent immigrant women, 87, 89

Treponemal diseases, 110

Triceps skin fold (TSF) measurement, 118

*Trichuris*, 107

Tricyclic antidepressants (TCAs), 215–216

Trinidad and Tobago, diabetes traditional treatment in, 158–159

Triple marker screens, 128

Tubal ligation, 122

Tuberculosis (TB), 98, 101, 103–104; assessment of immunization history for, 84; Class B, 92; comorbid with HIV, 91–92, 93, 98; denial of care to undocumented immigrants and, 73–74; drug-resistant, 91; immunosuppressive medications and, 111; incidence of, in United States, 98; screening and prophylaxis for, 91–92, 96, 98, 103–104, 127; stigma of, 16, 104

Tutsi women, rape of, 190

Twenty-four-hour diet recalls, 116

Typhoid fever, 101, 108

Typhoid vaccine, 96

Typhus, 101

**U**

Ukrainian immigrants, percentage of women, 5

Ultrasound, 128

Umbilicus binding, 133

Undifferentiated somatoform disorder, 234–235

Undocumented immigrants: California's Proposition 187 and, 72, 73–74; countries of origin of, 10;

defined, 7–8; denial of care to, 53; domestic violence and, 178, 182; emergency department utilization of, 50; infectious disease spread and, 73–74; issues of, 10; occupational issues of, 24; prevalence of, 10. *See also* Deportation

Unemployment, of Asian Pacific Islanders in Alameda County, 309

United Kingdom, men *versus* women immigrants from, 5

United Nations, 180, 190, 191

United States: cardiovascular disease in, 137; diet-disease relationship in, 113–114; domestic violence in, 179

U.S. Bureau of Population, Refugees, and Migration, 180

U.S. Census Bureau, 338; data limitations of, 13–14; race classifications of, 13

U.S. Congress, immigration and welfare reform and, 66, 68, 76–77, 340–341

U.S. Department of Health and Human Services (DHHS), 155, 200–201, 204, 266, 267, 319, 325

U.S. Preventive Services Task Force: guidelines of, 90; screening recommendations for breast and cervical cancer, 162

U.S. Public Health Service (USPHS), 3, 47

University of California, Berkeley, 295

University of California, San Francisco, 303

University of Michigan Composite International Diagnostic Interview Schedule, 207

University of Minnesota, 270

University of Washington Health Services Library, 337

Urinary tract infection, 101, 107, 197

Uterine cancer, hormone replacement therapy and, 146

Utilization: access and, 44–45, 51–53; in California, after Proposition 187 passage, 74–77; defined, 44; factors in, 44–45; of health services, 44–53; of mental health services, 54–64; stage model of, 55–64; studies on, limitations of, 45–46

Uvulectomy, 111, 112

**V**

Vaccines. *See* Immunizations

Varicella immunization, recommended primary schedule for, 94

Vietnam: sources of care in, 46; tuberculosis program in, 104

Vietnam War, rape in, 190

Vietnamese immigrants/Vietnamese Americans: boat migrant, rape of, 191; breast and cervical cancer screening behaviors of, 168; breast and cervical cancer screening program for, 302–303; breastfeeding among, 134; cardiovascular disease in, 141; cultural bereavement of, 224; health beliefs of, 28; health-seeking behaviors of, 30; hepatitis incidence in, 104; percentage of women, 5; posttraumatic stress disorder in, 226; tuberculosis incidence in, 103

Vinegar, 132–133

Violence Against Women Act, 182

Violence, posttraumatic stress disorder risk and, 220–222, 224–225. *See also* Domestic violence; Rape; War

Visa-mandated medical examinations, 90

Voluntary migrants: defined, 8; migration and, 9

Volunteer interpreters, 40–41, 265

Vouchers for mammograms, 303–304

## W

War: posttraumatic stress disorder and, 224–225; rape and, 190–193; stressor of, 9, 224–225
Washington: hospital interpretation programs in, 266–268; medical interpreter associations in, 39
Weight measurements, 118
Weight-bearing exercise, 173–174
Welfare reform, 66–71, 76–77, 310, 312, 340–341
West African immigrants, HIV-2 in, 109
Whipworm, 107
White magic, 31
Wisconsin, female genital mutilation legislation in, 200
Women immigrants. *See* Immigrant women
Women, Infants, and Children (WIC) food programs, 68–69
Women's health, advances in, 3
Women's health brochure, Korean, 296–297, 300
Women's Health Initiative, 3, 174
Women's shelters, for Asian Pacific Islanders, 179–180
*Wool hwa-byung,* 253–254

Work visas, temporary, 70
Workplace culture, 24
*World Guide to Infections, A* (Wilson), 51–52
World Health Organization: bone loss categorization of, 170, 171; female genital mutilation categorization of, 196
Written translation materials, 41, 43, 263, 264–265, 269, 306; for breast and cervical cancer screening, 297, 300, 302–303

## X

X rays, chest, for tuberculosis screening, 92, 93, 103
*Xiao-ke,* 159

## Y

Yemen, schistosomiasis in, 107
*Yerberos,* 30
Yin-yang balance, 28
Yoga, 280

## Z

Zen Buddhism, Morita therapy and, 244